Pediatric Ophthalmology for Primary Care

Pediatric Ophthalmology for Primary Care

Second Edition

Kenneth W Wright, MD, FAAP
Director, Pediatric Ophthalmology Research and Education
Cedars-Sinai Medical Center
Clinical Professor of Ophthalmology
University of Southern California—Keck
Los Angeles, California

American Academy of Pediatrics
DEDICATED TO THE HEALTH OF ALL CHILDREN™

AAP Department of Marketing and Publications Staff

Maureen DeRosa, Director, Department of Marketing and Publications

Mark Grimes, Director, Division of Product Development
Diane Beausoleil, Senior Product Development Editor
Kate Simone, Electronic Publishing Manager

Sandi King, Director, Division of Publishing and Production Services
Kate Larson, Manager, Editorial Services
Jason Crase, Editorial Specialist
Leesa Levin-Doroba, Manager, Print Production Services
Linda Diamond, Manager, Graphic Design

Jill Ferguson, Director, Division of Marketing and Sales

Natalie Arndt, Department Coordinator

Second Edition—2003
First Edition—© 1999 Williams & Wilkins as *Pediatric Ophthalmology for Pediatricians*

Library of Congress Control Number: 2002100844
ISBN: 1-58110-087-6
MA0199

The recommendations in this publication do not indicate an exclusive course of treatment or serve as a standard of medical care. Variations, taking into account individual circumstances, may be appropriate.

Dedication

This book is dedicated to the pediatricians and primary care physicians who devote their careers to preserving the health of our children.

AND

On a personal note, I would also like to acknowledge my younger brother, Dr Howard Weston Wright, for his love, inspiration, and infectious enthusiasm for life.

Preface

Pediatric ophthalmology is fundamentally different from adult ophthalmology, and it is much more than eye size! Visual development and nervous system plasticity sharply distinguishes pediatric ophthalmology from adult ophthalmology. A visually significant adult cataract does not affect neurodevelopment, and the cataract can be removed electively, without compromising the visual outcome. In a newborn, however, a visually significant cataract disrupts normal neurological development and can lead to irreversible amblyopia and even blindness if not treated within the first few weeks of life. Developmental ocular anomalies, genetic syndromes, retinopathy of prematurity, and learning disabilities are further examples of eye disorders distinct to pediatrics. Special skills are required for examining and treating children with eye disease. Something as easy as measuring visual acuity in an adult can be very challenging when working with a child in the "terrible twos."

This book was written specifically for the pediatrician to aid in the diagnosis and treatment of pediatric eye disorders. The style is intended to be lucid and easily understood with ample figures and photographs to demonstrate the pathology. This book covers a broad spectrum of important eye disorders, organized, for the most part, by the presenting signs and symptoms. This is distinct from other texts that typically base the organization on anatomy. Practical aspects of pediatric ophthalmology are provided, including chapters on ocular examination and vision screening, strabismus, dyslexia, and ocular trauma.

A variety of readers, including pediatricians, family physicians, nurses, and nurse practitioners will find this book useful. Care was taken to make the information brief, yet detailed and comprehensive enough, to thoroughly cover the broad subject of pediatric ophthalmology. Attendings should find this text an invaluable resource providing a quick synopsis on a specific clinical topic. Likewise, residents in training will find the length of this book manageable and use it as a basic text, as it can be read cover to cover.

As the author, I would personally like to thank Tina Kiss for her line by line editing of each chapter and her overall management of the entire project, keeping us on schedule. Her extraordinary organizational skills and editorial talents have made writing this book a pleasure.

I am also extremely fortunate to have true experts in the field of Pediatrics review this book. Special thanks go to Rena E. Falk, MD; Lloyd J. Brown, MD; Cathy Manuel, MD; and Kim Altamirano, MD. Thank you all for your hard work and dedication to make this book excellent.

It is my sincere hope that you, the reader, will find this book clear, informative, and enjoyable.

Kenneth W. Wright, MD

Special Thanks

I would like to personally thank Tina Kiss, our pediatric ophthalmology and adult strabismus coordinator. Her expertise, determination, and passion for the project made this book possible.

Tina Kiss, COT, CCRA
Coordinator, Research and Education
Pediatric Ophthalmology and Adult Strabismus Center
Cedars-Sinai Medical Center
Los Angeles, California

A special thanks is also extended to the following organizations for their overwhelming support in academic endeavors to promote research, education, and advancements in medicine.

Cedars-Sinai Medical Center
Los Angeles, California

The Henry L. Guenther Foundation and

The Discovery Fund for Eye Research
Los Angeles, California

Gustavus and Louise Pfeiffer Research Foundation
Denville, New Jersey

Contributors

M any thanks to my colleagues who authored special sections of this textbook. Their contributions were invaluable to its content, and I appreciate their hard work.

Sam Goldberger, MD
Oculoplastics, Reconstructive, and Cosmetic Plastic Surgery
Beverly Hills, California
Chapter 17—first edition

Jyoti Raina, MD
London, England
Chapter 24—first edition

In addition, I would also like to acknowledge the following contributors who spent numerous hours reviewing and editing the manuscript, and provided me with suggestions and comments that were critical to the success of this book.

Rena E. Falk, MD
Medical Genetics—Birth Defects Center
Director, Cytogenetics Laboratory
Cedars-Sinai Medical Center
Los Angeles, California

Lloyd J. Brown, MD
Associate Director, Pediatric Residency Training Program
Cedars-Sinai Medical Center
Associate Professor of Pediatrics, UCLA School of Medicine
Los Angeles, California

Catherine Manuel, MD
Canyon Country Pediatrics
Canyon Country, California

Kim Altamirano, MD
Staff, Cedars-Sinai Medical Center
Los Angeles, California

Contents

Ocular Anatomy and Physiology

The eye is a delicate structure protected by the bony orbit and cushioned by the surrounding orbital fat (**Figure 1-1**). It is a fluid-filled sphere whose outer wall consists of the optically clear cornea anteriorly and the white sclera posteriorly. These 2 structures, the cornea and sclera, have different radius of curvature, with the cornea representing a smaller sphere than the sclera. Consequently, it is a misconception that the eye is spherical. The junction between the cornea and the sclera takes on a bluish appearance, and is termed the limbus.

The interior of the eye consists of the lens, the anterior and posterior chambers, and the vitreous cavity. The lens is suspended behind the pupil by cord-like structures called zonules. Zonules are attached to the ciliary body, a muscle that controls lens focusing. The cornea and lens are the refractive elements of the eye. The cornea is a strong, fixed-focus lens structure, while the crystalline lens is less powerful but is able to change focus to fine tune image clarity. The anterior chamber is the space between the iris and cornea and the posterior chamber is the thin space between the lens and the back of the iris. The anterior and posterior chambers are in front of the lens and are filled with a clear nutrient fluid called the aqueous humor or "aqueous." Aqueous humor circulates around the lens and the posterior aspect of the cornea providing nutrition and oxygen to these avascular tissues. Behind the lens is the vitreous cavity, a large cavity filled with a clear gel called the vitreous humor or "vitreous" (**Figure 1-2**).

1

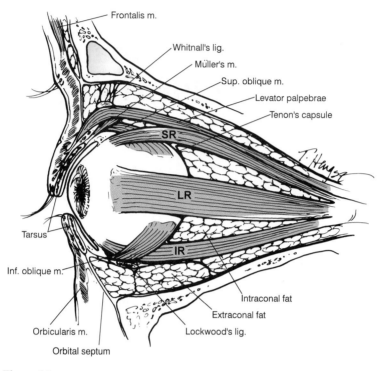

Figure 1-1.
Sagittal section of the eyebrow, upper and lower eyelid, as well as the globe and the extraocular muscles within the orbit. SR, superior rectus; LR lateral rectus; IR, inferior rectus.

The shape of the globe is maintained by the rigidity of the corneal-scleral wall and by aqueous fluid pressure of approximately 10-20 mm Hg. Epithelium lining the ciliary body produces aqueous to maintain intraocular pressure. Aqueous passes from the ciliary body, around the lens, through the pupil, and exits at the anterior chamber angle through a filterlike membrane called the trabecular meshwork (**Figure 1-3**). After passing through the trabecular meshwork, the aqueous enters Schlemm's canal, which in turn feeds aqueous veins that connect with systemic veins. Glaucoma is increased intraocular pressure (usually over 22 mm Hg) resulting from abnormalities in the drainage of aqueous that damages the optic nerve and can cause blindness.

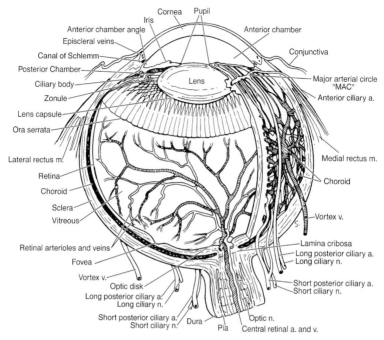

Figure 1-2.
Drawing of the eye showing important anatomic structures of the eye.

■ EYEBALL GROWTH

Eyeball growth is most dramatic during the first 2 years of life, and the eye is essentially adult size by 10 to 13 years of age. **Table 1-1** shows normal growth of the globe diameter (axial length) from birth to adulthood.

In addition to eyeball enlargement, there is also an increase in thickness and rigidity of the scleral wall with age. Scleral thickness in childhood is approximately 0.5 mm compared to 1 mm in adults. Children, especially infants, have elastic sclera that tends to collapse when intraocular pressure is low, and will stretch secondary to high intraocular pressure. This is why children with congenital glaucoma have large eyes.

■ CORNEA

The cornea is an amazing biological structure because of its optical clarity, allowing for clear transmission and focusing of light on to

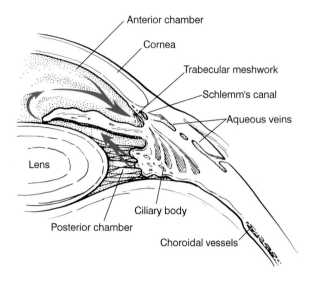

Figure 1-3.
Aqueous humor production and flow: Aqueous humor is produced by the ciliary body and released into the posterior chamber. In the normal eye, aqueous humor flows from the posterior chamber, between the lens and the iris, through the pupil and into the anterior chamber. Most of the aqueous humor outflow is through the trabecular meshwork (conventional outflow pathway).

the retina. Optical clarity is a result of relatively acellular tissue that consists of a dense, regular collagen matrix. Hydration of this collagen matrix is highly regulated and an increase in hydration results in corneal edema and loss of clarity. Since the normally transparent cornea does not contain blood vessels, it receives oxygen and nutrients from the aqueous humor and from tears. It also receives

Table 1-1.
Axial Length Growth (Gordon and Dunzs, 1985)

Age	Axial Length
Birth	15 mm
1 yr	17 mm
2 yrs	20 mm
3 yrs	21 mm
4 yrs	21.5 mm
5 yrs	22 mm
6 yrs	23 mm
Adult	24 mm

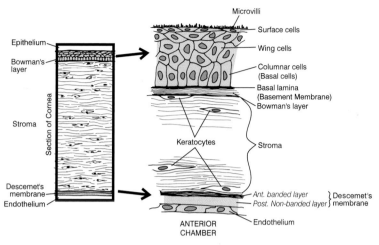

Figure 1-4.
Diagrammatic representation of the corneal ultrastructure through all 5 layers.

ambient oxygen from its surface. Because the central cornea is avascular, it tends to heal very slowly. Therefore, sutures used to repair a corneal laceration must be left in place for several months while the cornea heals.

At birth, the cornea averages 9.8 mm in diameter and increases to 11-12 mm by 1 year of age. Corneas in infants measuring less than 9 mm in diameter (**microcornea**) and corneas greater than 11 mm in diameter (**megalocornea**) should be considered abnormal. In childhood, corneas smaller than 10 mm in diameter and corneas larger than 13 mm in diameter are also considered abnormal.

On cross-section of the cornea, 3 major corneal structures can be identified: surface epithelium, stroma, and endothelium (**Figure 1-4**).

Corneal Epithelium

Corneal epithelium consists of non-keratinized, stratified, squamous epithelium approximately 8-10 cells thick. It is attached to its basement membrane by hemidesmosomes and provides a protective barrier against corneal infection. Traumatic removal of the corneal epithelium (corneal abrasion) is analogous to a tear of the skin. It causes extreme pain and provides an opportunity for corneal infection. Healing of a corneal epithelium abrasion first occurs by the sliding of adjacent corneal epithelium to fill the defect. Later, mitosis of basal epithelium cells replaces lost epithelium.

Corneal Stroma

Corneal stroma is made up of collagen fibers in a regular matrix with a uniform diameter. The few cells found within the corneal stroma are termed **keratocytes.** Keratocytes proliferate following corneal injury, and they secrete collagens and glycoproteins to repair the extracellular matrix. The new collagen matrix is disorganized and results in an opacification (corneal scar). Over several months to years, there is collagen remodeling and improved clarity, but the corneal scar almost always persists.

Corneal Endothelium

Corneal endothelium lines the interior surface of the cornea and consists of a single layer of hexagonal-shaped cells (**Figure 1-5**). These endothelial cells play an important role in active transport to pump fluid out of the corneal stroma, thus maintaining the normal condition of deturgescence and corneal clarity. Injury to the endothelium from disease or trauma results in hydration of the cornea (corneal edema), disruption of the well-organized corneal stromal collagen matrix, and opacification with the cornea appearing white.

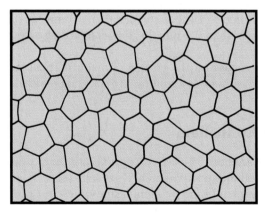

Figure 1-5.
Corneal endothelial pattern. A schematic drawing of the endothelial layer of the cornea demonstrating the hexagonal pattern of the cells, the slight difference in cell shape and size, and the continuous pattern of coverage.

Unlike the corneal epithelium, the corneal endothelium is almost completely amitotic soon after birth, so endothelial cells do not regenerate. Loss of corneal endothelial cells will not be replaced, but endothelial cells stretch and slide to cover defects. This process results in loss of the normal hexagonal cell morphology, decreased cell density, and eventually causes chronic corneal edema. The critical cell density, below which results in corneal edema, is approximately 400 to 700 cells per square millimeter. Treatment for endothelial cell loss and corneal edema is to perform corneal transplantation. Endothelial cell density and morphology are important indicators of the overall health of the cornea.

■ UVEA: IRIS, CILIARY BODY, CHOROID

The uvea is a densely pigmented vascular layer between the sclera on the outside and the retina on the inside. Moving from the anterior to the posterior, the uvea includes the iris, ciliary body, and choroid (**Figures 1-2 and 1-3**).

The **iris** is the most anterior part of the uvea and consists of a densely pigmented layer on the inside and a lighter pigmented stroma on the surface. The iris has 2 muscular layers: the iris sphincter near the pupil, and the dilator muscle toward the periphery of the iris. The iris sphincter muscle is innervated by parasympathetic fibers from the third cranial nerve, while the dilator muscle is innervated by sympathetic fibers from the superior cervical ganglion. Damage to the sympathetic innervation results in pupillary miosis (small pupil) called a Horner's pupil. Damage to the fibers from the parasympathetic third nerve results in pupillary mydriasis (dilation), causing the pupil to be unresponsive to light.

The **ciliary body,** a muscular structure located just posterior to the iris, consists of multiple radial folds called the ciliary processes. The ciliary body is covered with pigmented and non-pigmented epithelium and it is this epithelium that produces aqueous humor. Ciliary processes are connected to the lens by collagen fibers termed zonules. Ciliary muscle contractions cause the lens to change shape, which then changes the lens power, thus controlling lens focusing.

The **choroid** is a 0.25 mm-thick vascular structure with dense pigmentation and a capillary network called the choriocapillaris. The choroid has a spongy black appearance that can be seen as a jet-black tissue in a patient with a traumatic scleral rupture. This vascular tissue underlies the retina, providing oxygen and nutrients to the outer third of the retina. It has large capillaries that provide the highest perfusion rate of the body.

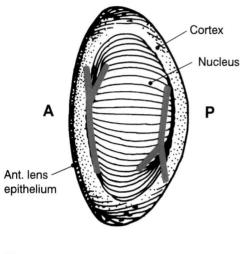

Cortex

Nucleus

A

P

Ant. lens epithelium

Figure 1-6.
Diagram of neonatal lens showing anterior lens epithelium; lens nucleus located between the Y-sutures and the cortex peripheral to the Y-sutures. A: anterior, P: posterior.

■ LENS

The lens, an avascular structure derived from surface ectoderm, functions to focus light onto the retina. It has a flexible capsule and a matrix of clear lens fibers. On the surface of the anterior lens capsule, there is a single layer of lens epithelium. At the equator, the lens epithelium differentiates into clear lens fibers and loses its nucleus and intracellular organelles. This process of lens fiber production continues throughout life. At birth, there are approximately 1.5 million fibers and, by age 80, there are 3.5 million fibers. There are 2 Y-shaped sutures that demarcate the fetal nuclear lens fibers located between the Y-sutures. The area within the Y-sutures is termed **fetal nucleus (Figure 1-6)**. In contrast to fetal nuclear lens fibers, lens fibers that develop after birth are found outside the Y-sutures. A **cataract** (lens opacity) located in the fetal nucleus usually indicates a congenital cataract that occurred prior to birth. Lens opacities peripheral to the fetal nucleus usually indicate a developmental cataract, an insult that occurred after birth. Lens flexibility and the ability to focus diminish with age and, by age 45, patients start to require reading glasses to focus on near objects.

■ VITREOUS

The vitreous is a transparent gel that fills the posterior chamber. Collagen type-2 is the major structural protein. The vitreous adheres most to the retina around the optic nerve and to the peripheral retina close to the ciliary body. The composition of the vitreous gel changes during the aging process. As a person ages, the gel becomes denser and loses its "jelly-like" consistency. Parts of the vitreous may break away and float around in the posterior aspect of the eye. Floaters are fairly common and do not necessarily indicate a retinal problem unless the patient also experiences the sensation of flashing lights.

■ FUNDUS

The **retina** is a highly organized structure consisting of alternating layers of neuron cell bodies and synaptic processes (**Figure 1-7**). The outer layer of the retina (layer closest to the sclera) consists of photoreceptors that are responsible for changing light energy into neuronal activity. There are 2 types of photoreceptors: rods, which are responsible for vision under dim illumination, and cones, which are responsible for fine, high resolution, and color vision. The ends of the rods and cones interdigitate with a basal single cell layer called the **retinal pigment epithelium (RPE).** The retinal pigment epithelium separates the retina from the vascular choroid. This single-cell layer has tight junctions and apical microvilli that extend around the tips of the rods and cones. The RPE functions to maintain a blood-retinal barrier, separating the retina from the choroid and choriocapillaris. The RPE selectively transports nutrients from the choriocapillaris to the outer retina. This active transport process maintains appropriate retina hydration. Breakdown of the RPE barrier results in fluid exudates within the retina causing retinal edema and decreased vision. The RPE cells also function to rejuvenate the rods and cones by phagocytizing debris from the tips of these photoreceptors. Rods and cones synapse with bipolar cells that, in turn, synapse with ganglion cells. Axons of the ganglion cells stream through the nerve fiber layer to exit the optic nerve. These same axons proceed uninterrupted to synapse with neurons in the lateral geniculate of the brain. Processes that damage the optic nerve actually damage the axons and subsequently affect the neurons in the inner aspect of the retina.

The **macula** is the central aspect of the retina, located within the vascular arcades, and the **fovea centralis** is the small pinpoint reflex in the center of the macula (**Figure 1-8**). The macula and fovea are almost entirely populated by cones; whereas, the peripheral

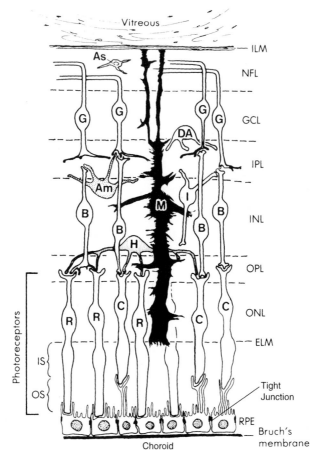

Figure 1-7.
Schematic diagram of the cell types and histologic layers in the human retina. Also shown are Bruch's membrane and the edge of the vitreous. The basic relationship between rod (R) and cone (C) photoreceptors as well as bipolar (B), horizontal (H), Amacrine (Am), inner plexiform cell (I), and ganglion (G) neurons are depicted. The Muller cell (M) extends almost the entire width of the retina. Astrocytes (As) are found primarily in the nerve fiber layer (NFL). Modified from Dowling JE, Boycott BB. In: Ryan, et al: *Retina.* 2nd ed. St Louis, MO: Mosby; 1994.

retina is populated mostly by rods. The fovea provides us with clear, central 20/20 vision. Loss of the fovea and macular retina results in legal blindness even though the peripheral retina is intact. The macula is an area of increased yellow pigmentation and is called the macula lutea (yellow spot). The macula can be visualized during

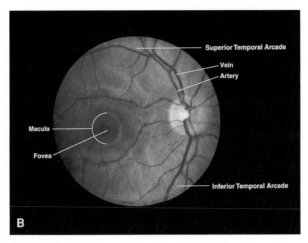

Figure 1-8.
Clinical fundus photograph showing normal optic disc macula and retina vessels. The macula is surrounded by the temporal retinal vascular arcade. The clinical macula is relatively ill-defined and represents the area inside the temporal arcade, which can be seen by the circular light reflex.

direct ophthalmoscopy by having the patient look directly at the light. In the center of the macula, the fovea is identified as a small indentation and may be visualized with a small light reflex.

The **optic disc,** which is the anterior aspect of the optic nerve, is located nasal to the macula. The optic disc is the exit point for the 1 million axons of the retinal ganglion cells that continue on to synapse with the lateral geniculate nucleus. There are no photoreceptors in the area of the optic disc. Therefore, the optic disc represents a blind spot of approximately 5 degrees in the visual field. The central aspect of the optic disc is excavated and is called the optic cup (**Figure 1-9**). The cup-to-disc ratio is the ratio of the diameter of the optic cup to the diameter of the optic disc. The normal cup-to-disc ratio is 0.3. A large cup may indicate glaucoma and increased intraocular pressure.

Retinal Vessels

Retinal vessels (eg, arteries and veins), emanate from the center of the optic disc and divide into the superior and inferior temporal arcades and the superior and inferior nasal arcades. The retinal vessels supply oxygen and nutrients to the inner layers of the retina while the choriocapillaris of the choroid supply the outer layers.

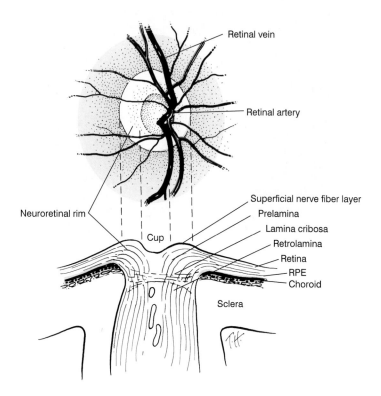

Figure 1-9.
Normal optic nerve (anterior optic nerve head and transverse view, right eye): note the central cup, neuroretinal rim, retinal vessels, 4 divisions of anterior optic nerve (superficial nerve fiber layer, prelaminar region, lamina cribrosa, retrolaminar region).

■ EXTRAOCULAR MUSCLES

There are 6 extraocular muscles: 4 rectus muscles and 2 oblique muscles (**Figures 1-1 and 1-10**). The 4 rectus muscles (superior, inferior, medial, and lateral recti) originate at the orbital apex and extend anteriorly to insert on the back of the globe. Horizontal rectus muscles (ie, medial and lateral recti) have relatively simple functions and pull the eye in the direction of the contracting muscle (**Figure 1-11**). **Adduction** is movement toward the midline (to the nose) and **abduction** is movement away from the midline (toward the ear). Note that the vertical rectus muscles (ie, superior and infe-

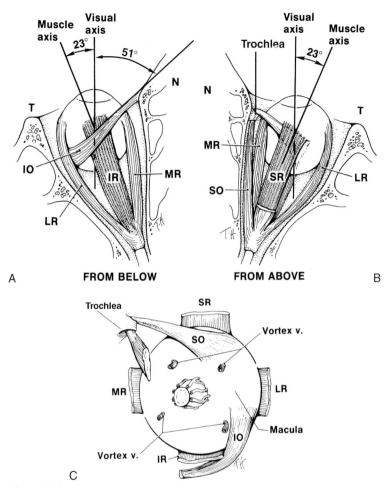

Figure 1-10.

Drawing of extraocular muscles. Notice that the visual axis is 23° off the vertical muscle axis (inferior rectus [IR] and superior rectus [SR]) and 51° off oblique muscle axis (inferior oblique [IO] and superior oblique [SO]) (Figure 1-10 A and B). **A,** The inferior oblique muscle view seen from below the eye. **B,** The superior oblique muscle view from above. Notice the superior oblique parallels the inferior oblique with the functional origin being the trochlea. **C,** View behind the eye shows relationship of the extraocular muscle. Notice that both oblique muscles lie below their corresponding rectus muscles (superior oblique is below the superior rectus and the inferior oblique is below the inferior rectus). LR = Lateral rectus muscle; MR = Medial rectus muscle. (From Wright K. *Color Atlas of Ophthalmic Surgery: Strabismus.* Philadelphia, PA: JB Lippinoctt; 1991.)

Table 1-2.
Extraocular Muscle Measurements

Muscle	Origin	Insertion: Distance From Limbus (mm)	Approximate Muscle Length (mm)	Tendon Length (mm)	Arc of Contact (mm)	Action From Primary Position
Medial rectus	Annulus of Zinn	5.5	40	4	6	Adduction
Lateral rectus	Annulus of Zinn	7.0	40	8	10	Abduction
Superior rectus	Annulus of Zinn	8.0	40	6	6.5	Elevation, intorsion, adduction
Inferior rectus	Annulus of Zinn	6.5	40	7	7	Depression, extorsion, adduction
Superior oblique	Orbit apex above annulus of Zinn	From temporal superior rectus insertion to 6.5 mm from optic nerve	32	26	12	Intorsion, depression, abduction
Inferior oblique	Larcimal fossa	Macular area	37	1	10	Extorsion, elevation, abduction

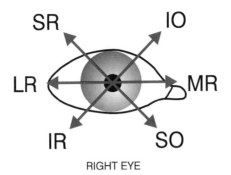

RIGHT EYE

Figure 1-11.
Field of action of the extraocular muscles. Diagram shows right eye, and the arrows point to the direction of gaze where a specific muscle is the major mover. To test a specific muscle, have the patient look in the direction of the arrow. **SR** = Superior rectus; **IO** = Inferior oblique; **MR** = Medial rectus; **SO** = Superior oblique; **IR** Inferior rectus; **LR** = Lateral rectus.

rior rectus muscles) and the oblique muscles (ie, superior and inferior oblique muscles) have more than one function, as the muscle axis is different than the visual axis of the eye (**Figure 1-10** and **Table 1-2**). **Figure 1-11** shows the field of action of the extraocular muscles. The field of action is the gaze position where a specific muscle contributes most and is the major mover. For example, the superior oblique (SO) muscle is the major contributor in moving the eye down and in. Therefore, as noted in **Figure 1-11,** the arrow relating to the superior oblique points down and in.

Table 1-3 lists the relationship of the muscles to each other, including the agonist-antagonists and synergists. Agonist-antagonist muscles work against each other to maintain smooth eye movements; the agonist muscle contracts, while the antagonist muscle relaxes. For example, when the eye moves inward toward the nose (adduction), the medial rectus (MR) contracts and the lateral rectus (LR) is inhibited (**Figure 1-12**). This physiologic relationship is termed **Sherrington's law of reciprocal innervation** (agonist/antagonist). Synergists move the eye in the same direction.

The 4 horizontal rectus muscles (one medial and one lateral rectus per eye) carry arterial supply that nourishes the anterior aspect of the cornea and iris. Surgical removal of 3 or more of the rectus muscles may result in decreased perfusion to the anterior part of the eye, causing **anterior segment ischemia.** Anterior segment is-

Table 1-3.
Monocular Movements

	Agonist-Antagonist
Medial rectus	Lateral rectus
Superior rectus	Inferior rectus
Superior oblique	Inferior oblique

	Synergists	
Duction	*Primary Mover*	*Secondary Mover*
Supraduction	Superior rectus	Inferior oblique
Infraduction	Inferior rectus	Superior oblique
Adduction	Medial rectus	Superior rectus/inferior rectus
Abduction	Lateral rectus	Superior oblique/inferior oblique
Extorsion	Inferior oblique	Inferior rectus
Intorsion	Superior oblique	Superior rectus

chemia is very unusual in children because of the tremendous perfusion capacity in the young. However, it can occur in older adults with compromised circulation.

The superior oblique muscle originates at the orbital apex and courses supranasally to enter the trochlea and then reflects posteriorly to insert under the superior rectus onto the globe. The functional origin of the superior oblique muscle is the trochlea, located in the superior nasal quadrant of the orbit. When the superior oblique muscle contracts, it pulls the back of the eye up and in, therefore depressing the front of the eye. The inferior oblique muscle originates in the lacrimal fossa located in the inferior nasal quadrant of the anterior aspect of the orbit. The inferior oblique parallels the course of the superior oblique tendon and inserts on the posterior temporal aspect of the globe. When the inferior oblique contracts, it pulls the back of the eye down and in, thus elevating and abducting the eye.

The third cranial nerve innervates the superior rectus, inferior rectus, medial rectus, and inferior oblique muscles. The lateral rectus is innervated by the sixth cranial nerve and the superior oblique is innervated by the fourth cranial nerve. A congenital paresis of the fourth cranial nerve is fairly common, and affected children present with torticollis (head tilt) to compensate for the weak superior oblique muscle.

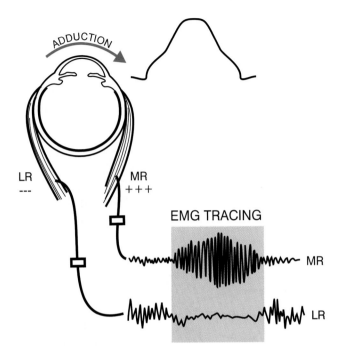

Figure 1-12.
Sherrington's law of reciprocal innervation (agonist/antagonist). Diagram shows left eye moving in adduction with the left medial rectus muscle the agonist and firing on EMG recordings while the left lateral rectus is the antagonist and relaxes as shown by EMG recording.

■ EYELIDS

The eyelids represent specialized structures of the face designed to protect, moisten, and cleanse the ocular surfaces (**Figure 1-13**). The eyelids close by contracture of the orbicularis oculi muscle, which is innervated by the facial nerve (seventh cranial nerve) and courses in a circumferential pattern within the eyelids. The levator and Müller's muscle are responsible for elevating the upper lid (**Figure 1-13**). The levator muscle is innervated by the third cranial nerve, while Müller's muscle is innervated by sympathetic nerves. In Horner syndrome (sympathetic nerve palsy causing miosis, anhydrosis, and ptosis), the ptosis is secondary to denervation of Müller's muscle.

Tarsal plates are firm, dense, fibrous, connective tissue (not cartilage) structures that provide strong structural integrity of the upper

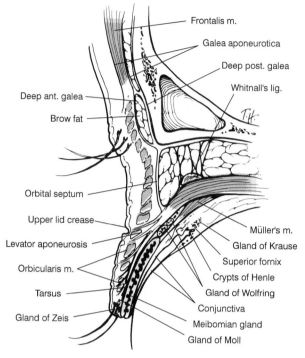

Figure 1-13.
Sagittal section of the upper lid containing the various tear-secreting glands along with the eyebrow and the superior fornix. The basal secretory tear glands reside near the surface of the posterior eyelid in addition to the eyelid margin and the superior fornix.

and lower eyelids. The inside surface of the tarsal plate is lined with conjunctiva (tarsal conjunctiva). Within the tarsal plate are specialized sebaceous glands called **meibomian glands.** Blockage of the orifice of the meibomian gland can result in inspissation of the sebaceous material with secondary inflammation and is referred to as a **sty (chalazion).** Meibomian glands are present in both the upper and lower lids, and the orifices can be seen as they exit at the lid margins (**Figure 1-13**). Glands that are located anterior to the tarsal plate include the glands of Zeis and Moll. An infection of the Zeis gland results in an **external hordeolum.** The upper and lower eyelids join nasally to form the medial canthal area and laterally to form the lateral canthal area.

■ LACRIMAL SYSTEM

Aqueous tears are secreted from the lacrimal gland soon after birth, at approximately 2 to 4 weeks of age. Tears exit the lacrimal gland, then course across the surface of the eye and exit through the upper and lower puncta located in the nasal aspect of the upper and lower lids (**Figure 1-14**). The puncta are connected to canaliculi that course through the upper and lower lids to come together as they enter the nasolacrimal sac. The nasolacrimal sac extends inferiorly to become the nasolacrimal duct. The nasolacrimal duct exits in the posterior aspect of the nose under the inferior turbinate. A series of small valves are present in the duct, with the most important being Hasner's valve 8 at the distal aspect of the lacrimal duct. This valve is usually closed at birth, but opens during the first few weeks of life. If the valve does not open, it will obstruct normal tear flow and will result in a **nasolacrimal duct obstruction** and infantile tearing.

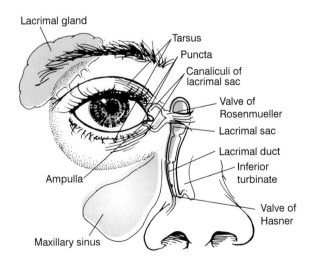

Figure 1-14.
Nasolacrimal excretory system with a portion of the maxillary bone removed. The nasolacrimal duct can be seen emptying under the inferior turbinate in the lateral nose.

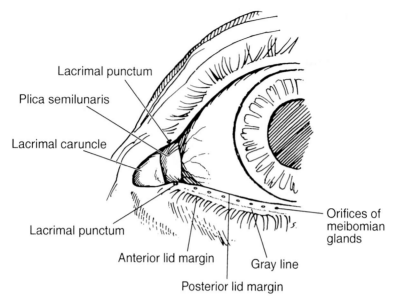

Figure 1-15.
Drawing of medial canthal area showing lacrimal caruncle, lacrimal punctum orifice or meibomian glands, and gray line. Note that the gray line is just anterior to the meibomian gland orifices.

■ MEDIAL CANTHAL AREA

The medial canthal area is important, as the punctum and canaliculi are located here (**Figure 1-15**). A lid laceration in the medial canthus can disrupt the canaliculi and result in tearing. Canalicular tears must be carefully sutured to avoid this complication.

■ BIBLIOGRAPHY

1. Gordon RA, Donzis PB. Refractive development of the human eye. *Arch Ophthalmol.* 1985;103:785–789

2 Amblyopia and Strabismus

■ VISUAL DEVELOPMENT

At birth, our visual acuity is quite poor, probably in the range of 20/200 to 20/800 (legal blindness). For the most part, this is due to immaturity of the visual centers in the brain responsible for vision processing. Visual acuity rapidly improves during the first 3 to 4 months of life as clear, in-focus retinal images stimulate functional and structural development of visual centers such as the lateral geniculate nucleus and the striate cortex (**Figure 2-1**). Normal visual development is therefore dependent on appropriate visual stimulation during the developmental period. Requirements for normal visual development include equal retinal stimulation, with clearly formed images, and proper eye alignment (**Table 2-1**).

Visual development is most critical during the first 3 to 4 months of life and this stage is termed the **critical period of visual development.** Note that, in **Figure 2-1,** the curve of visual acuity improvement is steepest during the first 4 months of life, but development continues to 8 or 9 years of age. Early treatment of pediatric eye disease is important to promote normal visual development.

Table 2-1.
Requirements for Normal Visual Development

Clear retinal image
Equal image clarity
Proper eye alignment (no strabismus)

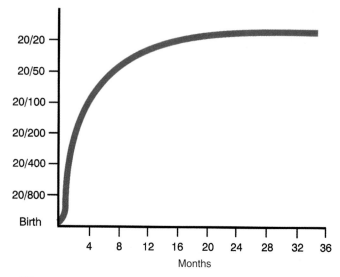

Figure 2-1.
Curve represents visual acuity development, with age on the horizontal axis and Snellen acuity on the vertical axis. Note the exponential improvement in visual acuity during the critical period of visual development (birth to 4 months).

■ BINOCULAR VISION

Binocular vision requires integration of retinal images from 2 eyes into a single, 3-dimensional perception. This process of merging 2 separate images into one binocular image is termed **binocular fusion.** Binocular fusion is required to maintain proper eye alignment and provide stereopsis (depth perception). Animal studies by **Wiesel and Hubel** have shown that binocular cortical connections are present from birth. Normally, around 70% of visual cortex neurons are binocular and respond to visual stimulation of both eyes. The minority of visual cortical cells are monocular, responding to only one eye. Even though binocular anatomy is present at birth, appropriate visual input from each eye is necessary to refine and maintain these binocular neural connections. The presence of strabismus (eg, ocular misalignment) or a unilateral blurred retinal image (eg, congenital cataract or anisometropia) will disrupt normal binocular visual development and cause a partial or complete loss of binocular fusion and stereopsis.

■ VISUAL DEVELOPMENTAL MILESTONES

For the first 4 to 6 weeks of life, eye movements are inaccurate, fast, and jerky, without the smooth coordination of normal visual fixation. During the first several weeks after birth, infants develop accurate, smooth, pursant eye movements and central fixation. A key developmental milestone for normal infants is the ability to visually fixate and accurately follow small objects accurately by 2 to 3 months of age. Normal infants may occasionally show delayed visual maturation; however, poor fixation past 6 months of age is usually pathologic and should be fully investigated with a complete ophthalmologic examination.

Eye alignment also changes after birth. At birth, eye alignment is variable with approximately 70% of infants showing a small variable exotropia, 30% having essentially straight eyes (orthotropia), and esotropia is rare. By 2 to 3 months of age, the majority of normally developing infants have established proper alignment. The persistence of a strabismus after 2 months of age may indicate ocular pathology, and these patients and should be referred for ophthalmological evaluation. Primitive binocular vision begins in early infancy, as human studies have documented binocular fusion at 2 to 3 months of age. Stereopsis (depth perception) and higher grade binocular fusion, however, develops later, between 3 and 6 months of age. **Table 2-2** outlines the visual developmental milestones from birth to visual maturity.

Table 2-2.
Visual Developmental Milestones

Birth to 2 months	Poor and sporadic fixation
	Jerky, fast eye movements (saccades)
	Exotropia 70%, Orthotropia 30% (straight eyes), Esotropia is rare
2 months to 6 months	Accurate fixation (locks on target)
	Precise smooth pursuit eye movements
	Orthotropia (straight eyes)
3 to 4 years	Visual Acuity 20/40
5 to 6 years	Visual Acuity 20/30
7 to 9 years	Visual Acuity 20/25 to 20/20

■ ADAPTATIONS TO ABNORMAL VISUAL STIMULATION

As stated previously, normal visual development requires clear retinal images and proper eye alignment. Abnormal visual stimulation by a unilateral or bilateral blurred retinal image or ocular misalignment can disrupt normal visual development and cause poor vision, which is called **amblyopia.**

Strabismus

Strabismus is the condition of ocular misalignment including esotropia (eye turned in), exotropia (eye turned out), or vertical deviation (eye turned up or down). If strabismus occurs early, before 4 to 6 years of age, the child will cortically turn off, or **suppress,** the image from the deviated eye. This defense mechanism (suppression) prevents bothersome double vision. Alternating strabismus is a switch in fixation from one eye to the other (**Figure 2-2**) and is associated with alternating suppression. This alternating fixation allows for equal monocular visual development with no amblyopia, however, suppression disrupts binocular development and causes loss of binocular fusion and stereopsis. In contrast, strong fixation preference for an eye and prolonged suppression of the fellow eye can lead to amblyopia with loss of vision in the suppressed eye. A constant strabismus, with strong fixation preference for an eye, results in both loss of binocular fusion and amblyopia of the non-preferred deviated eye (ie, strabismic amblyopia).

Amblyopia

Amblyopia occurs in approximately 2% of the general population and is the most common cause of decreased vision in childhood. The term *amblyopia* is derived from the Greek language and means dull vision: amblys = dull, ops = eye. Generally speaking, amblyopia can refer to poor vision from any cause but, in this text and in most medical literature, amblyopia refers to poor vision caused by abnormal visual development secondary to abnormal visual stimulation. Abnormal visual stimulation can be caused by a blurred image (cataract or severe refractive error) or strabismus with strong preference for one eye and constant suppression of the non-preferred eye (see Pathophysiology and Classification of Amblyopia on page 26). Other terms for amblyopia include *functional amblyopia* and *amblyopia ex anopsia.*

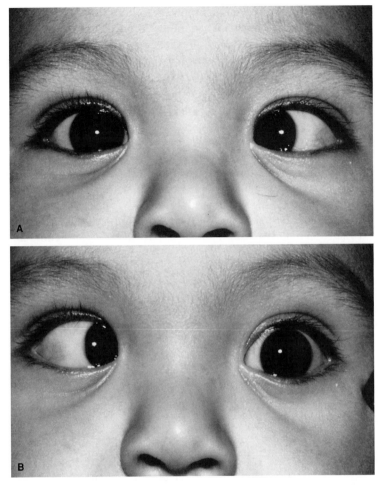

Figure 2-2.
Infant with congenital esotropia and alternating fixation. In figure A, patient is fixing right eye. In figure B, patient has switched fixation to the left eye. Alternating fixation indicates equal visual preference, no amblyopia.

Children are susceptible to developing amblyopia between birth and 7 years of age. The earlier the onset of abnormal stimulation, the greater is the visual deficit. For practical purposes, amblyopia is defined as at least 2 Snellen lines difference in visual acuity between the eyes, but amblyopia is truly a spectrum of visual loss, ranging from missing a few letters on the 20/20 line to hand motion vision.

Functional amblyopia, or amblyopia, should be distinguished from *organic amblyopia*, which is poor vision caused by structural abnormalities of the eye or brain that are independent of sensory input, such as optic atrophy, a macular scar, or anoxic occipital brain damage.

Pathophysiology and Classification of Amblyopia

Hubel and Wiesel were awarded the Nobel Prize for their work demonstrating that amblyopia is caused by abnormal visual stimulation during early visual development, and abnormal stimulation results in anatomical changes in visual centers of the brain (**Figure 2-3**). There are 3 basic types of abnormal visual stimulation that can cause amblyopia: *strabismus* with constant suppression of one eye, *monocular blurred image*, and *binocular blurred image* (**Table 2-3**).

RIGHT EYE

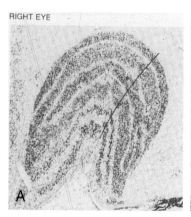

LEFT EYE

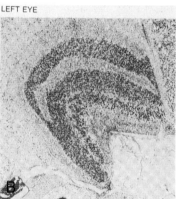

RIGHT EYE

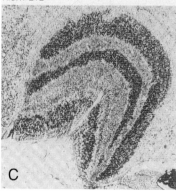

Figure 2-3.
Pathology of amblyopia (LGN). **A,** Cross section of lateral geniculate nucleus (LGN) from a normal monkey. **B and C,** Vs amblyopic monkey caused by a unilateral blurred image. Note that the normal LGN, **A** has 6 nuclear layers (darkly stained cell layer), and the amblyopic LGN, **B and C** only have 3 layers and they are thicker than normal. (from Wiesel and Hubel)

Table 2-3.
Classification of Amblyopia

A. Strabismic Amblyopia
   1. Congenital esotropia
   2. Acquired esotropia in childhood
B. Monocular Blurred Image
   1. Anisometropia (difference in refractive error)
      a. Hypermetropic
      b. Myopic
      c. Astigmatic
   2. Media Opacity
      a. Unilateral cataract
      b. Unilateral corneal opacity (eg, Peters anomaly)
      c. Unilateral vitreous hemorrhage or vitreous opacity
C. Bilateral Blurred Image
   1. Refractive error
      a. Bilateral high hypermetropia
      b. Astigmatism
   2. Media opacity
      a. Bilateral congenital cataracts
      b. Bilateral corneal opacities (eg, Peters anomaly)
      c. Bilateral vitreous opacity (hemorrhages)

Pathological changes associated with amblyopia occur in the lateral geniculate nucleus (LGN) and the visual cortex of the occipital lobe. **Figure 2-3** shows the pathological changes in the LGN of a monkey raised with a monocular blurred retinal image. Normally, there are 6 nuclear layers of the LGN—3 layers corresponding to the right eye and 3 layers corresponding to the left eye. Because of the blurred retinal image, only 3 layers corresponding to the eye with the clear retinal image developed. Due to the increased visual stimulation of the good eye, these 3 layers are darker stained and larger than normal. Ocular dominance columns in the visual cortex are also damaged as a result of a unilateral blurred image during early development, as shown in **Figure 2-4.** Thus, there is strong evidence to show that the poor vision found with amblyopia is caused by anatomical changes in the visual areas of the brain.

Monocular Blurred Image Amblyopia

Clinically, mild image blur (eg, blur associated with a mild refractive error) causes mild amblyopia, but allows for the development of some degree of binocular fusion and stereopsis (ie, peripheral fu-

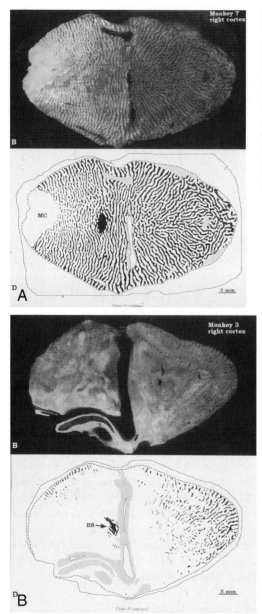

Figure 2-4.
Pathology of amblyopia
(striate cortex).
Histopathology of monkey
striate cortex (visual
cortex). **A,** Well-defined
cortex columns are on
seen in the normal
specimen. **B,** cortex
columns are
underdeveloped in
specimen from the
amblyopic monkey. (from
Horton and Hocking)

sion). A severely blurred image during infancy (eg, unilateral congenital cataract or corneal opacity), however, can result in profound vision loss and strabismus.

Anisometropic amblyopia, one of the most common types of amblyopia, is caused by a difference in refractive errors that results in a monocular or asymmetric image blur. Most patients with anisometropic amblyopia have straight eyes that appear normal, so the only way to identify these patients is through vision screening. Stereo acuity testing has had limited value in screening for anisometropic amblyopia because most patients have relatively good stereopsis (between 70 and 3000 seconds arc). Myopic anisometropia is generally less amblyogenic than hypermetropic anisometropia. As little as + 1.00 hypermetropic anisometropia and -2.00 myopic anisometropia can be associated with amblyopia. Astigmatic anisometropic amblyopia does not occur unless there is a unilateral astigmatism greater than 1.50 diopters. Myopic anisometropic amblyopia is often amenable to treatment even in late childhood, whereas hypermetropic amblyopia is often difficult to treat past 4 or 5 years of age. This is probably due to the fact that high myopia is usually acquired after the critical period of visual development, and the more myopic eye is in focus for near objects (a baby's world is up close). In contrast, patients with hypermetropic anisometropia always use the less hypermetropic eye because it requires less accommodative effort. This causes the more hypermetrophic eye to become blurred, and is constantly suppressed.

Bilateral Blurred Image Amblyopia

Bilateral amblyopia occurs when there is bilateral symmetrical retinal image blur and no strabismus. Clinically, the effects of pure image blur are seen in cases of bilateral high hypermetropia (>6.00 diopters), bilateral symmetrical astigmatism (>3.00 diopters), or with bilateral severe ocular opacities such as dense bilateral congenital cataracts. The severity of the visual deficit depends on the extent of the image distortion. If severe image blur occurs during the neonatal period so that essentially no pattern stimulation is provided, extremely poor vision and **sensory nystagmus** develops. Bilateral amblyopia and sensory nystagmus will occur in cases of dense bilateral congenital opacities. Other causes of sensory nystagmus include organic causes of congenital blindness such as macular or optic nerve pathology. Sensory nystagmus does not occur with cortical blindness because extra striate visual pathways anterior to the occipital cortex supply the fixation reflex. Acquired opacities after 6 to 12 months of age usually do not cause sensory nystagmus, as the motor component of fixation has already been established. The presence of sensory nystagmus indicates severe bilateral visual loss during the first few months of life and has a poor prognosis.

Amblyopic Vision

The visual deficit associated with amblyopia has certain unique characteristics, including the *crowding phenomenon* and *eccentric fixation*. The crowding phenomenon relates to the fact that patients with amblyopia have better visual acuity reading single optotypes than reading multiple optotypes in a row (linear optotypes). Often, patients with amblyopia will perform 1 or 2 Snellen lines better when presented with single optotypes versus linear optotypes. This crowding phenomenon may have something to do with the relatively large receptive field associated with amblyopia. Crowding bars can be placed around a single optotype to provide a more sensitive test for amblyopia.

Eccentric fixation is a characteristic of severe amblyopia. Patients with mild amblyopia (20/40-20/100) fixate so close to the fovea, they appear to fixate centrally. Severe amblyopia, usually 20/200 to count fingers, is associated with parafoveal viewing or eccentric fixation. When the good eye is occluded and the amblyopic eye is forced to view, patients with eccentric fixation demonstrate roaming eye movements and cannot "visually lock" on the target. The presence of eccentric fixation is a clinical sign of severe amblyopia and has a poor visual prognosis.

■ AMBLYOGENIC PERIOD

The severity of the amblyopia depends on when the abnormal stimulus began, the length of exposure to abnormal stimulation, and the severity of the image blur. The more severe the image blur, the earlier the onset, and the longer the duration of a malapropos stimulus, the more severe the visual loss. Children are most susceptible to amblyopia during the critical period of visual development, which is the first few months of life. Stimulation of a severely blurred retinal image during the critical period of visual development results in dense, often irreversible, amblyopia. This is why visually significant congenital cataracts must be operated and visually rehabilitated within the first few weeks of life for best visual results. Amblyopia can occur, however, in older children. Acquired strabis-

Table 2-4.
Visual Development and Amblyopia

Critical period:	One week to 3 to 4 months (most susceptible to amblyopia)
Visual plasticity:	Birth to 7 or 8 years (susceptible to amblyopia)
Extended plasticity:	Ten years to adulthood—may retain limited plasticity (not susceptible to amblyopia and amblyopia therapy is ineffective)

mus, or an acquired media opacity such as a cataract, can cause some amblyopia, even up to 7 or 8 years of age, albeit of lesser severity. **Table 2-4** lists the major periods of visual plasticity and susceptibility to amblyopia.

■ DETECTION OF AMBLYOPIA

Early detection and early intervention is critical to the treatment of amblyopia. In preverbal children and infants, the best method for vision screening is the simultaneous red reflex test or "Bruckner" test. This test will detect amblyopic refractive errors and optical media opacities such as cataracts. Older children ($2\frac{1}{2}$ years to 3 years of age) should be able to cooperate with some form of visual acuity testing, usually a type of picture card, such as Wright figures or the "E" game. Details on detecting amblyopia are covered in the next chapter (Chapter 3).

■ TREATMENT OF AMBLYOPIA

The first step to treating amblyopia is to make sure that there is a clear retinal image. Refractive errors are corrected with spectacle or contact lenses, and visually significant opacities, such as cataracts, must be surgically removed. The next step is to correct ocular dominance in patients with unilateral amblyopia by occluding the good eye. Patients with strabismus and amblyopia may or may not require optical correction, but virtually all require occlusion therapy to correct the ocular dominance. Occluding or patching the sound eye forces use of the amblyopic eye to stimulate visual development. Young children, especially under 1 year of age, may develop occlusion amblyopia of the "good eye" so part-time occlusion is often prescribed for young children.

The earlier the intervention, the better the prognosis for amblyopia. Children with visually significant congenital cataracts are best treated during the first weeks of life, while delaying treatment past 3 or 4 months of age carries a relatively poor visual prognosis. Patients with less severe forms of amblyopia, such as anisometropic amblyopia (difference in refractive error), will have a better prognosis even when treated between 3 and 7 years of age. After 8 to 9 years of age, however, the chance of significantly improving the amblyopia is small. Even so, patients who present late with amblyopia are often treated. Even patients with presumed congenital cataracts may show some visual improvement with aggressive amblyopia management. Adults with amblyopia, who lose vision in their good eye, may even show some limited improvement of vision in the amblyopic eye.

Atropine Drops for the Treatment of Amblyopia (Penalization)

Topical atropine 1% dilates the pupil and paralyzes accommodation (focusing). Atropine drops can be used in patients with amblyopia to blur the vision of the good eye to force use of the amblyopic eye, and this is called penalization. The blurring effect of atropine is greatest for near vision and for eyes that are hyperopic. Atropine will not significantly blur the vision if the eye is myopic or if there is no refractive error. Thus, atropine penalization will not work unless the good eye is significantly hyperopic. Most patients with amblyopia are best treated with occlusion of the good eye, but in selected cases atropine may be useful.

■ BIBLIOGRAPHY

1. Horton JC, Hocking DR. Timing of the critical period for plasticity of ocular dominance columns in macaque striate cortex, *J Neurosci.* 1997 17:3684–3709
2. Sondhi N, Archer SM, Helveston EM. Development of normal ocular alignment. *J Pediatr Ophthalmol Strabismus.* September/October 1988; 25:210–211
3. von Noorden GK, Crawford ML, Levacy RA. The lateral geniculate nucleus in human anisometropic amblyopia. *Invest Ophthalmol Vis Sci.* 1983; 24:788–790
4. Wiesel TN, Hubel DH. Ordered arrangement of orientation columns in monkeys lacking visual experience. *J Comp Neurol.* December 1974; 158:307–318
5. Wright KW, Matsumoto E, Edelman PM. Binocular fusion and stereopsis associated with early surgery for monocular congenital cataracts. *Arch Ophthalmol.* 1992;110:1607–1609

3 Ocular Examination and Vision Screening

Early detection and treatment of pediatric ocular disease is critical. Diseases such as congenital cataracts, retinoblastoma, and congenital glaucoma require early treatment during infancy. Delay in diagnosis may result in irreversible vision loss and, in the case of retinoblastoma, potentially death. It is therefore imperative to provide effective vision screening of all children from newborns to older children.

■ VISION SCREENING

Vision screening examinations should start at birth and continue as part of routine check-ups. The acronym **I-ARM** (**I**nspection, **A**cuity, **R**ed reflex, and **M**otility) can be a helpful reminder of the essential parts of a pediatric screening examination. **Table 3-1** summarizes the I-ARM screening eye examination for neonates, babies, and children. The most important test for the newborn is the **red reflex test.** If an abnormal red reflex is present, then an immediate referral to an ophthalmologist is required. Infant screening examinations take less than a minute, but these brief examinations are quite powerful, and if performed properly, can detect the vast majority of eye pathology including the important diagnoses mentioned above. Equipment needed for the I-ARM screening examination include the direct ophthalmoscope and a visual chart such as the E-game, Wright figures **(Figure 3-1),** or Snellen letters (for literate children).

Table 3-1.

Screening Eye Examination: I-ARM

	Neonate (Birth to 2 months)	Babies (3 months to 2 years)	Childhood (3 years and older)
Inspection	Ocular symmetry	Ocular symmetry; Face turn or head tilt	Ocular symmetry; Face turn or head tilt
Acuity	Sporadic fixation; Pupillary response	Good fixation and smooth pursuit. Test each eye separately.	Optotype acuity: Wright figures, E-game, and Snellen acuity
Red reflex	Red reflex test	Binocular red reflex (Bruckner)	Bilateral red reflex test (Bruckner)
Motility	Gross alignment; (70% small exotropia—but esotropia is probably abnormal)	Good alignment; Light reflex and Bruckner (Strabismus is considered abnormal after 2 months)	Good alignment; Light reflex and Bruckner

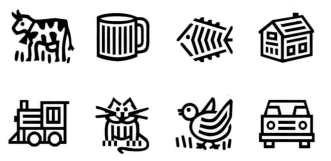

Figure 3-1.
Wright Figures for visual assessment of preverbal children. The figures are made up of white and black bars, with the overall footprint being approximately 2 times the size of a normal Snellen letter, but the resolution is equivalent to Snellen letters. (Copyright 2000 Kenneth W. Wright, MD)

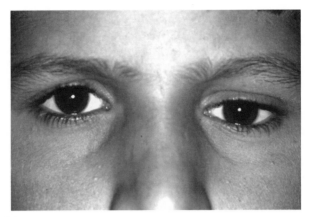

Figure 3-2.
Inspection. Look for symmetry. Thirteen-year-old boy. Note the left ptosis and downward displacement of the left eye. A dermoid cyst located on the roof of the left orbit is causing the inferior displacement of the left eye.

Inspection

Simple inspection of the eyes and lids for abnormalities of symmetry can be very helpful. **Figure 3-2** shows a patient with a left orbital dermoid cyst. At first glance, the patient appears to have no gross abnormality. However, as one compares the right eye to the left eye, it becomes obvious that this patient has a left ptosis and the left eye is displaced down. Also, inspect for a face turn or head tilt because this can be compensatory mechanism to reduce strabismus or damp nystagmus. If the onset of an ocular abnormality is in question, look at family photographs for documentation. **Table 3-2** outlines the 3 major categories for ocular inspection.

Acuity

Visual acuity testing for preverbal and verbal children is described in the following paragraphs. **Table 3-3** shows the normal visual acuity expected at specific ages.

Table 3-2.
Ocular Inspection

1. Symmetry—compare fellow eyes, look at pupils, eyelids, and lid fissures
2. Check for face turn or head tilt
3. Ocular irritation (pink eye, squinting)

Preverbal Children

It is important to try to obtain a visual acuity on every child, even infants. From birth to approximately 2 months of age, there may only be sporadic fix and follow. Between 2 and 6 months of age, patients should have the ability to fix and follow on a small toy or the human face. Cover one eye and move a target (eg, your face or a toy) right, left, up, and down to observe if the eyes will accurately follow the motion. It is important to test each eye individually, as with both eyes open, the eyes will track together even if one eye is blind. Also, use a compelling target. In infants, the human face is probably the most compelling target, while in toddlers and young children, a small toy or a finger puppet is a good target. Observe for **central fixation** with the presence of accurate smooth pursuit. Central fixation means that the patient looks directly at the target, not off-center, and will smoothly and accurately follow the target. If the patient has trouble locking on the target and appears to be looking off-center, this indicates poor fixation and poor vision (**Figure 3-3**).

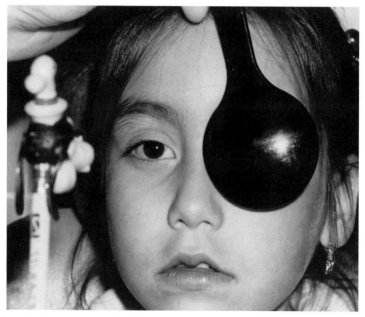

Figure 3-3.
A child being tested for central fixation right eye. Check for accurate and smooth pursuit eye movements. Does the patient lock on the target? Test each eye individually by covering the opposite eye.

Verbal Children

By 2½ to 3 years of age, most children should be able to cooperate with optotype visual acuity testing using either a picture (E-game, Wright figures) or Snellen letters. It is important to test each eye separately and make sure that the occluded eye is truly covered. Many examiners prefer occluding one eye with an adhesive patch, rather than a paddle occluder, to prevent the child from peeking. Most vision charts are calibrated at 10 or 20 feet from the patient. Examine patients with their customary eyeglasses or contact lenses. If patients forget their corrective lenses, first test the vision without correction and then retest using a pinhole.

Pinholes

Pinholes are commercially available; however, you can make your own pinhole by taking a 3″ x 5″ card and placing several small pinholes in the card. If the patient's visual acuity improves after viewing through the pinhole, this indicates that a refractive error is the cause of the decreased vision. A pinhole is useful when a patient presents without his or her spectacle correction to estimate visual acuity with optical correction. A pinhole will improve vision to around 20/30, even when patients have large refractive errors.

Criterion for Referral

If a 3- to 5-year-old has a visual acuity of 20/50 or worse, or >2 lines difference between fellow eyes, then this patient should be referred. Children 6 years or older should be referred if visual acuity is 20/40 or worse or if there is >2-line difference between fellow eyes (**Table 3-3**). Many young children will give inconsistent re-

Table 3-3.
Visual Acuity Milestones

Age	Normal Acuity*
0-2 months	Pupillary response, sporadic fix and follow, jerky eye movements (saccades)
2-6 months	Central fix and follow, smooth eye movements
6 months to 2 years	Grabs for toy, central fixation, accurate and smooth pursuit eye movements
3 years to 4 years	20/40 and not more than 2 lines difference
≥5 years	20/30 and not more than 2 lines difference

* If patient's vision does not meet these standards, then an ophthalmology referral is indicated.

sponses and, in these cases, visual acuity should be re-tested, or the patient referred for a complete ophthalmic examination. In children with very poor vision, visual acuity is measured by the ability to (1) count fingers at 1 to 2 feet, (2) see hand motions at 1 foot, or (3) ability to perceive any light. The ability to see light is called **light perception (LP)** and no light vision is called **no light perception (NLP).** Most states define **legal blindness** as 20/200 or worse visual acuity.

Red Reflex Test

The red reflex test is the single best vision screening examination for infants and young children. It is best performed using the **Bruckner test,** which is simply a simultaneous bilateral red reflex. Use the direct ophthalmoscope and view the patient's eyes at a distance of approximately 2 feet. Use a broad beam so that both eyes are illuminated at the same time. Have the child look directly into the ophthalmoscope light and dim the room lights. Start with the ophthalmoscope on low illumination, and then slowly increase the illumination until a red reflex is seen. You will observe a red reflex that fills the pupil, and a small (approximately 1 mm) white light reflex that appears to reflect off the cornea (**Figure 3-4**). The light reflex is actually a reflex coming from just behind the pupil; however, it is commonly called the **corneal light reflex** or the "Hirschberg Reflex." Thus, the Bruckner test will give both a red reflex and the corneal light reflex simultaneously.

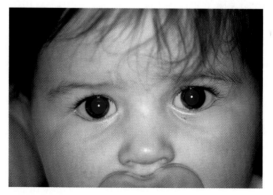

Figure 3-4.
Normal Bruckner test with symmetric red reflexes and centered corneal light reflexes.

An opacity in the optical media or large area of retinal pathology will result in an abnormal red reflex (**Figures 3-5 A through D**). A cataract can either block the red reflex or reflect light to give a white reflex (**Figure 3-5A**). Retinoblastoma has a yellowish white color and will produce a yellow reflex (**Figure 3-5B**). Anisometropia (ie, asymmetric refractive error) will result in an unequal red reflex (**Figure 3-5C**). Strabismus will cause a brighter red reflex in the

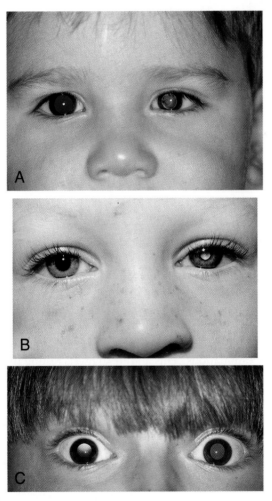

Figure 3-5.
Abnormal reflex. **A,** Cataract and esotropia—left eye. **B,** Retinoblastoma—left eye. **C,** Anisometropia—brighter reflex right eye.

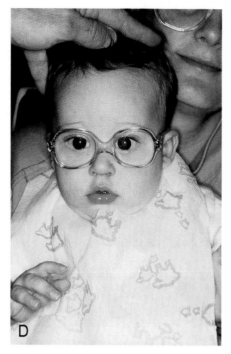

Figure 3-5. (continued)
D, Strabismus—esotropia with brighter reflex from deviated left eye (Note this is the author's youngest son. The author subsequently performed strabismus surgery, and is happy to report the eyes have remained straight.)

deviated eye and the corneal light reflex will be decentered (**Figure 3-5D**). The key sign of a normal examination is symmetry. Asymmetry or an abnormality of the reflex indicates a need for an immediate ophthalmology referral (**Table 3-4**).

Use of Mydriatic Drops

Some physicians have recommended the use of mydriatics for vision screening examinations. This author suggests testing the red reflex

Table 3-4.
Abnormal Red Reflex — (Asymmetry indicates pathology)

Cataract	May block the red reflex (dark or dull reflex) or may look white (leukocoria).
Vitreous hemorrhage	Blocks red reflex (dark or dull reflex).
Retinoblastoma	Appears as a yellow or white reflex (leukocoria).
Anisometropia	Results in an unequal red reflex.
Strabismus	The corneal light reflex will be decentered and cause a brighter red reflex in the deviated eye.

without mydriatics, but using low-light illumination and low oph-thalmoscope illumination to keep the pupil dilated. If dilation is desired, Mydriacyl 1% or cyclopentolate ½% with phenylephrine 2.5% may be used. For infants younger than 1 year of age, ½% Mydriacyl or Cyclomydril, which is a low concentration of Cyclogyl and phenylephrine, can be used.

Ocular Motility and Eye Alignment

Ocular motility is assessed by having the patient follow a target right, left, up, and down, observing for full ocular rotation. Patients with a muscle weakness show limited eye movement. If a limitation of eye movement is identified, an ophthalmology consult is indicated.

Ocular alignment is best assessed by the use of the corneal light reflex, or **Hirschberg,** test. As described previously, the corneal light reflex can be obtained when performing the Bruckner test. Alternatively, any light source that produces a beam broad enough to illuminate both eyes can elicit a corneal light reflex. Proper procedure is to use a muscle light or flashlight held at the examiner's nose and pointed toward the patient's nose, having the child look directly at the light (**Figure 3-6**). The light reflex should be symmet-

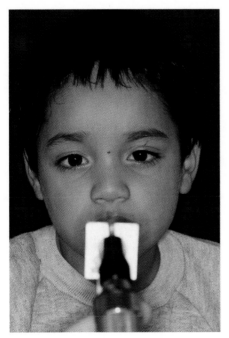

Figure 3-6.
Demonstration of the corneal light reflex test (Hirschberg test). Note that the fixation target (white square is a cartoon picture) is in line with the light and the child is looking at the fixation target. The examiner should be situated directly behind the muscle light.

rically centered or slightly nasally deviated. The key is that the light reflex is symmetric. Displacement of the light reflex indicates strabismus. Examples of the Hirschberg test are shown in **Figure 3-7 A through C**. Make sure the patient maintains fixation on the light source; otherwise, the light will appear to be off-center. Some authors have suggested the cover test be used to identify strabismus;

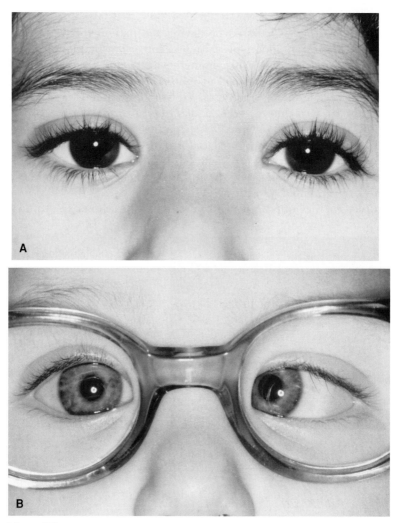

Figure 3-7.
Corneal Light Reflex. **A,** Orthotropia (light reflexes centered). **B,** Esotropia (left light reflex temporally displaced).

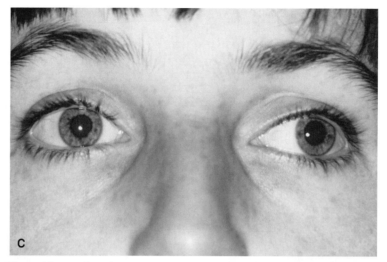

Figure 3-7. (continued)
C, Exotropia (left light reflex medially displaced).

however, this test is complex and even a normal patient may show a shift on cover test. This author prefers the light reflex and does not suggest the cover test for routine vision screening.

Cover test—The cover test is probably not necessary for vision screening, since the Bruckner test (bilateral red reflex test) and the corneal light reflex test are more specific for a true strabismus with a manifest deviation (ie, tropia). Many normal children show an eye movement shift with alternate cover testing, thus making the test difficult to interpret. The cover test entails covering one eye for 3 to 4 seconds then removing the cover. If there is a tendency for an eye to drift, the eye under the cover will drift **(Figure 3-8 A through C)**. If there is a history of intermittent strabismus (especially intermittent exotropia), yet the eyes appear well aligned, then the cover test may be helpful, although a referral to an ophthalmologist is indicated by the history alone.

Other Tests

Pupils

Pupils should be evaluated for size, shape, symmetry, and reaction to light. The swinging flashlight test identifies an afferent pupillary

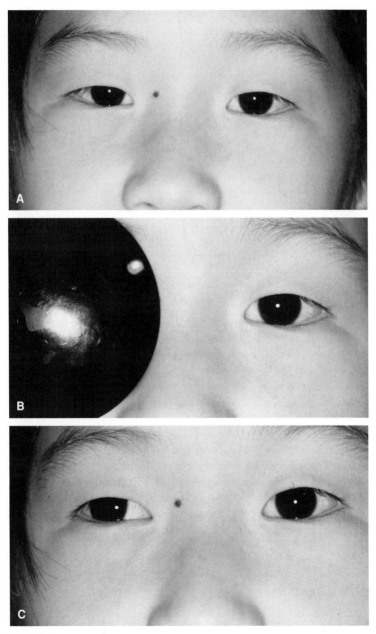

Figure 3-8.
Cover test; Intermittent Exotropia. **A,** Straight eyes—patient fusing. **B,** One eye covered. **C,** Right exotropia manifest after disrupting binocular fusion by covering the right eye (B).

defect (ie, pathology of retina or optic nerve). This test is based on the fact that both pupils will constrict to a light shined in one eye. If there is an optic nerve lesion or a large retinal lesion in one eye, light directed toward that eye results in minimal pupillary reaction and both eyes remain dilated. When the light is briskly moved to the fellow "good" eye, this results in increased pupillary reaction and miosis. Moving the light back to the eye with the pathology results in pupillary dilatation. Patients with equal pupillary responses show little change in pupil size when the flashlight is moved from eye to eye (see also Chapter 11).

Fluorescein Staining

Fluorescein staining is used to identify a corneal or conjunctival epithelial defect. The corneal epithelium is only approximately 5 to 8 cell-layers thick. A scratch or abrasion of the corneal epithelium results in positive staining by fluorescein. Use a premixed fluorescein solution, or use a fluorescein strip and add a drop of sterile saline or topical anesthetic to moisten the strip, and place a drop of fluorescein on the eye. Then have the patient blink several times and observe for a staining defect. Too much fluorescein will cloud the entire cornea and make identification of the staining defect very difficult. A wood's light or blue light causes the fluorescein to fluoresce and facilitates identification of the epithelial defect. A blue light, however, is not absolutely necessary as one can often see the fluorescent even with natural white light.

Fundus Examination

Direct ophthalmoscopy (hand-held ophthalmoscope) allows visualization of the optic nerve, retinal vessels, and fovea. The optic nerve will be visualized just nasal to the fovea. The fovea can be visualized by having the patient looking directly into the light while direct ophthalmoscopy is performed. One can usually visualize a small reflex at the center of fixation, which is the foveal pit. The optic nerve should be pink with sharp margins. Blurred optic disc margins, especially if associated with hemorrhages, may indicate papilledema. The optic cup is the central area of the optic disc that is delineated by the retinal vessels. In patients with glaucoma, the retinal vessels exit the optic nerve, separate, and are splayed out widely with an enlarged cup (see Chapter 12, Figure 8). The normal cup-to-disc ratio should be 0.3 or less (see Chapter 1, Figures 1-8 and 1-9).

Automated Vision Screening

There are 2 major types of automated vision screening devices for pre-verbal children: automated refractors and photoscreeners. In general, these devices should not be used to replace a good clinical examination, but only to be used as a supplement for early screening of pre-verbal children.

Automated Refractors

Automated refractors use infrared light to measure the optical power of the eye and identify refractive errors. Automated refractors are used in general ophthalmology practice to prescribe glasses, with the hand-held version marked for vision screening (Sure-Sight™ by Welch Allyn). Clinical studies have shown that automated refractors are most sensitive for detecting anisometropic amblyopia. Automated refractors have inherent limitations; they have a high rate of over-referrals, do not test visual function, and do not identify strabismus because they test one eye at a time. Since automated refractors do not test visual function, they will not identify vision loss secondary to optic nerve lesions or retinal lesions.

Photoscreening

Photoscreening uses a special linear streak of light that records a bilateral red reflex to screen for eye pathology. This method identifies large refractive errors, ocular opacities (eg, cataracts), and strabismus. Questions remain regarding their screening sensitivity and specficity in young children. Like the automated refractors, photoscreeners also do not test visual function. Photoscreening will not identify patients with optic nerve or small retinal lesions that do not disrupt the red reflex.

4 Common Types of Strabismus

■ COMITANT VERSUS INCOMITANT STRABISMUS

Strabismus is a misalignment of the eyes and can be classified into 2 basic types: comitant and incomitant. **Comitant** strabismus means the deviation is the same in all fields of gaze. Even though the eyes are misaligned, they move normally without restriction or muscle paresis. Most childhood strabismus is a comitant strabismus associated with normal muscle function. **Incomitant** strabismus means there is limited eye movement and the size of the deviation is different in different fields of gaze. Limited eye movement may be caused by a restriction (periocular scarring or tight extraocular muscles) or a muscle paresis (sixth, third, or fourth nerve paresis). Comitant strabismus usually is not associated with neurologic disease, whereas incomitant strabismus is often secondary to a neurologic disease or muscle pathology.

Suppression and Diplopia

One might expect children with strabismus to have a difficult time dealing with confusing double vision (diplopia). Actually, if strabismus occurs early before 4 to 6 years of age, the child will cortically turn off, or suppress, the image in the deviated eye. This defense mechanism, known as **suppression,** prevents bothersome double vision. Prolonged suppression of one eye, however, can lead to am-

Table 4-1.
Red Flags for Dangerous Strabismus

- Acquired strabismus
- Diplopia
- Limited eye movements
- Ptosis or other neurological signs
- Poor vision or abnormal red reflex

blyopia of the suppressed eye (see Chapter 2). Acquired strabismus after 6 to 7 years of age, on the other hand, results in diplopia, because the more mature visual system cannot suppress the double image. The clinical symptom of diplopia, therefore, is an important clue indicating that the strabismus is acquired. Acquired strabismus may indicate a more dangerous cause, such as a neurologic process or acquired visual loss. **Table 4-1** lists important characteristic red flags indicating that the strabismus may be secondary to a potentially dangerous disease process. These red flags should prompt an urgent ophthalmology consult.

■ COMITANT STRABISMUS

Infantile Esotropia (Congenital Esotropia)—uncommon

- Onset within the first 6 months of life
- Usually associated with large-angle strabismus
- Best treated with early surgery
- Amblyopia in 50% of patients
- Poor prognosis for high-grade stereo acuity

Infantile esotropia, or congenital esotropia as it is often termed, is defined as a large esotropia with onset prior to 6 months of age (**Figure 4-1**). The esotropia may present at birth although, in many cases, the esotropia is acquired during the first 6 months of life (**Archer, et al**). Small transient exodeviations are common in normal neonates, but esodeviations in newborns are rare. Persistent, large-angle esotropia that is present after 2 months of age is probably pathologic and usually does not resolve spontaneously.

No consistent inheritance pattern for infantile esotropia has been established, but it does tend to run in families. Some pedigrees appear to be autosomal recessive and others autosomal dominant;

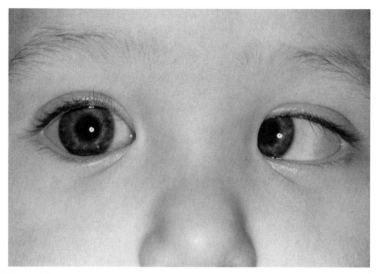

Figure 4-1.
Eight-month-old with infantile esotropia. Note the large-angle deviation, which is typical of infantile esotropia.

however, there is no family history of strabismus in many cases. The variability of inheritance patterns suggests heterogeneity for the phenotype of infantile esotropia. Thus, it is not surprising that the pathogenesis of infantile esotropia is probably multifactorial. In some cases, farsightedness (hypermetropia) is causative (see infantile accommodative esotropia below) and spectacle correction is required. In other cases, infantile esotropia is associated with developmental delay, cerebral palsy, or other diseases including as Down syndrome.

Patients may show strong fixation preference for one eye, which is an indication of amblyopia, or may alternate fixation. Amblyopia occurs in approximately 50% of children with infantile esotropia. There is often some limitation of abduction in voluntary version testing; however, doll's-head maneuver reveals normal abduction and normal lateral rectus function.

Associated motor anomalies frequently related to infantile esotropia include vertical strabismus (**inferior oblique overaction** in 70% and **dissociated vertical deviation** [DVD] in 75%). Nystagmus is unusual in children with congenital esotropia, but latent nystagmus is seen in approximately 50% of cases. **Latent nystagmus** is a nystagmus that is manifest when one eye is covered. It causes vision to appear poor when doing standard vision testing (testing with one eye covered). Children with latent nystagmus obtain best visual acuity by testing with both eyes open (binocular vision) to avoid inducing latent nystagmus. Interestingly, these associated motor anomalies present late at age 1 or 2 years, often several months after the esotropia has been surgically corrected.

Differential Diagnosis

Differential diagnoses of infantile esotropia include Duane syndrome (discussed later in this chapter), congenital fibrosis of extraocular muscles, congenital sixth nerve palsy, Möbius syndrome associated with sixth nerve paresis, and infantile myasthenia gravis. These disorders are associated with limited abduction and, therefore, can be differentiated from infantile esotropia where the ductions are full. Esotropia in an infant also may be an important sign of vision loss. Disorders such as congenital cataracts and retinoblastoma often first present as infantile esotropia.

Pseudoesotropia

Pseudoesotropia is a common condition that also needs to be distinguished from infantile esotropia. With pseudoesotropia, the infant has a wide nasal bridge and prominent epicanthal folds, giving the appearance of esotropia; however, the eyes are aligned (orthotropic) (**Figure 4-2**). It is important to document proper eye alignment using the Hirschberg corneal light reflex test. It can be difficult to convince parents that the eyes are truly straight, so it may be helpful to show the parents that the light reflex is well centered in each eye. Follow-up is important in patients with pseudoesotropia, as a small percentage will develop a true esotropia.

Treatment of Infantile Esotropia

In most cases, the treatment of infantile esotropia is surgical, usually a recession of the medial rectus muscles of both eyes. In patients with farsightedness (hypermetropia of > +3.00), spectacles should be prescribed first, as spectacles alone may correct the deviation. If amblyopia is present, it should be treated with patching of the dominant eye prior to surgery. This is important because, after surgery, parents often feel the problem is solved and may not return

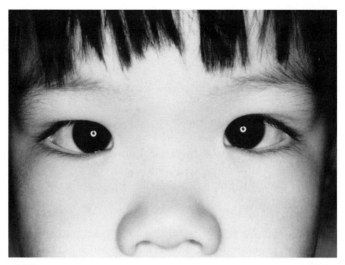

Figure 4-2.
Three-year-old with pseudoesotropia. Patient was referred with a question of right esotropia.

for follow-up visits. Patching does not correct eye misalignment but improves the vision of the non-dominant eye.

Timing of Surgery for Infantile Esotropia

The standard approach has been to operate between 6 months and 2 years of age. This is based primarily on a study by **Ing** that showed peripheral fusion can be achieved if the eyes are aligned before 2 years of age. However, peripheral fusion is subnormal binocular vision, and approximately half of the children with congenital esotropia will require multiple surgeries. Poor binocular fusion results may be due to the fact that even brief periods of strabismus during the early period of visual development result in permanent loss of binocularity. **Crawford and von Noorden** showed that even 3 weeks of prism-induced esotropia in infant monkeys resulted in irreversible loss of binocular cortical cells. This author has shown that excellent fusion with high-grade stereopsis and good alignment can be obtained when surgery is performed prior to 6 months of age (**Wright 1997**). Surgery should be considered as early as 3 months of age if the following criteria are met: large-angle esotropia (40 prism diopters or more), constant or increasing deviation documented by 2 visits 1 month apart, and the infant is a good anesthesia risk. Spontaneous resolution of the esotropia can occur; however, it is rare if the previously stated criteria are met (**Wright 2002**).

Accommodative Esotropia—common

- Associated with farsightedness.
- Acquired between 3 months and 5 years of age.
- Treatment is to prescribe spectacles; however, many will require spectacles AND eye muscle surgery.
- Relatively good prognosis for stereo acuity and binocular fusion with early surgery.

Children who are farsighted (hypermetropic) must increase focusing effort (accommodate) to see clearly. Since accommodation is linked to convergence, increased accommodation will result in increased convergence of the eyes. In farsighted children, this increased convergence will result in esotropia, termed **accommodative esotropia.** Hypermetropic spectacle correction is useful in these cases to decrease accommodation, thereby reducing convergence and correcting the esotropia (**Figure 4-3**). The presence of a combined mechanism of accommodative esotropia and a basic esotropia is termed **partially accommodative esotropia.** Patients with this diagnosis improve with hypermetropic spectacle correction, but still require surgery for the residual esotropia (**Figure 4-4**).

Clinical Features

Accommodative esotropia is acquired and can present any time between infancy (infantile accommodative esotropia) to late childhood, but most often presents between 12 months to 5 years of age. Initially, the deviation is small and intermittent. The esotropia is seen mostly at near fixation or when the child is tired, and may be manifested by the child squinting or closing one eye. Over time, sometimes after only a few weeks, the deviation may increase to become constant and amblyopia may develop.

Differential Diagnosis

The differential diagnosis of acquired esotropia includes any neurologic cause of a sixth nerve palsy including intracranial tumor, hy-

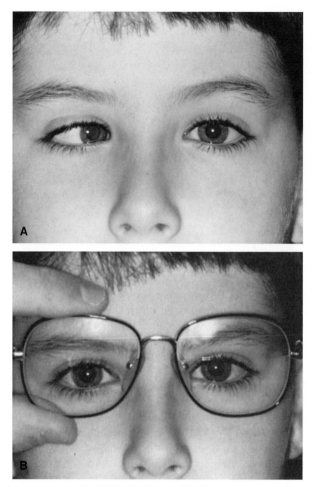

Figure 4-3.
An 8-year-old child with accommodative esotropia. **A,** Note the large-angle esotropia associated with accommodation for farsightedness. Patient is squinting, as she is forcibly accommodating to see clearly. Increased accommodation results in increased convergence. **B,** Patient is given hypermetropic spectacle correction that focuses the retinal image without increased accommodation and convergence. With spectacle correction, accommodation and convergence diminish, thereby allowing the eyes to straighten.

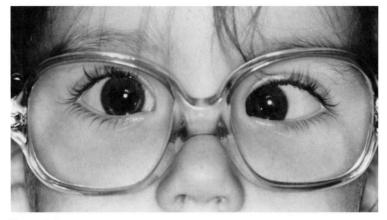

Figure 4-4.
A 3-year-old with partially accommodative esotropia. Patient is wearing full hypermetropic correction of +3.00 in both eyes; however, a residual esotropia persists.

drocephalus, mastoiditis, post viral sixth nerve palsy, Arnold-Chiari malformation and myasthenia gravis.

Treatment of Accommodative Esotropia

Immediate referral is important in patients with acquired esotropia to provide early treatment, to establish binocular vision, and to rule out ocular or neurologic disease. The treatment of accommodative esotropia is based on prescribing full hypermetropic correction as soon as possible via spectacles or contact lenses. Patients who are corrected to proper alignment with glasses for distance viewing, but still cross at near, can be corrected at near by prescribing bifocal glasses. If spectacles do not correct the esotropia, then surgery is needed in addition to spectacles. In most cases, these children require hypermetropic spectacles postoperatively to maintain good alignment.

Another less common form of treatment is to prescribe **miotic drops** such as Phospholine Iodide (echothiophate iodide) to both eyes. Miotics block cholinesterase, enabling acetylcholine to last longer. This reduces the accommodative effort needed to focus and clear the retinal image. Less accommodative effort results in less accommodative convergence, therefore decreasing the esotropia. Miotics can occasionally be successful in treating patients with relatively small-angle accommodative esotropia, but hypermetropic spectacle correction is the treatment of choice. In addition, miotics have significant side effects including iris pupillary cysts, lens opacities, retinal detachment, and angle closure glaucoma. Topical Phospholine Iodide also has a systemic effect, lowering cholinesterase activity in the blood for several weeks. Patients on miotics who are undergoing general anesthesia should avoid succinylcholine, or be off miotics for at least 4 to 6 weeks before having succinylcholine anesthesia. Miotics such as Phospholine Iodide prolong the effect of succinylcholine, which may result in prolonged respiratory paralysis postoperatively. Because of the side effects and relatively poor results, miotics are rarely used.

Prognosis for Binocular Fusion

Unlike children with congenital esotropia, patients with acquired accommodative esotropia have had straight eyes during early visual development; thus, they retain relatively good fusion potential. The earlier the eyes are straightened, the better the chances for recovering fusion. This and the fact that acquired esotropia may have a neurologic cause are 2 important reasons to immediately refer patients with acquired esotropia. This author has personal experience with infantile accommodative esotropia because one of his 5 children developed a small, variable angle esotropia at 2-1/2 months of age with a refractive error of +5.00 sphere OU. Early prescription of glasses at 3 months of age and early surgery at 6 months of age resulted in excellent eye alignment and high-grade stereopsis, both of which are still present after 13 years.

Sensory Esotropia—uncommon

Loss of vision may cause an eye to drift. Sensory esotropia is an esodeviation caused by unilateral blindness. The general teaching has been that if the visual loss occurs prior to 2 years of age, then patients develop esotropia. This is only a general rule, as there are many exceptions, and the presence of an esotropia is not a good marker for the onset of blindness. The treatment of sensory esotropia is a recession/resection procedure of the blind eye, avoiding surgery on the eye with good vision.

Intermittent Exotropia–common

- Most commonly occurring between ages 2 to 8 years.
- Intermittent strabismus: the exotropia occurs when the child is tired or daydreaming.
- Patient may squint one eye.
- Good stereopsis and binocular fusion are present when the eyes are aligned.
- Treatment is usually strabismus surgery if the deviation is poorly controlled.

A **phoria** is a tendency for the eyes to drift apart, but alignment is maintained by binocular fusion. A **tropia** is a manifest deviation of the eyes without binocular fusion. Small exophorias (the eye tends to drift out but binocular fusion controls the eye alignment) are common in the general population and are easily controlled. Large exophorias, however, may be difficult to control. Intermittent exotropia is an exodeviation that is controlled part of the time by fusional convergence, but becomes manifest some of the time (**Figure 4-5**). This is, by far, the most common type of exodeviation. The pathogenesis of intermittent exotropia is unknown.

Clinical Manifestation of Intermittent Exotropia

Intermittent exodeviation usually occurs between 2 and 8 years of age, but may present any time between infancy and adulthood. Initially, an exotropia may only be seen when the patient is fatigued or ill. Covering an eye will manifest the exotropia (Chapter 3, Figure 3-8). Thus, this is a form of strabismus best detected by the cover test rather than the corneal light reflex test. Symptoms include blurred vision, asthenopia (vague visual discomfort such as eyestrain or brow ache), visual fatigue, and photophobia with squinting. The photophobia and squinting is thought to be a mechanism for eliminating diplopia or visual confusion. The natural history of intermittent exotropia is variable. Approximately 70% will show an increasing frequency of the exotropia and progressive loss of fusion, 20% will stay the same, and a very small percentage will improve over time.

During the exophoric phase, patients have bifoveal fusion with excellent stereo acuity. When exotropia (manifest strabismus) is present, most patients demonstrate suppression. Occasionally, patients with late-onset intermittent exotropia (after 5 or 6 years of age) will experience diplopia. Significant amblyopia is rare in patients with intermittent exotropia.

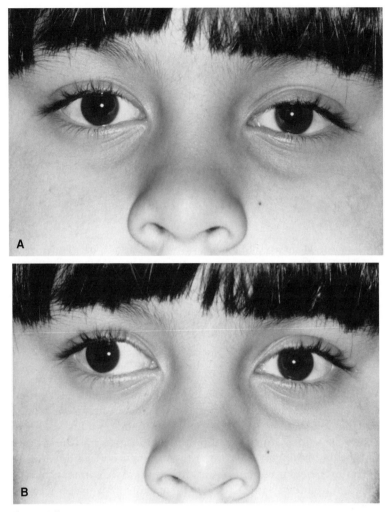

Figure 4-5.
Six-year-old with intermittent exotropia. **A,** Patient in the phoric phase with straight eyes and high-grade stereopsis. **B,** Patient in the tropic phase with large right exotropia. Patient is suppressing right eye and does not have diplopia.

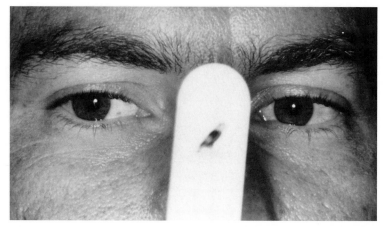

Figure 4-6.
Adult patient with convergence insufficiency. Note the left eye is fixing on the fixation target and the right eye is exotropic. The patient had no significant deviation for the distance. Convergence insufficiency is best treated with convergence exercises.

Treatment of Intermittent Exotropia

In contrast to esotropia, which requires urgent intervention, the treatment of intermittent exotropia is elective. These children have binocular fusion and are well aligned most of the time. Eye muscle surgery is the treatment of choice for most forms of intermittent exotropia. Indications for surgery include increasing exotropia, exotropia present more than 50% of the time, and poor fusion control of the exotropia. Nonsurgical treatments include part-time occlusion of the dominant eye, prescribing myopic correction, and eye exercises. These interventions act as temporary treatments at best, except for patients with a special type of exotropia termed "convergence insufficiency" (described as follows).

Convergence Insufficiency

The type of intermittent exotropia where there is an exotropia at near but straight eyes with distance fixation is called **convergence insufficiency (Figure 4-6)**. There is a lack of appropriate near convergence. Convergence insufficiency is the one form of strabismus that is best treated with eye exercises instead of surgery. Convergence insufficiency is a common cause of reading fatigue in older children and adults.

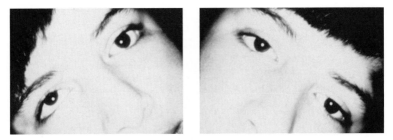

Figure 4-7.
Right superior oblique muscle paresis. Note the right hypertropia when the patient's head is tilted to his right shoulder. This patient maintained a compensatory head tilt to the left to keep his eyes aligned.

■ INCOMITANT STRABISMUS

Fourth Nerve Palsy

The superior oblique muscle is a depressor and intortor (twists the eye nasally). A weak superior oblique muscle (fourth nerve palsy) will cause strabismus consisting of hypertropia (vertical strabismus) and extorsion (temporal twisting of the eye). The hypertropia is worse when the patient's head tilts to the side of the weak superior oblique muscle (**Figure 4-7**). Thus, patients with a superior oblique paresis usually present with a compensatory head tilt to the opposite side of the paresis to help keep their eyes aligned. The most common types of superior oblique palsies are congenital and traumatic.

Congenital Superior Oblique Palsy—common

Congenital superior oblique muscle palsy is the most common cause for a vertical strabismus in childhood. The etiology of congenital superior oblique palsies is unknown. The child will invariably present with a compensatory head tilt, often misdiagnosed as a musculoskeletal problem of the neck (**Figure 4-8**). Examine the family photo album to document the onset of the head tilt.

A patient with a congenital superior oblique palsy tilts his or her head to the opposite side of the palsy to keep the eyes aligned. Patients with congenital superior oblique paresis typically have good stereopsis and manifest the hyperdeviation intermittently when fatigued. Most have the ability to suppress so they do not to

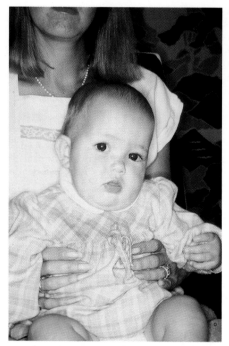

Figure 4-8.
Right congenital superior oblique muscle paresis with compensatory head tilt to the left to keep the eyes aligned. Note the facial asymmetry with left side of the face smaller than the right.

experience diplopia when the deviation is manifest. A subtle finding in most children with a congenital superior oblique palsy is facial asymmetry. The dependent side of the face is more shallow (**Figure 4-8**). This is possibly due to the effects of gravity on facial development.

Even though the paresis is present at birth, symptoms may present in late childhood or even adulthood. Over time, the fusional control weakens and results in a vertical deviation and, in these cases, strabismus surgery is indicated.

Other Causes of Superior Oblique Paresis

Closed head trauma is a common cause of acquired superior oblique paresis. Traumatic palsies tend to be bilateral, and patients present with vertical and torsional diplopia. In many cases, the palsy will spontaneously resolve; however, if diplopia persists after 6 months, then strabismus surgery is indicated. Other causes of acquired superior oblique paresis include vascular disease with brain stem lacunar infarcts, multiple sclerosis, intracranial neoplasm, herpes zoster

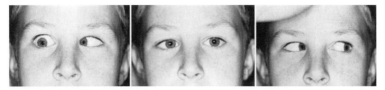

Figure 4-9.
Right sixth nerve palsy. Patient demonstrates an inability to abduct the right eye. Note the esotropia in primary position and that it increases in right gaze because the right eye cannot abduct. In left gaze, the eyes are straight.

ophthalmicus, and diabetes with an associated mononeuropathy. These disorders, however, usually occur in adults and not children.

Sixth Nerve Palsy—uncommon

Sixth nerve palsy results in limited abduction and an esotropia that is worse on the side of the palsy (**Figure 4-9**). Neonates can have a transient sixth nerve palsy often associated with a facial palsy that resolves spontaneously by 4 to 8 weeks. One of the more common causes of an acquired sixth nerve palsy in childhood is post-viral or post-immunization neuropathy, usually occurring between 2 and 6 years of age. Most of the patients in this group show resolution of the palsy within 8 to 10 weeks. If there is no sign of improvement, or if there are other neurologic signs, then a full neurologic evaluation is indicated. Head trauma is another cause of a sixth nerve palsy. About half of the traumatic sixth nerve palsies show resolution over a 6-month observational period. Other causes include intracranial tumors, meningitis, mastoiditis (Gradenigo syndrome), post-lumbar puncture, hydrocephalus, or migraine.

Duane Syndrome—uncommon

- Congenital absence of sixth nerve nucleus with aberrant innervation of the lateral rectus muscle by part of the medial rectus nerve
- Contralateral face turn to align eyes
- Limited abduction (rarely binocular)
- Lid fissure narrowing on adduction and lid fissure widening on abduction

Duane syndrome is caused by a congenital absence of the sixth nerve nucleus with misdirection of the medial rectus nerve, in-

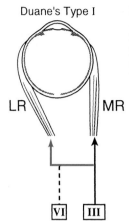

Duane's Type I

LR   MR

VI   III

Figure 4-10.
Diagrammatic representation of misdirection of nerve fibers in Duane syndrome. The aberrant nerve pathway is shown in red, and the dotted lines represent hypoplasia or agenesis. (Modified from Wilcox, et al. *Am J Ophthalmol.* 1981;91:1–7)

nervating both the medial rectus and the lateral rectus muscles (**Figure 4-10**). Since both the medial and lateral rectus muscles are innervated by the nerve to the medial rectus muscle, both muscles fire and contract simultaneously on attempted adduction. This co-contraction of the medial and lateral rectus muscles causes globe retraction and lid fissure narrowing on attempted adduction (**Figure 4-11**). Most children with Duane syndrome adopt a compensatory face turn to keep their eyes straight (**Figure 4-12**). Strabismus surgery is very effective for correcting the face turn and improving abduction slightly, but does not provide full abduction capabilities (**Figure 4-12 C**). Duane syndrome may be associated with a variety of systemic diseases including Goldenhars syndrome and prenatal exposure to the teratogen thalidomide. Duane syndrome, however, is most often isolated, sporadic, and of unknown cause.

Möbius Syndrome—rare

Möbius syndrome is characterized by a combination of facial palsy, sixth nerve palsy often with a partial third nerve palsy, and distal limb abnormalities such as syndactyly or even amputation defects. Craniofacial anomalies can occur and include micrognathia, tongue abnormalities, and facial or oral clefts. Ocular motility abnormalities include failure of the eyes to abduct and the presence of lid retraction on adduction, typical in some patients with Duane syndrome. The facial palsy usually spares the lower face, although orbicularis function is weak. Skeletal abnormalities also include pec-

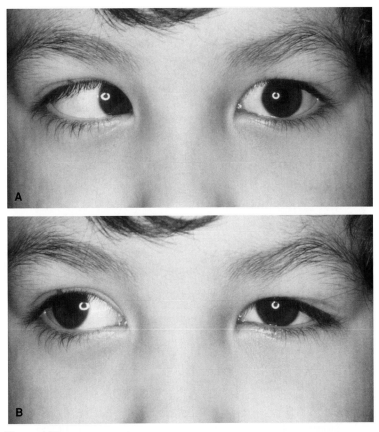

Figure 4-11.
Duane retraction syndrome in the left eye. **A,** Left eye shows limited abduction and widening of palpebral fissures on attempted abduction. **B,** On adduction, there is narrowing of palpebral fissures, left eye.

toralis muscle deficits. The inheritance pattern is variable and may be familial, but most cases are sporadic.

Third Nerve Palsy—uncommon

Third nerve palsy involves all the extraocular muscles (ie, medial rectus, superior rectus, inferior rectus, and inferior oblique muscles) except the lateral rectus (sixth cranial nerve) and the superior oblique (fourth cranial nerve). Since both major vertical muscles are weak, the eye does not move up or down and is exotropic due to the weak medial rectus muscle. The levator muscle of the upper

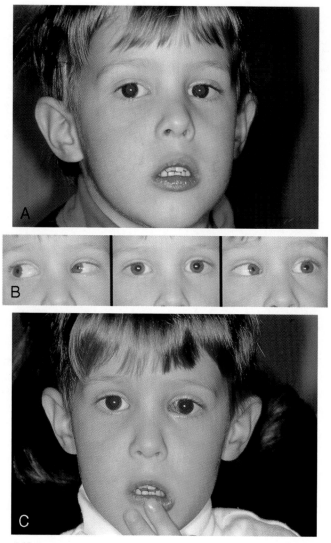

Figure 4-12.
Left Duane syndrome. **A,** Compensatory face-turn to the left and eyes in right gaze to place eyes where they are aligned. **B,** Limited abduction left eye and large esotropia as patient looks to his left. On right gaze, the left eye fully adducts, eyes are aligned, but note the lid fissure narrowing left side. **C,** One day post-operative after a left medial rectus recession. Note the head turn has resolved, and eyes are well aligned.

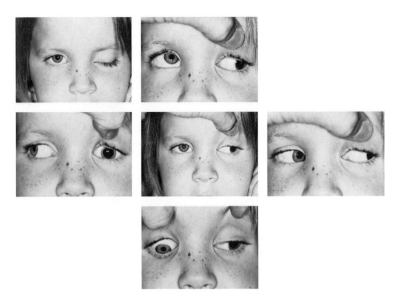

Figure 4-13.
Left third nerve palsy. Patient with a left third nerve palsy illustrating inability to adduct, elevate, or depress the left eye. Note complete ptosis and dilated pupil on the left.

eyelid is also innervated by the third cranial nerve and ptosis is usually present (**Figure 4-13**) in a third nerve palsy. The pupil is large and nonreactive in complete third nerve palsy. Causes of third nerve palsy include congenital (unknown etiology), traumatic, or migraine related. Other rare causes include intracranial tumor, viral illness, posterior communicating aneurysm, and post-immunization.

Brown Syndrome—uncommon

Brown syndrome consists of an inability to elevate an eye when the eye is in adduction (**Figure 4-14**). The most common cause is a congenitally tight superior oblique muscle tendon complex, termed **true congenital Brown syndrome.** Clinical findings include limited elevation in adduction, an exodeviation in attempted up-gaze, and an ipsilateral hypotropia that increases in up-gaze. Most patients with Brown syndrome have good binocular vision with a compensatory chin elevation and slight face turn away from the Brown eye.

The management of true congenital Brown syndrome is conservative unless there is a significant vertical deviation in primary posi-

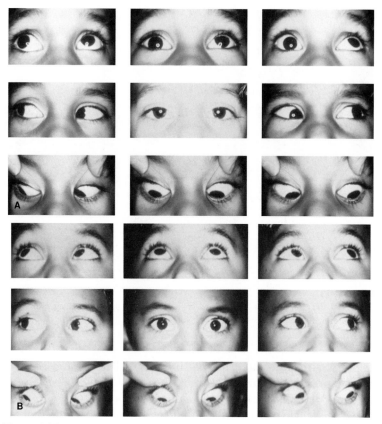

Figure 4-14.
Patient with Brown syndrome in the right eye. **A,** Composite preoperative photographs show defective elevation in adduction. **B,** Postoperative photographs showing normal eye movements after Wright superior oblique silicone tendon expander insertion.

tion. In most cases, it is better to wait until the child is visually mature before performing surgery because an induced strabismus after surgery is not uncommon and can lead to the loss of binocular vision. If surgery is indicated, the procedure of choice is superior oblique tenotomy with insertion of a segment of silicone (Wright's silicone tendon expander procedure invented by this author) (**Figure 4-15**).

Acquired Brown syndrome is usually caused by an inflammation around the superior oblique tendon and trochlea. There may be pain and tenderness in the superior nasal quadrant, with the condition often being intermittent. Treatment of inflammatory Brown

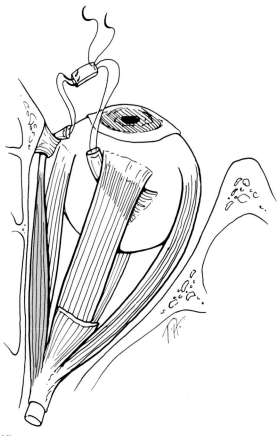

Figure 4-15.
Wright's superior oblique silicone tendon expander: A segment of a retinal 240
band is sewn between the cut ends of the superior oblique tendon. The procedure
lengthens the tendon in a graded fashion, separating the tendon end by a specific
amount. The silicone keeps the ends from growing back together.

syndrome is the use of oral nonsteroidal anti-inflammatories (ie,
ibuprofen) or, in severe cases, local corticosteroid injections, but
surgery is usually contraindicated. Other causes of acquired Brown
syndrome or pseudo-Brown syndrome include floor fracture, peri-
trochlear scarring or superior oblique tendon sheath syndrome,
trochlear inflammation (rheumatoid arthritis), glaucoma implant
under superior oblique tendon in the superior nasal quadrant, or
fat adherence syndrome. Virtually any periocular condition that
results in limited elevation in adduction can look like Brown syndrome.

Double Elevator Palsy—rare

Double elevator palsy is the congenital limitation of elevation of one eye, occurring sporadically without an inheritance pattern. The term "double elevator" implies paresis of the superior rectus muscle and inferior oblique muscle. This, however, is a misnomer, as in 70% of all cases the deficient elevation is due to restriction, secondary to a tight inferior rectus muscle. A better term, therefore, is **monocular elevation deficit syndrome**. Double elevator palsy may be mistaken for Brown syndrome, though the limited elevation in Brown syndrome is worse in adduction than in abduction.

Congenital Fibrosis Syndrome—rare

Congenital fibrosis syndrome of the extraocular muscles is usually inherited as an autosomal dominant trait. The etiology is unknown, but the syndrome is associated with fibrotic replacement of extraocular muscle tissue.

Because of the tight fibrotic muscles, ductions are limited. The medial rectus muscle is most commonly affected producing an esotropia, though the fibrosis can be generalized and affect virtually all of the rectus muscles. Treatment is surgical recession of the fibrotic muscles. These cases can be technically difficult because exposure of the muscle is limited, especially in cases with a fibrotic medial rectus muscle.

Graves Ophthalmopathy—rare in children

Graves ophthalmopathy is an autoimmune disease related to thyroid dysfunction, despite the fact that thyroid function studies may be normal. It is usually an adult disease, although it may be present in childhood. There is an initial acute inflammatory phase with lymphocytic infiltration of the extraocular muscles, resulting in extraocular muscle enlargement and proptosis (**Figure 4-16**). This active phase usually lasts several months to a year. Orbital imaging studies show thickened extraocular muscles, especially posteriorly. Later (6 months to a year after onset), there is a cicatricial phase with quiescence of inflammation and secondary contracture of the muscles. All extraocular muscles are usually involved, but the inferior rectus and medial rectus are most often affected (**Figure 4-17**). Strabismus develops in the cicatricial phase, with hypotropia and a

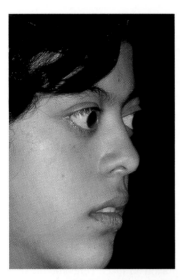

Figure 4-16.
Ten-year-old boy with Graves ophthalmopathy, bilateral proptosis, and vertical strabismus.

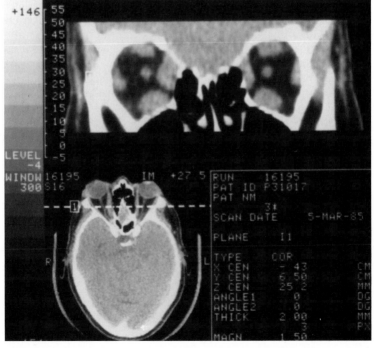

Figure 4-17.
CT scan of thyroid myopathy. Note enlargement of all the extraocular muscles, especially the inferior and medial recti.

restrictive esotropia being the most common signs. The management of Graves ophthalmopathy is careful observation during the acute inflammatory phase. Treatment with systemic steroids, and even external beam radiation, may be indicated for severe cases where there are signs of optic nerve compression from inflamed extraocular muscles. Orbital decompression surgery is also useful if vision is compromised or if there is severe proptosis. Treatment is rarely indicated for children. After the inflammatory phase has subsided and strabismus measurements have stabilized, strabismus surgery may be considered.

■ BIBLIOGRAPHY

1. Archer SM, Sondhi N, Helveston EM. Strabismus in infancy. *Ophthalmology*. 1989;96:133–137
2. Crawford MLJ, von Noorden GK. Optically induced concomitant strabismus in monkeys. *Invest Ophthalmol Vis Sci* 1980;19:1105
3. Crawford MLJ, von Noorden GK. The effects of short-term experimental strabismus on the visual system in macaca mulatta. *Invest Ophthalmol Vis Sci*. 1979;18:496–505
4. Ing MR. Early surgical alignment for congenital esotropia. *Ophthalmology* 1983;90:132–135
5. Pediatric Eye Disease Investigator Group. Spontaneous resolution of early-onset esotropia: experience of the Congenital Esotropia Observational Study. *Am J Ophthalmol.* 2002;133:109-1198
6. Pediatric Eye Disease Investigator Group. The clinical spectrum of early-onset esotropia experience of the Congenital Esotropia Observational Study. *Am J Ophthalmol.* 2002;133:102–108
7. Wright KW, Edelman PM, Terry A. McVey J, Lin M. High grade stereo acuity after early surgery for congenital esotropia. *Archiv Ophthalmol.* 1994;112:913–919

5 Refractive Errors and Spectacles in Children

■ THE EYE AS AN OPTICAL SYSTEM

The cornea and lens are the refractive elements of the eye. The cornea accounts for approximately two-thirds of the optical power and the lens makes up the remaining third. Together, the combined power of the cornea and lens equals approximately 60 diopters. This strong "plus" lens converges light on the retina at a distance of about 23 mm from the cornea.

In contrast to the lens, the cornea cannot change refractive power and cannot change focus. The lens is secured to a sphincter-type muscle called the ciliary body muscle. When this muscle contracts, the sphincter closes and slackens the tension of the lens' zonules that connect to the lens. This results in the steepening of the lens curvature and increases the lens power, which is called **accommodation.** The mechanism for increasing the lens power is used when focusing at near. Children have great accommodative amplitudes. These accommodative amplitudes, however, start decreasing at around after 20 years of age. At age 10 years, the accommodative amplitude is approximately 14 diopters. By age 40 years, accommodative amplitudes are down to 4.5 diopters, and reading glasses may be needed for near vision. Large accommodative amplitudes are what allow children to see details on a penny at a distance of only a few centimeters. Accommodation is physiologically linked to pupillary miosis and ocular convergence (both eyes turning in towards midline). Thus the classic triad for **near response** is convergence, miosis, and accommodation.

71

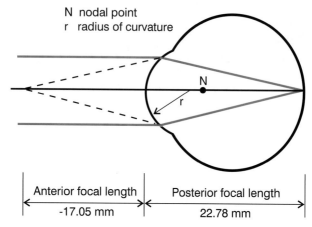

N nodal point
r radius of curvature

Anterior focal length
-17.05 mm

Posterior focal length
22.78 mm

Figure 5-1.
Posterior focal length is approximately 23 mm. This drawing shows "emmetropia" with the parallel light focused on the retina.

If the eye is naturally in focus when accommodation is at rest, the retinal image will be in focus for distance, and this is called **emmetropia** (**Figure 5-1**). Emmetropia is the normal state and glasses are not required. Most children, especially infants, are actually slightly farsighted at birth and become emmetropic as the eye grows. A description of refractive errors including hypermetropia, myopia, astigmatism, and anisometropia follows.

■ REFRACTIVE ERRORS

Hypermetropia (Hyperopia)

Hypermetropia (farsightedness), or hyperopia as it is also termed, occurs when the cornea and lens power are not sufficient to bring the image clearly in focus on the retina because of the relatively short length of the eye. With hyperopia, the light theoretically focuses behind the retina (**Figure 5-2 top**). Small amounts of hypermetropia are normal in infants and young children (**Figure 5-2 bottom**). Children with small to moderate amounts of hyperopia have 20/20 vision for distance and near, as they can correct for the refractive error by lens accommodation. Over time, the eye grows and the hyperopia improves.

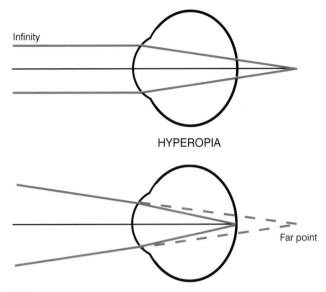

Figure 5-2.
Drawing of hyperopia. Top, note that lens power is too weak for the relatively short length of the eye and parallel light rays entering the eye are focused behind the eye. Bottom, note that the lens is steeper as the eye accommodates (focuses) to converge and focus the light rays on the retina.

Children with moderate hypermetropia (greater than 3.00 diopters) can accommodate to keep retinal images clear, but this amount of accommodation often results in the eyes over-converging (turning in) and can lead to accommodative esotropia (see Chapter 4). Prescribing hyperopic spectacle correction relaxes accommodation and consequently relaxes convergence. In many cases, hyperopic spectacles will straighten the eyes without the need for eye muscle surgery. Large amounts of hyperopia (6 diopters), can result in bilateral amblyopia. This happens because infants cannot fully accommodate for high hypermetropia, which then results in bilateral blurred retinal images. Unilateral or asymmetric hyperopia is very amblyogenic, as the child accommodates for the eye with the lesser amount of hyperopia, thus leaving the more hyperopic eye constantly out of focus (anisometropic amblyopia).

Myopia

Myopia (nearsightedness) occurs when the cornea and lens power are too great for the length of the eye and light focuses in front of

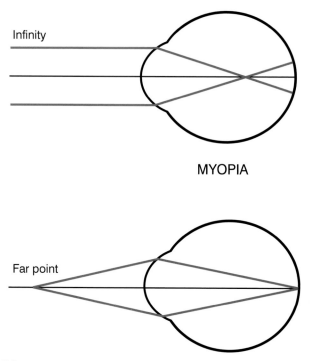

MYOPIA

Figure 5-3.
Drawing of myopia. Top shows parallel light converging in front of the retina, as the eye is too long for the power of the cornea and lens. Bottom shows that an object close to the eye gives off divergent light that is focused more posteriorly on the retina.

the retina. Another way to think of myopia is that the eye is too long for the relatively strong cornea-lens power (**Figure 5-3 top**). Near objects, however, are naturally in focus for a myopic eye, as near objects reflect divergent light that is focused more posteriorly (**Figure 5-3 bottom**). Thus, the layman uses the term nearsightedness for this refractive error, as patients with myopia can see up close.

Myopia runs in families and the inheritance pattern is variable; some being autosomal dominant or autosomal recessive, and others apparently sporadic. Myopia tends to develop in school-age children and tends to increase during the growth spurt period as the eye increases in size. In most cases, myopia will stabilize by the mid- to late-teenage years. Patients with myopia usually do not have amblyopia, since myopia develops after the critical period of visual development. Because infants with myopia can see clearly up close, this provides clear retinal images necessary for normal visual development.

Astigmatism

Astigmatism is a condition in which the power of the lens or cornea is different at different axes. Instead of the cornea and lens being symmetrically round and spherical like a basketball, they are shaped more like a football. Thus, light is not focused on a single point and the image is blurred. The word astigmatism is derived from Greek and means without point, (a = without and stigma = point). In some cases, astigmatism produces both myopia and hypermetropia, with one of the images being focused in front of the retina and the other image being focused behind the retina **(Figure 5-4)**. Moderate to large amounts of astigmatism (3 diopters or more) distort the retinal image sufficiently to cause amblyopia. Astigmatism tends to change in children, and follow-up eye examinations are important to monitor vision.

Anisometropia

Anisometropia is a condition in which each eye has a different refractive error. Myopic anisometropia usually does not produce significant amblyopia; however, hypermetropic anisometropia is very amblyogenic.

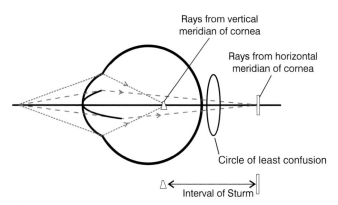

Figure 5-4.
Diagram showing astigmatism. Note there are 2 corneal curvatures shown. Each corneal curvature focuses light at a different point. The vertical curve is steeper and focuses light in front of the retina, while the horizontal curve focuses light behind the retina.

Aphakia

Aphakia means without lens. This occurs after cataract surgery if an intraocular lens is not implanted. The spectacle power correction of aphakia is a high plus, usually over 10.00 diopters. **Pseudophakia** is the term for an intraocular lens (IOL) that has been implanted to replace a cataract.

■ CORRECTING REFRACTIVE ERRORS

There are 2 ways to correct refractive errors in children: (1) the use of contact lenses or (2) the use of spectacles. Spectacles have the advantage of being easy to use, providing protection for the eyes with no chance of corneal problems. Contact lenses, on the other hand, are cosmetically desirable, and they do not magnify or minify the image as glasses can. However, there is a risk of corneal infection, especially with soft contact lenses, and contact lenses can also be difficult for children to use. Contact lenses are very important in the treatment of aphakia (patients without the natural lens), as they provide a constant, clear image without significant distortion or magnification. Even infants can be fit with contact lenses if necessary.

■ WHY DO WE USE CYCLOPLEGIC DROPS TO TEST FOR REFRACTIVE ERRORS?

Since children have great accommodative amplitudes, they can change the measurement of the refraction. A child who is emmetropic or only slightly myopic appears significantly myopic if he or she accommodates. Changing accommodation results in the appearance of astigmatism. The only way to obtain an accurate refraction in children is to control accommodation by using cycloplegic drops.

6 Neonatal and Infantile Blindness
"My Baby Doesn't See"

At birth, visual acuity is very poor and newborns show only sporadic fixation. By 2 months of age, smooth pursuit eye movements have developed and visual acuity will have improved significantly. Two-month-old infants should show some visual attentiveness, and by 4 to 6 months of age, an infant should show visual behavior such as following mother's face. Lack of visual attentiveness by 2 to 4 months of age requires an ophthalmology consultation. As discussed in Chapter 3, all newborns should have a red reflex screening test.

■ DELAYED VISUAL MATURATION

One of the most common causes of poor visual attentiveness in infancy is delayed visual maturation. Delayed visual maturation may be an isolated finding or may be associated with a neurologic abnormality. Patients with an isolated finding of delayed visual maturation with normal neurologic function generally have an excellent visual prognosis and show normal fixation and visual attentiveness by approximately 6 to 12 months of age. Those patients who have delayed visual maturation in association with neurologic defects and/or seizures show slower visual development and less complete visual recovery. Children with seizures often show poor vision when seizures are active and display better vision when the seizures are under control.

Sensory Nystagmus

Children who are born bilaterally blind, or develop blindness in the first few months of life, will develop **sensory nystagmus,** except in cases of cortical blindness. In this chapter, we describe causes of bilateral neonatal blindness that are almost always associated with nystagmus. If the disease process is asymmetrical or unilateral and spares the vision of one eye, then the patient will not have nystagmus. Causes of neonatal blindness can be divided into the following 5 categories:

Causes of Neonatal Blindness

1. Blurred Retinal Image (bilateral amblyopia)
   A. Congenital cataract
   B. Glaucoma with corneal edema
   C. Congenital corneal opacity (Peters anomaly)
   D. Vitreous opacity (hemorrhage)
   E. Large refractive error (hyperopia)
2. Retinal Disease
   A. Leber amaurosis
   B. Congenital toxoplasmosis (bilateral macular scars)
   C. Albinism
   D. Joubert syndrome
   E. Alstrom syndrome
   F. Aniridia (Chapter 11)
   G. ROP (retinopathy of prematurity) (Chapter 19)
   H. Retinal dysplasia (Norrie disease)
   I. Achromatopsia
3. Optic Nerve Disorders
   A. Optic nerve hypoplasia
   B. Optic nerve coloboma
   C. Hereditary optic atrophy
4. Cortical Blindness
   A. Neonatal anoxia
   B. Congenital occipital anomalies
   C. Hydrocephalus
5. Neurodegenerative Disease
   A. Zellweger syndrome
   B. Neonatal adrenoleukodystrophy
   C. Infantile Refsum disease
   D. Infantile neuronal ceroid-lipofuscinosis (NCL)
   E. Leigh disease

F. Canavan disease

G. Pelizaeus-Merzbacher syndrome

Retinal and optic nerve disorders may or may not present with an abnormal red reflex. If there are large areas of pathology, such as in retinoblastoma or optic nerve coloboma, an abnormal red reflex occurs. Diseases that involve less disruption of retinal anatomy, such as retinal dystrophies and optic nerve hypoplasia, show a normal red reflex. Cortical blindness has a normal red reflex examination with no nystagmus. Poor vision in infancy may also be due to a neurodegenerative process that results in retinal, optic nerve, or cortical damage. In this chapter, we cover those diseases that present with visual loss in infancy and a normal-appearing eye to inspection. Disorders that are associated with a distinctly abnormal red reflex (eg, cataracts) are covered in Chapter 22, under Leukocoria.

■ BLURRED RETINAL IMAGE

Disorders that cause a blurred retinal image include congenital cataracts, congenital corneal opacities (Peters anomaly), congenital glaucoma causing corneal edema, large refractive error, and vitreous hemorrhage. A bilaterally blurred retinal image during the neonatal period results in disruption of normal visual development and severe bilateral amblyopia if not treated promptly. Neonates with ocular opacities demonstrate an abnormal red reflex and can be identified by using the direct ophthalmoscope to perform the red reflex test. Profound hypermetropia can cause visual inattentiveness. The red reflex may or may not be abnormal, and delays in referrals often occur. Fortunately, patients with large refractive errors respond well even if optical correction is given in late infancy to early childhood. The best treatment is to prescribe full optical correction as soon as possible, even in the first few months of life.

■ RETINAL DISEASE

The macula provides high visual resolution and central visual acuity. Scars within the macular area can cause significant visual loss and blindness. Peripheral retinal lesions may diminish the peripheral visual field but will not affect central acuity.

Leber Amaurosis

Leber amaurosis is a congenital dystrophy that causes blindness at birth. These patients have nystagmus and very poor visual function, and show a phenomenon called the **oculodigital sign.** Children with this disorder rub their eyes intensely in an attempt to stimulate the retina. Over time, this leads to atrophy and disfiguring sunken orbits (enophthalmos), cataracts, and abnormal corneal molding (keratoconus). In most cases, Leber congenital amaurosis is inherited in an autosomal recessive pattern. Associated neurological abnormalities may occur in approximately 20% of cases; however, most children have normal intelligence and the psychomotor retardation may be secondary to visual deprivation. Rarely, Leber congenital amaurosis is associated with systemic abnormalities such as polycystic kidney disease, osteopetrosis, deafness, and cardiomyopathy.

Initial ophthalmic examination in early infancy may be normal. Over time, the retina degenerates and retinal pigment epithelial changes occur similar to retinitis pigmentosa, including optic atrophy and attenuated retinal vessels. The most important ocular laboratory test is an electroretinogram (ERG) that measures generalized retinal activity. The ERG is typically extinguished in Leber congenital amaurosis. One important note is that the ERG may be normally reduced and non-recordable in neonates, so the ERG should be repeated at 6 months of age.

Macular Toxoplasmosis

Congenital toxoplasmosis is an important cause of macular scarring in neonates. Congenital infection of toxoplasma gondii can occur from maternal transmission to the fetus. Transmission to the fetus occurs in approximately 33% to 44% of neonates born to mothers with toxoplasmosis acquired during pregnancy. Of those infants congenitally infected, however, only 10% have clinical manifestations of toxoplasmosis at birth. The classical triad of congenital toxoplasmosis includes hydrocephalus, chorioretinitis, and intracranial calcifications. There is a large spectrum of presentations from infants with severe microcephaly and mental retardation to infants who are asymptomatic and only have ophthalmic involvement often discovered in late childhood.

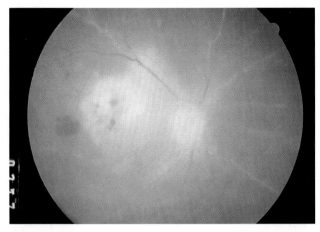

Figure 6-1.
Active toxoplasmosis causing retinochoroiditis with vitritis and retinal vasculitis. The white lesion left of the optic nerve represents the focal area of retinal inflammation.

Ocular findings at birth may consist of an abnormal red reflex caused by a retinochoroiditis and secondary vitreous inflammation (vitritis) (**Figure 6-1**). In most cases, however, the eye is not inflamed and the patient presents with a quiescent retinal scar (chorioretinal scar) (**Figure 6-2**). If the scarring involves both maculas, then the patient will be blind. Fortunately, in most cases, the scars are either unilateral or do not directly involve the center of the macula (fovea). Toxoplasmosis chorioretinal scars can be quite large and can measure up to 5 optic disc diameters in size. Toxoplasmosis cysts can lay dormant within the retinal scar and reactivate in later childhood, causing retinal inflammation, vitritis, and visual loss.

Ocular Albinism

With the advent of molecular biology and gene sequencing, various forms of albinism have recently been described. For clinical purposes, however, it is best to think of 2 forms: ocular albinism and oculocutaneous albinism. Both forms are associated with reduced visual acuity, nystagmus, transillumination defects of the iris, fovea hypoplasia, and reduced retinal pigmentation. Patients with ocular albinism will have pigmentation of skin and hair and otherwise appear normal. Ocular albinism is usually inherited as an X-linked recessive trait. Oculocutaneous albinism associated with hypopigmentation of skin and hair is inherited as an autosomal recessive trait and can be divided into many types, but are classified in 2 general categories:

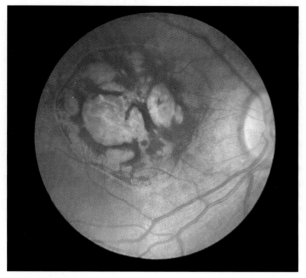

Figure 6-2.
Congenital toxoplasmosis scar of the macula. This scar has areas of hyperpigmenta-
tion and hypopigmentation and involves all retinal layers (ie, chorioretinal scar).
This is an inactive scar; however, the fovea is involved. Vision was 20/400.

1. Tyrosinase-positive with significant increase in hair and skin pigmentation over time, and
2. Tyrosinase-negative, where hair and skin hypopigmentation remains relatively constant with little improvement.

Visual acuity is quite variable in ocular albinism. The severe
Tyrosinase-negative types usually have very poor visual acuity in
the range of 20/200. See also Chapter 21 for further discussion of
albinism.

Joubert Syndrome

This is a rare autosomal recessive syndrome consisting of poor vision, cerebellar vermis hypoplasia, nystagmus, and irregular breath-
ing. The patient has jerky eye movements and retinal dystrophy.
The decreased vision seems to be secondary to the retinal dystrophy, and the diagnosis is made by documenting cerebellar vermis
hypoplasia and decreased ERG amplitudes.

Alström Syndrome

This is a rare autosomal recessive multisystem disorder associated with poor vision and nystagmus in infancy. Diabetes mellitus (75%), obesity, deafness, and with normal mentation are the basic features of the disorder. By 7 years of age, most patients are legally blind secondary to a progressive pigmentary retinopathy. It is similar to Bardet-Biedl syndrome (see Chapter 7); however, Alström syndrome does not have polydactyly, syndactyly, or mental retardation and the onset of visual loss in Alström syndrome occurs in early infancy. Other systemic associations include renal disease (common cause of death), alopecia, hypogonadism, hypothyroidism, acanthosis nigricans, and hypertriglyceridemia.

Norrie Disease (retinal dysplasia)

This is a rare X-linked recessive disease (affecting only males) that includes bilateral retinal dysplasia, progressive deafness (30%), and progressive mental retardation (60%). Infants are usually blind at birth; but, in rare cases, children retain some vision into the teens. If the retina is detached at birth, the ocular findings may mimic persistent hyperplastic primary vitreous (PHPV), retinopathy of prematurity, or retinoblastoma. Life span is normal.

Achromatopsia

Achromatopsia is an autosomal recessive condition that consists of abnormal retinal development with no functioning cones present; the retina consists solely of rods. The complete form of achromatopsia is associated with extremely poor visual acuity (20/200 or worse) and causes legal blindness. Because cones are absent, patients have no color vision and are very photophobic. Fundus examination is usually normal. Patients with the complete form of achromatopsia have nystagmus, but no other neurological disorders. The condition is stationary, in contrast to the metabolic diseases described previously where there is systemic neurological involvement, a progressive retinal dystrophy, and progressive visual loss.

■ OPTIC NERVE DISORDERS

Optic Nerve Hypoplasia

Optic nerve hypoplasia is a nonprogressive congenital anomaly affecting one or both optic nerves. It is the most common developmental anomaly of the optic nerve and may be associated with multiple central nervous system and endocrine malformations as listed in **Table 6-1.** Optic nerve hypoplasia may be sporadic; however, teratogenic factors have been implicated including phenytoin, quinine, lysergic-acid-diethylamide (LSD), phencyclidine (PCP), alcohol (50% of fetal alcohol syndrome), intrauterine infection, cytomegalovirus (CMV), and possibly maternal diabetes. Optic nerve hypoplasia is bilateral in 60% of all cases; however, when bilateral, it often presents with nystagmus and neonatal blindness. Visual potential is determined by the integrity of the central retinal axons and does not necessarily correlate with the size of the optic disc. Unilateral cases usually present with strabismus, as the eye with the optic nerve hypoplasia tends to drift causing either esotropia or exotropia.

The red reflex will appear normal; however, ophthalmoscopic examination reveals a small optic nerve and a ring of hypopigmentation (**double ring sign**) (**Figure 6-3A**). The hypopigmented ring represents bare sclera, as the optic nerve is not large enough to fill the surrounding area. The retinal vessels are usually normal, but their pattern may be distorted.

Optic nerve hypoplasia (especially the bilateral form) is frequently associated with multiple CNS malformations. The triad of nystagmus, poor vision, and short stature (pituitary hypoplasia) is termed **septo-optic dysplasia,** or **de Morsier syndrome.** Intracra-

Table 6-1.
Optic Nerve Hypoplasia Associated Endocrine Abnormalities

1. Growth hormone deficiency
2. Congenital hypothyroidism
3. Diabetes insipidus
4. Infantile hypoglycemia
5. Hyperprolactinemia
6. Sexual precocity
7. Adrenal insufficiency

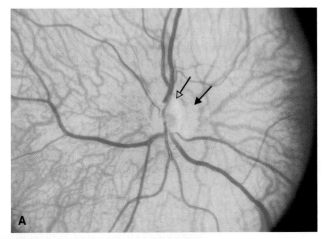

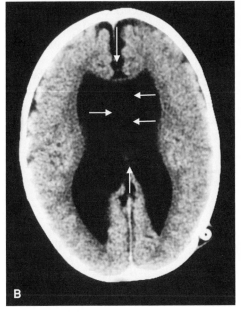

Figure 6-3.
A, Optic nerve hypoplasia. Notice the double-ring sign due to small optic disc (open arrow) within normal scleral canal (closed arrow). **B,** Septo-optic dysplasia. Axial CT scan demonstrates absence of septum pellucidum and hypoplasia of the corpus callosum (arrows).

nial anomalies include absence of the septum pellucidum, hypoplasia or agenesis of the corpus callosum, dysplasia of the anterior third ventricle (holoprosencephaly), and anomalies of the hypothalamic-pituitary axis (**Figure 6-3B**). Sudden death has been reported following relatively benign illness, presumably from adrenal crisis and hypopituitarism. Patients with optic nerve hypoplasia and hypopituitarism may require supplemental corticosteroids during times of stress. Magnetic resonance imaging (MRI) findings of posterior pituitary ectopia and cerebral hemispheric abnormalities are highly predictive of pituitary hormone and neuro-developmental defects. The endocrine abnormalities associated with optic nerve hypoplasia are treatable, and an endocrine work-up, including provocative tests, should be obtained on patients with optic nerve hypoplasia. There is no specific treatment for the optic nerve anomaly.

Optic Nerve and Macular Colobomas

Optic nerve and macular colobomas result from failure of the embryonic fissure to properly close at 5 to 6 weeks' gestation (**Figure 6-4**). The embryonic fissure normally closes at the center, then zippers up in an anterior and posterior direction. Two of the most common locations for colobomas are at the anterior aspect of the eye (iris) and the posterior aspect of the eye (macula and optic nerve).

Optic nerve and macular colobomas can be unilateral, bilateral, or asymmetric. Visual acuity is often severely affected; however, even significantly distorted optic nerves can be associated with good visual acuity. By ophthalmoscopy, the optic nerve appears very

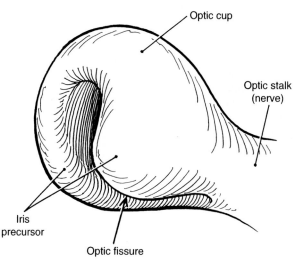

Figure 6-4.
Developing eye. Embryonal fissure located inferiorly.

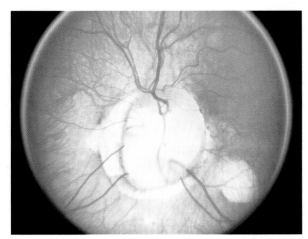

Figure 6-5.
Optic disc coloboma. Excavation of nerve inferiorly with normal retinal vessels.

large, and careful examination will show that the retinal vessels are distorted and widely separated as they exit the optic nerve (**Figure 6-5**). **Macular colobomas** involve all retinal layers including the choroid. The coloboma is white and represents bare sclera (**Figure 6-6**). Macular colobomas will usually reflect light and produce an abnormal red reflex test.

Genetic syndromes may be associated with optic nerve colobomas, such as **CHARGE Association** (*c*oloboma, *h*eartdefect, *c*hoanal *a*tresia, *r*etarded growth and development, *g*enital hypoplasia, and *e*ar anomalies), Lenz syndrome, Trisomy 13, Cat's Eye syndrome, and Meckel-Gruber syndrome, among others. A chromosomal abnormality should be considered when optic nerve colobomas occur in association with multiple congenital anomalies, mental retardation, or growth failure. Optic nerve colobomas have been associated with various CNS abnormalities including basal encephaloceles.

Systemic Syndromes and Colobomas

1. CHARGE syndrome: **C**olobomatous microphthalmia, **H**eart defect, **A**tresia choanal, **R**etarded growth, **G**enital hypoplasia, **E**ar anomalies (deafness).
2. Meckel-Gruber syndrome: colobomatous microphthalmia, occipital encephalocele, heart defect, renal and hepatic disease.

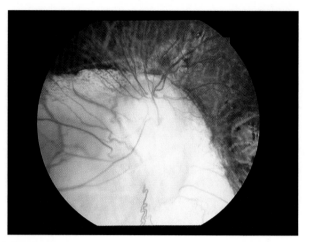

Figure 6-6.
Photograph of optic nerve coloboma. Notice that the optic nerve is disrupted and the retinal vessels are splayed out and disorganized. Inferiorly, the white area represents a choroidal coloboma. Choroidal colobomas are typically found inferiorly.

3. Lenz syndrome: colobomatous microphthalmia.
4. Rubinstein-Taybi syndrome: coloboma, cataract, ptosis, mental retardation, broad fingers and toes, short stature, cardiac and renal abnormalities.
5. Basal Cell Nevus syndrome: iris coloboma, cataract, hypertelorism, basal cell nevus (prone to carcinoma) over torso, mental retardation.
6. Cat's Eye syndrome: colobomatous microphthalmia, anal atresia, preauricular skin tags, abnormal chromosome 22.
7. Trisomy 13: microphthalmia, coloboma, cataract, intraocular cartilage, cleft lip/palate, polydactyly, central nervous system malformations.

Hereditary Optic Atrophy

Hereditary optic atrophy with blindness in the neonatal period is usually autosomal recessive optic atrophy. This is a rare form of bilateral severe optic atrophy often causing nystagmus in half of the patients. Ophthalmoscopic examination shows pale optic nerves and vascular attenuation. Retinal functions are normal, as the electroretinograph shows normal amplitudes. **Behr syndrome** may be associated with mental retardation, spasticity, and cerebellar ataxia.

Other forms of optic atrophy have a later onset in late infancy or early childhood (see Chapter 7).

■ CORTICAL BLINDNESS

Cortical blindness is due to injury to the optic radiations or the visual cortex in the occipital lobe. The occipital cortex is extremely sensitive to hypoxia, as it is in the watershed area of the cerebral vessels. Neonatal hypotension and birth asphyxia are important causes of neonatal cortical blindness. Hydrocephalus, stroke, intracranial hemorrhages, direct trauma, and congenital aplasia in the occipital cortex are other causes. In contrast to the previously listed causes for neonatal blindness, cortical blindness is usually associated with normal ocular examination, and nystagmus is not present. Stimulation with an **optokinetic nystagmus stimulus,** even in cortically blind children, usually produces a response. In addition, pupillary responses are brisk in contrast to pupillary responses associated with optic nerve or retinal diseases. If the occipital damage is severe and widespread and occurs within a few weeks of birth, retrograde transsynaptic degeneration of optic nerve axons can occur and result in optic atrophy. Acute hypoxia associated with cardiac bypass surgery can result in transient cortical blindness. The majority of these patients will show spontaneous improvement over several weeks. An MRI scan of the visual pathways and cortex often aids in the diagnosis of cortical blindness.

■ NEURODEGENERATIVE DISORDERS ASSOCIATED WITH VISUAL LOSS

Neurodegenerative disease can cause visual loss through retinal degeneration, optic neuropathy, or cortical blindness.

Peroxisomal Disorders

Peroxisomes are small single-membrane bound organelles that contain enzymes responsible for catabolism of long-chain fatty acids. There are 3 peroxisomal disorders that can cause blindness in the neonate. These are **Zellweger syndrome, Neonatal Adrenoleukodystrophy,** and **Refsum disease.** All are autosomal recessive and are associated with progressive pigmentary retinopathy, optic atrophy, and neurological deterioration secondary to massive and progressive white matter degeneration. Over time, quadriparesis, dysphagia, and, finally, death occur. Adrenal Leukodystrophy and Zellweger syndrome both have an onset during early infancy, while Infantile Refsum disease has a later onset and is discussed in Chapter 7.

Zellweger Syndrome

Zellweger syndrome causes the most rapid deterioration of vision of all the peroxisomal diseases. Patients are born with dysmorphic features including prominent forehead, hypertelorism, epicanthal folds, hypoplastic supraorbital ridge, and a high-arched palate. Neonates have hypotonia, seizures, severe psychomotor retardation, deafness, and spastic contracture of the limbs. Ocular features include pigmentary retinopathy and optic atrophy that result in early visual loss. Cataracts, corneal clouding, and glaucoma also occur. Visceral involvement includes polycystic kidneys, cardiac ventricular septal defects, and intrahepatic biliary dysgenesis. Currently, there is no treatment, and death often occurs in the first year of life.

Neonatal Adrenoleukodystrophy

Neonatal adrenoleukodystrophy is associated with early visual loss secondary to retinal pigment epithelial degeneration. At birth, infants are severely hypotonic and develop uncontrollable infantile seizures. Adrenal insufficiency occurs late in the disease and causes increased pigmentation of the skin. Death usually occurs by 3 years of age.

X-linked Adrenoleukodystrophy

X-linked adrenoleukodystrophy has a later onset in life and is discussed in Chapter 7, under Acquired Visual Loss in Childhood.

Neuronal Ceroid-Lipofuscinosis

Neuronal ceroid-lipofuscinosis (NCL) refers to a group of lysosomal storage disorders of lipopigments with secondary neuronal degeneration. Neonates are not blind at birth, but start losing visual milestones between 6 months and 3 years of age. These disorders are covered more fully in Chapter 7, under Acquired Visual Loss in Childhood. Infantile NCL (**Haltia-Santavuori**) is an infantile form characterized by normal development until 6 months of age, then progressive regression with loss of psychomotor milestones, onset of seizures, pigmentary retinal degeneration, and optic atrophy. Patients are usually blind by 2 to 3 years and death occurs around 6 to 7 years of age.

Leigh Disease

Leigh disease is a progressive disorder presenting in the first 2 years of life with feeding difficulties, seizures, and ataxia. Severe psychomotor regression is associated with hypotonia, involuntary movements, and respiratory dysfunction. Ocular findings include ophthalmoplegia, nystagmus, optic atrophy, and visual loss. This disorder is caused from deficiencies in various mitochondrial enzymes. Lactate and pyruvate are almost always elevated in the serum and cerebrospinal fluid (CSF). Spongiform lesions in the basal ganglia can be seen on neuroimaging. This disease causes rapid neurodegeneration, and death usually occurs by 2 years of age.

Canavan Disease

Canavan disease is an autosomal recessive disease that rapidly progresses during the first 2 months of life. Patients present with hypotonia, nystagmus, and seizures. Visual loss is secondary to early optic atrophy that occurs during the first few months of life. Cystic spaces occur in the white matter, giving a characteristic spongiform appearance on histopathology. These cystic spaces represent coalescence of vacuoles within swollen astrocytes. Mitochondria within the astrocytes have a pathognomonic elongation on electromicroscopy. There is a paucity of myelin, but no evidence of demyelination. The primary enzyme defect is aspartoacylase deficiency and patients excrete urinary N-acetylaspartic acid. Prenatal diagnosis can be made by assay of aspartoacylase activity in chorionic villus samples and possibly through urinary N-acetylaspartic acid levels in the pregnant mother. Neuroimaging can be helpful in demonstrating small ventricles and increased signal on MRI. The neuroradiologic changes are similar to that of the leukodystrophies.

Pelizaeus-Merzbacher Disease

There are 4 types of this extremely rare disease, with the classic form beginning in the first year of life. The early onset forms are X-linked recessive, although autosomal recessive pedigrees have been described. The first presenting feature is often nystagmus associated with poor fixation. Neurologically, the infants are hypotonic and progress to develop spasticity and hyperreflexia. The early onset form is associated with severe developmental delay, and death usually occurs at 4 to 6 years of age secondary to respiratory complications. Ataxia is usually present along with choreoathetosis. The disease is a problem of *dys*myelination, not *de*myelination. Histopathologically, there are patchy areas of myelination and areas of white matter gliosis. It has also been associated with a deficiency in the proteolipid apoprotein lipophilic (PLP). The PLP represents approximately half of the protein content of normal central nervous system (CNS) white matter, and is believed to be important in forming CNS myelin. With polymerase chain reaction amplification of the PLP gene, prenatal diagnosis may be available.

Acquired Visual Loss in Childhood

In this chapter, causes of acquired visual loss after 1 year of age, associated with a red reflex, are discussed. Disorders are classified as follows: optic nerve disease, retinal disease, and neurodegenerative disorders.

■ OPTIC NERVE DISEASE

Juvenile Onset Glaucoma

Glaucoma is increased intraocular pressure (IOP >22 mm Hg) that causes optic nerve atrophy. Glaucoma is rare in children but, when present, can cause visual loss and blindness. Juvenile onset glaucoma is usually asymptomatic, in contrast to congenital glaucoma (see Chapter 12), which is almost always associated with large corneas, corneal edema, and tearing. In some cases, if the IOP is extremely high (over 35 to 40 mm Hg), then symptoms of tearing, corneal edema, red eye, and pain may occur. There are various forms of juvenile onset glaucoma, some hereditary and others sporadic. See Chapter 12 for systemic diseases associated with pediatric glaucoma.

Leber Hereditary Optic Neuropathy

This is inherited through a mitochondrial DNA point mutation that results in defective oxidative phosphorylation. Over time, this meta-

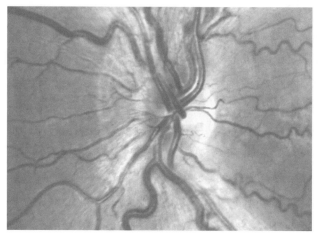

Figure 7-1.
Leber hereditary optic neuropathy.

bolic abnormality results in optic neuropathy with acute or subacute severe, painless visual loss. Visual loss can start in one eye and then subsequently go to the other eye, or the patient may present with bilateral simultaneous visual loss. Visual loss is in the range of 20/200 or worse, and is associated with poor red/green color vision. Patients are usually male and lose vision between 10 and 13 years of age. Visual acuity has been reported to improve in anywhere from 5% to 30% of patients after the acute episode.

The classic fundus appearance of the acute phase consists of telangiectatic microangiopathy around the optic disc and blurred disc margins (pseudopapilledema) (**Figure 7-1**). Later, the optic disc will turn pale and lose its normal pink appearance (**Figure 7-2**). Leber hereditary optic neuropathy has been associated with cardiac arrhythmia syndromes such as Wolff-Parkinson-White. A definitive diagnosis can be made by genetic analysis of leukocyte mitochondrial DNA. At this time, there is no effective treatment for Leber hereditary optic neuropathy.

Dominant Optic Atrophy

Dominant optic atrophy is associated with slow, insidious, bilateral visual loss, usually beginning around 10 years of age. In some cases, visual acuity can remain quite good, even in the range of 20/25 or 20/30. In other cases, visual acuity is as poor as 20/100. Color vision

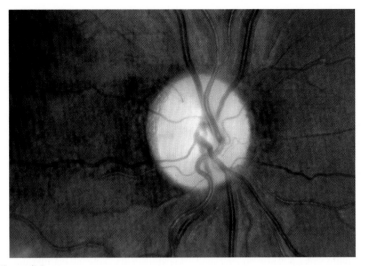

Figure 7-2.
Optic atrophy. Note the optic nerve is pale, especially in the temporal area of the disc.

is significantly affected. Direct ophthalmoscopy reveals temporal optic disc pallor.

Recessive Optic Atrophy

Recessive optic atrophy is associated with severe bilateral visual loss, often with nystagmus. Vision loss occurs before age 5, often in infancy.

Optic Neuritis

Optic neuritis is inflammation of the optic nerve and/or chiasm. Inflammation is usually caused by autoimmune postviral syndrome associated with a systemic infection such as measles, mumps, chickenpox, nonspecific viral disease, or immunizations. Children often present with a headache, nausea, pain on eye movements, bilateral optic disc swelling (**papillitis**) (**Figure 7-3**), and acute visual loss (20/200 or worse) (also see Chapter 9). If the inflammation is isolated to the posterior optic nerve, the optic disc may appear normal; however, vision will be affected. Spontaneous recovery with visual im-

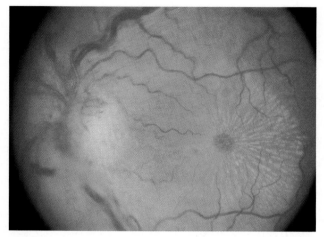

Figure 7-3.
Papillitis with optic disc swelling similar to papilledema. Note the macular star pattern that represents fluid and lipid exudates.

provement usually occurs after 1 to 2 weeks; however, permanent visual loss can occur. In children, the majority of cases are secondary to an autoimmune post-viral syndrome; however, there is a risk for developing demyelinating disease (multiple sclerosis [MS]). Unilateral optic neuritis has a higher risk of being associated with MS than bilateral optic neuritis. Initial evaluation should include full physical examination, Venereal Disease Research Laboratory test (VDRL), and fluorescent treponemal antibody absorption test (FTA-ABS)—both for syphilis; cat scratch skin test and magnetic resonance imaging (MRI) if the diagnosis is in question and to rule out MS. Treatment with high-dose intravenous (IV) corticosteroids may speed up visual acuity recovery, but probably does not have an effect on the final visual acuity outcome. A multicenter adult trial showed that IV corticosteroids may decrease the incidence of late multiple sclerosis; however, oral corticosteroids may increase the incidence of the development of demyelinating disease. If visual improvement does not start within the first 3 weeks or if vision worsens after treatment, then neuro-imaging and a work-up for sarcoidosis, Lyme disease, and autoimmune vasculitis (lupus) are indicated.

Macular Stellate Neuroretinitis

Optic disc edema may be extensive enough to leak into the macula and cause macular edema and exudates, producing a macular star

(**Figure 7-3**). This form of optic neuritis is called macular stellate neuroretinitis. It is unilateral in 80% of cases and is associated with viral illness, cat scratch disease, leptospirosis, Lyme disease, sarcoidosis, and toxoplasmosis.

Devic Neuromyelitis Optica

This is bilateral optic neuritis followed by a transverse myelitis.

Optic Nerve Glioma

In contrast to the rare malignant glioblastoma in adults, optic nerve gliomas in children are histologically very benign and are termed **juvenile pilocytic astrocytoma.** They occur along the optic nerve and, more commonly, in the chiasm, causing a fusiform enlargement of the optic nerve as it diffusely replaces normal neuronal architecture. Posterior tumors can bring about a slow diencephalic syndrome with diabetes insipidus, failure to thrive after a normal growth period, hyperactivity, changes in skin pallor, hypotension, and hypoglycemia. Tumors can occur anywhere along the optic nerves, chiasm, and optic tract (**Figure 7-4**). Optic nerve and chiasmal gliomas are slow growing, and patients present with proptosis, unilateral or bilateral visual loss, strabismus, optic atrophy, or nystagmus. The nystagmus is similar to *spasmus,* a unilateral or asymmetrical shimmering pendular nystagmus (see Chapter 8). Optic nerve gliomas are most common in children under 10 years of age and represent two thirds of all primary optic nerve tumors.

There is an important association with neurofibromatosis, as it is reported that anywhere from 10% to 70% of optic nerve gliomas are associated with neurofibromatosis type 1 (NF1). Likewise, approximately 15% of patients with NF1 will develop an optic nerve glioma. The treatment of optic nerve gliomas remains controversial, as the natural history is unknown. Some studies have reported an overall benign course; however, other studies indicate that 50% show progressive enlargement with visual loss. Obtaining serial ocular examinations and neuroimaging are important to monitor the tumor progress. Neuroimaging should be performed at least every 6 months and visual acuity with visual field testing at approximately 3-month intervals, at least for the first year after the tumor is diagnosed. Progressive visual loss and enlargement of the tumor are indications for therapy. If the tumor is localized to one optic nerve, many advocate removal of the optic nerve. Bilateral optic nerve

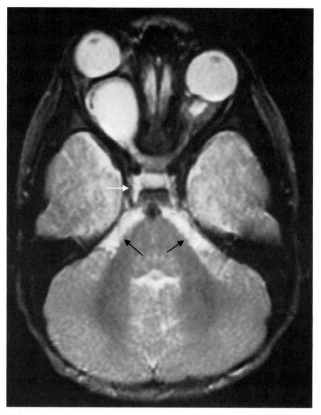

Figure 7-4.
MRI scan of patient with right optic nerve glioma; note extensive involvement of the contralateral nerve, chiasm (white arrows), and the optic tract (black arrows).

involvement and chiasmal involvement are usually treated with radiation therapy. In children younger than 4 years of age, chemotherapy of vincristine and carboplatin is often preferred over radiation therapy. Usually a biopsy is not necessary; however, a biopsy may be performed in cases of chiasmal glioma when there is a need to debulk an exophytic portion of the tumor because of secondary compression of surrounding structures.

Craniopharyngioma

Craniopharyngioma comes from squamous epithelial cells that are remnants from Rathke's pouch. It is the third most common brain tumor found in children. These tumors may be solid or cystic, often containing necrotic blood, epithelium, and cholesterol crystals (machine oil) fluid. Children often present with nonspecific complaints of headaches or progressive visual loss of unknown etiology. It is important to consider the diagnosis of craniopharyngioma in children who have decreased vision of unknown cause. Children may also present with endocrine dysfunction consisting of pituitary deficiency. Optic atrophy occurs in 60% of patients, and papilledema in 65% of patients. Acquired nystagmus (see-saw nystagmus) and bitemporal hemianopsia may result from large parasellar tumors expanding within the third ventricle. The treatment of craniopharyngioma involves removing the tumor completely, if possible. Often, complete resection is not possible. Repeat neuroimaging is important to follow the progress of the tumor. Unfortunately, most children with visual loss and optic atrophy at the time of their presentation will not show significant vision acuity improvement after surgery; however, decompression stops further visual loss. Recurrences usually occur 1 to 2 years after the primary procedure. Radiotherapy may be employed in older children and teenagers.

■ RETINAL DISEASE

Retinal Toxicosis

Several medications have retinal toxicity as a side effect. These medications include chloroquine (Aralene), hydroxychloroquine (Plaquenil), thioridazine (Mellaril), chlorpromazine (Thorazine), tamoxifen (Nolvadex), nicotinic acid (Niacin), and canthazanthine.

Chloroquine and hydroxychloroquine were first used in the treatment of malaria and are currently used for treating connective tissue diseases. Both drugs produce identical retinopathies that progress from mild macular pigmentary abnormalities to severe central maculopathies with loss of central vision. The classic appearance of the maculopathy is that of a bull's-eye, consisting of a central foveal area of hyperpigmentation surrounded by hypopigmentation (**Figure 7-5**). Toxicosis usually does not occur until the cumulative dose is greater than 100 grams. Follow-up ocular examinations should be obtained on patients undergoing chloroquine or hydroxychloroquine therapy. Ocular examinations should occur every 4 to 6 months and include testing visual acuity, checking the central visual field with an amsler grid, and performing fundoscopic exami-

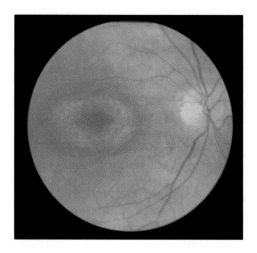

Figure 7-5.
Bull's-eye macular lesion in a 28-year-old patient who had received a cumulative dose of almost 700 g chloroquine over 6 years. The pigmentary changes in the macular remain, even after discontinuation of the drug.

nation. It is important to note that once toxicosis is diagnosed, progression can be seen even after discontinuing the medication.

■ HEREDITARY RETINAL DISORDERS

Stargardt Disease-Fundus Flavimaculatus

The most common hereditary macular dystrophy is Stargardt disease-Fundus Flavimaculatus. Typically, it is inherited as an autosomal recessive trait that results in a progressive macular degeneration. Stargardt disease begins in adolescence with complaints of slowly progressive, decreased visual acuity and mild loss of color vision. In its late stages, visual acuity drops to a range of 20/200 and patients may complain of poor night vision (**nyctalopia**). Macular appearance is that of beaten bronze, then changes to show areas of retinal pigment epithelial atrophy, which are seen as whitish yellow flecks (**Figure 7-6**). Unfortunately, there is no treatment.

Best Disease

Best disease is an autosomal dominant retinal dystrophy that affects central vision and causes dystrophic changes in the macula. During

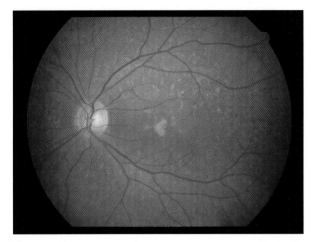

Figure 7-6.
Fundus flavimaculatus in a 42-year-old patient with 20/100 vision. Color photograph showing multiple yellow flecks at the level of the RPE, visible throughout the posterior pole.

early childhood to the mid-teens, patients develop a yellowish macular lesion. This is a well-circumscribed round lesion in the macula, approximately 1 to 2 disc diameters in size. The lesion has a distinct appearance, that of an "egg yolk," and is termed vitelliform macular lesion (**Figure 7-7**). Over time, the lesion represents abnormal accumulation of lipofuscin granules within the retinal pigment epithelium. The yellowish "egg yolk" lesion breaks up and creates a "scrambled egg" appearance that will ultimately result in an area of retinal atrophy. Visual acuity is fairly well preserved, in the range of 20/40 to 20/100. Late complications of retinal scarring and retinal vascularization, however, can lead to legal blindness.

X-Linked Retinoschisis

X-linked retinoschisis is an X-linked recessive retinal dystrophy that affects both the fovea and peripheral retina. This disorder consists of a splitting of the retina (schisis) at the level of the nerve fiber layer (inner retina). Unlike the previously described retinal dystrophies, this retinal dystrophy does not primarily affect the retinal pigment epithelium (outer pigment layer). In the fovea, there are small cystic cavities that form a spoke-like pattern (**Figure 7-8**). Fine folds in the area of the fovea occur overlying these microcysts. In

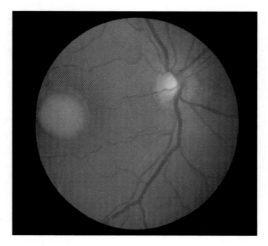

Figure 7-7.
The vitelliform macular lesion of Best disease is an accumulation of lipofuscin with the RPE. At a later stage, the "egg yolk" may be partially reabsorbed, producing a scrambled egg appearance.

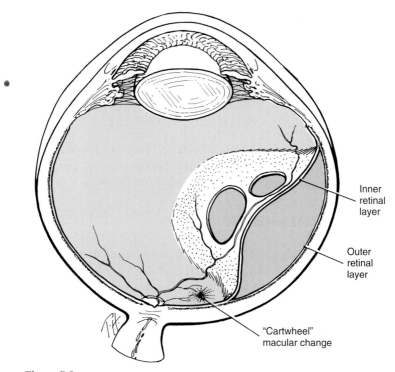

Inner retinal layer

Outer retinal layer

"Cartwheel" macular change

Figure 7-8.
Drawing—X-linked retinoschisis. The splitting occurs at the nerve fiber layer.

the periphery, large areas of retinoschisis occur, usually involving the inferior temporal quadrant. Schisis can be difficult to see if the retinal separation is shallow. Late in the disease, secondary retinal pigment epithelial changes can occur, and pigment can sometimes take on the appearance of retinitis pigmentosa. Vision often remains in the range of 20/70; however, vitreous hemorrhages can occur in areas of schisis, and the retina can detach in some patients, resulting in very poor vision.

Congenital Stationary Night Blindness

Congenital stationary night blindness is a hereditary, nonprogressive disorder of night vision. It can be inherited as autosomal dominant, autosomal recessive, or X-linked. The autosomal recessive pattern is rare and usually associated with consanguineous relationships or found in Jewish families. Visual acuity may be normal, although many cases have poor vision. Poor vision can be secondary to myopia, as patients with congenital night blindness are highly myopic. The night blindness usually occurs during the first decade of life as an isolated complaint. Color vision, visual field, and fundus examinations are normal. There are 2 distinct variants, however, that have fundus findings. These are Oguchi disease and Fundus albipunctatus, both autosomal recessive. They are stable, nonprogressive disorders and have no known treatment.

Cone Dystrophy

Cone dystrophy is a rare retinal dystrophy that preferentially affects cones more than rods. It is typically an autosomal dominant disorder; however, autosomal recessive and X-linked varieties have been described. This cone dystrophy usually presents during the first 3 decades of life, causing decreased central visual acuity. Other symptoms include photophobia (hypersensitivity to light), dark to light adaptation difficulty, and a history of better vision at night versus during the day. Color vision is significantly affected early in the development of the disorder. Visual fields demonstrate a central scotoma. Cone dystrophy, in most cases, is isolated to the retina without systemic involvement; however, renal-retinal dysplasia, which preferentially involves cone photoreceptors, has been described. The course of the disease is progressive and can be quite variable even among members of the same family. Vision often declines to the 20/200 level by the end of the third decade. For those experiencing photophobia, tinted lenses may help reduce the symptoms.

Retinitis Pigmentosa

Retinitis pigmentosa (RP) is an overall description for a large group of inherited disorders that affect the retinal pigment epithelium (outer pigmented layer of the retina). The retinal pigment epithelium is critical to the health of the neurosensory retina, as the retinal pigment epithelium nourishes and revitalizes the outer segments of the rods and cones. Diseases of the outer segments of the rods and cones and the retinal pigment epithelium result in decreased function of the rods and cones and ultimately, over time, can cause blindness. These inherited diseases may be confined to the eye; however, many are associated with systemic abnormalities. Retinitis pigmentosa is a major health problem, as approximately 1 in 4,000 individuals are affected. The inherited pattern is 20% autosomal dominant, 20% autosomal recessive, 10% X-linked recessive, and 50% sporadic. The autosomal recessive and X-linked recessive forms tend to develop early in childhood or adolescent years and have a rapid, progressive course. Autosomal dominant cases tend to occur later in adulthood and have a slower, milder course.

The cause of progressive, retinal, pigmentary, epithelial atrophy has undergone intensive study. Recent molecular biological breakthroughs have shown the primary defect in many types of retinitis pigmentosa is a point mutation in the rhodopsin gene. Rhodopsin is a critical protein in the outer segments of the rods. Over time, the abnormal protein builds up and results in rod death and secondary retinal pigment epithelial atrophy. Retinitis pigmentosa is mostly a rod disease and first affects the peripheral retina where the rod concentration is very high. Some types of retinitis pigmentosa affect both rods and cones, while other inherited retinal diseases preferentially affect cones.

Symptoms associated with retinitis pigmentosa include poor night vision with abnormal dark adaptation. Rods are responsible for our night vision (scotopic vision), and loss of rods first affects our ability to adapt to dark conditions. Patients also experience peripheral visual field loss and develop tunnel vision. Late in the disease, the tunnel vision can be so severe that it greatly restricts

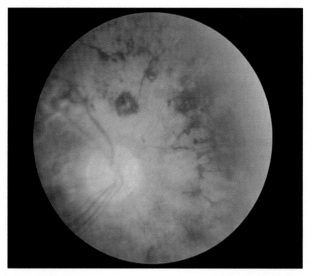

Figure 7-9.
Usher syndrome. Fundus photograph showing typical retinitis pigmentosa findings of bone spicule hyperpigmentary changes, attenuated retinal vessels, and optic disc pallor (atrophy).

patient activity. Central visual acuity loss can occur late in the disease.

Ophthalmoscopic findings are peripheral bone spicule hyperpigmentation (**Figure 7-9**). This is an area of clumped pigmentation with adjacent areas of hypopigmentation and retinal pigment epithelial atrophy. The optic nerve will take on a waxy pallor and the retinal vessels will be significantly attenuated. Electrophysiological testing is important to document decreased electroretinogram from poor dark adaptation.

Systemic Diseases Associated With Retinitis Pigmentosa (Table 7-1)

Usher Syndrome
Usher syndrome is an autosomal recessive form of retinitis pigmentosa (**Figure 7-9**) associated with sensorineural deafness. In some cases, the deafness is associated with abnormal vestibular function. The combination of both visual and auditory deprivation has devastating social implications, and affected individuals often have severe psychological problems.

Table 7.1
Neurologic Disorders Accompanying Retinitis Pigmentosa

Errors in Lipid Metabolism
   3-Hydroxydicarboxylic aciduria
   Abetalipoproteinemia
   Refsum disease
   Neuronal ceroid lipofuscinoses
     Infantile form
     Late infantile form
     Juvenile form
Errors in Mucopolysaccharid Metabolism
   Hurler disease (MPS IH)
   Hunter disease (MPS II)
   Scheie disease (MPS IS)
Peroxismal Disorders
   Zellweger disease
   Neonatal adrenoleukodystrophy
   Infantile Refsum disease
Mitochondrial Disorders
   Kearns-Sayre syndrome
Heredodegenerative Disease
   Friedreich ataxia
   Cerebellar ataxia, dominant
   Familial spastic paraplegia
   Hallervorden-Spatz disease
   Cockayne syndromes
   Chédiak-Higashi syndrome
   Hallgren syndrome
Other Hereditary Disorders
   Gyrate atrophy due to ornithine aminotransferase deficiency
   Sjögren-Larsson syndrome
   Laurence-Moon syndrome
   Allström syndrome
   Usher syndrome

Refsum Syndrome

Refsum syndrome is an autosomal recessive defect in fatty acid metabolism that results in increased phytanic acid throughout the body. This metabolic defect results in peripheral neuropathy, cerebellar ataxia, deafness, and retinitis pigmentosa. The time of onset is usually in the third decade. The diagnosis is confirmed by the presence of elevated levels of phytanic acid in the serum. Restricting dietary phytanic acid early in life may slow the progression of the disease.

Bassen-Kornzweig Syndrome (Abetalipoproteinemia)

Bassen-Kornzweig syndrome is a rare autosomal recessive disorder caused by malabsorption of intestinal fat. Patients have decreased serum levels of cholesterol, triglycerides, and fat-soluble vitamins A, E, and K. Diagnosis is confirmed by very low serum cholesterol. Patients present with steatorrhea, acanthocytosis (ichthyosis-abnormal scaling and dryness), ataxia, and childhood onset retinitis pigmentosa. Dietary supplementation with vitamin E can be helpful.

Laurence-Moon-Bardet-Biedl Syndrome

Laurence-Moon-Bardet-Biedl syndrome is a disorder consisting of obesity, mental retardation, hypogenitalism, and retinitis pigmentosa. This syndrome has been divided into 2 forms: the **Laurence-Moon syndrome,** which is associated with spinocerebellar ataxia, hypogonadism, and spastic paraplegia, and the **Bardet-Biedl syndrome,** which includes polydactyly. Bardet-Biedl syndrome is autosomal recessive. These patients may have subtle findings, and the diagnosis may be overlooked. Examination of feet and hands may require radiography to determine polydactyly or brachydactyly. Recently, the genotype of Bardet-Biedl syndrome has been mapped to chromosome 16.

Renal-Retinal Syndromes

Retinitis pigmentosa is associated with certain renal diseases including **Senior-Loken syndrome** and **Maldino-Mainzer syndrome.** These are usually autosomal recessively inherited and feature retinal pigment epithelium degeneration. Senior-Loken syndrome consists of juvenile renal failure, often leading to transplantation and progressive retinitis pigmentosa.

■ NEURODEGENERATIVE DISORDERS ASSOCIATED with VISION LOSS (Tables 7-2 and 7-3)

Neuronal Ceroid-Lipofuscinosis (NCL)

Batten Disease

Neuronal ceroid-lipofuscinosis (NCL) refers to a group of lysosomal storage disorders of lipopigments with secondary neuronal degen-

Table 7.2
Neurodegenerative Conditions With Onset in Late Infancy or Early Childhood

Defective Organelle	Condition	Principal Ophthalmic Manifestation	Principal Systemic Manifestations	Biochemical Defect
Lysosome sphingolipidoses	Metachromatic leukodystrophy	Optic atrophy, nystagmus	Weakness, ataxia, dementia	Arylsulfatase A
	Gaucher disease type 3	Abducens palsy, ocular motor apraxia	Dysphagia, spasticity, dementia, myoclonus organomegaly, osseous lesions	Glucocerebrosidase
	Nieman-Pick type IS (formerly type B)	Pigmentary maculopathy	Organomegaly, mental retardation	Sphingomyelinase
	Niemann-Pick type IIS (formerly type C)	Vertical gaze palsy	Organomegaly, psychomotor retardation	Unknown
Lysosome oligosaccharidoses	Aspartylglycosaminuria	Crystalline cataracts	Coarse facies, mental retardation, diarrhea, recurrent infections	Aspartylglycosaminidase
	Fucosidosis	Tortuous conjunctival vessels	Coarse facies, psychomotor deterioration, dysostosis multiplex, angiokeratoma	α-L-fucosidase
	Mannosidosis type II	Spoke-like cataracts, corneal opacities	Coarse facies, psychomotor deterioration, dysostosis multiplex, deafness, recurrent infections	α-mannosidase
	Schindler's neuroaxonal dystrophy	Optic atrophy, nystagmus	Weakness, peripheral neuropathy, psychomotor retardation	α-N-acetylogalactosaminidase

Lysosome mucolipidoses	Mucolipidosis III (Pseudo-Hurler polydystrophy)	Corneal clouding, pigmentary retinopathy, hyperopic astigmatism	Dysostosis multiplex, mental retardation, coarse facies (mild)	UPD-N-acetylglucosamine: lysosomal enzyme N-acetylglucosaminyl-l-phosphotransferase
Lysosome mucopolysaccharidoses	MPS 1H (Hurler)	Corneal clouding, pigmentary retinopathy	Dysostosis multiplex, organomegaly, coarse facies, mental retardation	α-L-iduronidase
	MPS II (Hunter)	Pigmentary retinopathy, corneal clouding (rare)	Dysostosis multiplex, organomegaly, coarse facies, psychomotor retardation	Iduronate sulfatase
	MPS III (Sanfilippo)	Pigmentary retinopathy	Severe mental retardation, mild dysostosis multiplex, deafness	Heparan N-sulfatase (MPS IIIA) α-L-acetylglucosaminidase (MPS IIIB) Acetyl-CoA: α-glucosaminide acetyltransferase (MPS IIIC) N-acetylglucosamine 6-sulfatase (MPS IIID)
Lysosome ceroidoses	Late infantile NCL (Jansky-Bielschowsky)	Pigmentary retinopathy, optic atrophy	Seizures, ataxia, spasticity, loss of speech	Unknown
Mitochondria	MELAS syndrome	Hemianopsia, cortical visual loss	Seizures, lactic acidosis, hemiparesis	Mitochondrial tRNA

(continued)

Table 7.2 *(continued)*
Neurodegenerative Conditions With Onset in Late Infancy or Early Childhood

Defective Organelle	Condition	Principal Ophthalmic Manifestation	Principal Systemic Manifestations	Biochemical Defect
Peroxisome	Adrenoleukodystrophy	Cortical blindness, optic atrophy	Quadriparesis, dysarthria, cognitive, decline, Addison's disease	Lignoceroyl CoA ligase
Unknown	Riley-Day syndrome (familial dysautonomia)	Dry eyes, corneal hypoesthesia, band keratopathy, optic atrophy	Vomiting, motor delay, poor temperature control, postural hypotension, emotional lability	Unknown
	Chédiak-Higashi syndrome	Iris transillumination, foveal hypoplasia, nystagmus	Oculocutaneous albinism, recurrent infections, ataxia, polyneuropathy	Unknown
	Neuroaxonal dystrophy	Optic atrophy, cortical blindness, nystagmus, esotropia	Weakness, peripheral neuropathy, spasticity	Unknown
	Ataxia telangiectasia (Louis-Bar syndrome)	Conjunctival telangiectasia, dysmetric saccades, nystagmus, optic atrophy	Ataxia, polyneuropathy, immunologic impairment	Unknown

Table 7-3
Neurodegenerative Conditions With Onset in Late Childhood or Adolescence

Defective Organelle	Condition	Principal Ophthalmic Manifestation	Principal Systemic Manifestations	Biochemical Defect
Lysosome sphingolipidoses	Metachromatic leukodystrophy (late onset)	Optic atrophy	Personality changes, ataxia, incontinence, gallstones	Arylsulfatase A
Lysosome oligosaccharidoses	Sialidosis (type I)	Cherry red spots, nyctalopia, cataracts	Myoclonus, ataxia	Neuroaminidase (oligosaccharide sialidase)
Lysosome ceroidosis	Juvenile NCL (Spielmeyer-Vogt)	Pigmentary maculopathy	Behavioral problems, cognitive decline, seizures, spasticity	Unknown
Peroxisome (presumed)	Refsum's disease	Pigmentary retinopathy, nyctalopia, cataracts	Ataxia, hearing loss, cardiac arrhythmia	Phytanic acid α-hydroxylase
Mitochondria	Fukuhara's disease (MERRF)	Optic atrophy	Myoclonus, ataxia, weakness	Mitochondrial tRNA^{lys}
	Chronic progressive external ophthalmoplegia (CPEO)/Kearns-Sayre	Ptosis, ophthalmoplegia, pigmentary retinopathy, nystagmus	Weakness, heart block, ataxia, hearing loss, endocrine problems	Unknown

(continued)

Table 7-3 *(continued)*
Neurodegenerative Conditions With Onset in Late Childhood or Adolescence

Defective Organelle	Condition	Principal Ophthalmic Manifestation	Principal Systemic Manifestations	Biochemical Defect
None	SSPE	Macular chorioretinitis, optic atrophy, papilledema	Cognitive decline, myoclonus, epilepsy, rigidity	Immune response to measles virus
Unknown	Hallervorden-Spatz disease	Vertical gaze palsy, saccadic pursuit, eyelid apraxia, pigmentary retinopathy	Rigidity, choreoathetosis, dysarthria, dysphagia, dementia	Unknown
	Wilson disease	Kayser-Fleischer rings, sunflower cataracts, saccadic pursuit	Liver failure, choreoathetosis, renal stones, cardiomyopathy	Unknown
	Myotonic dystrophy	Ptosis, blepharospasm, cataracts, pigmentary retinopathy	Myotonia, muscle atrophy	Unknown
	Friedreich's ataxia	Optic atrophy, nystagmus	Ataxia, dysarthria, pes cavus, kyphoscoliosis, proprioceptive loss, hyporeflexive joints, hearing loss	Unknown

eration. Neonates are not blind at birth, but start losing milestones between 6 months and 3 years of age. These are autosomal recessive generalized disorders with progressive psychomotor delay, seizures, and choreoathetosis. Patients develop a retinal degeneration that leads to blindness and an attenuated or extinguished electroretinogram. Intracellular inclusions can be seen by electronmicroscopy in neurons, pericytes, macrophages, smooth muscle cells, lipocytes, and capillary endothelial cells. Diagnosis is made by biopsy of the skin and rectum. Conjunctival biopsy may also be helpful.

Haltia-Santavuori

Haltia-Santavuori is an infantile form of NCL characterized by normal development until 6 months of age. Then, progressive regression with loss of psychomotor milestones, onset of seizures, pigmentary retinal degeneration, and optic atrophy occur. Patients are usually blind by 2 to 3 years of age, and death occurs around 6 to 7 years of age.

Jansky-Bielschowsky

Jansky-Bielschowsky disease is an NCL that has a later onset, between 2 and 4 years of age, with patients often presenting with seizures. This progresses with visual loss (optic atrophy and retinal pigmentary degeneration), ataxia, loss of developmental milestones, and eventually decerebrate rigidity and death.

Spielmeyer-Batten-Vogt

Spielmeyer-Batten-Vogt disease is an NCL that differs because of its later onset and that visual loss (retinal degeneration) often presents before neurologic deterioration occurs. Visual loss first occurs between 3 and 7 years of age, and death from progressive neurologic deterioration occurs by age 20.

■ PEROXISOMAL DISEASE (ALSO SEE CHAPTER 6)

X-linked Adrenoleukodystrophy

X-linked Adrenoleukodystrophy is a peroxisomal disease occurring in males between 4 to 8 years of age. As with any leukodystrophy, there is massive and progressive white matter degeneration. It is associated with adrenal insufficiency and with bronzing of the skin, personality changes, and intellectual decline. Neurological deterioration is progressive, with dysphagia, quadriparesis and death occurring around age 8 to 12 years. Initial visual loss is from cortical pathology and, later, optic nerve involvement leads to optic atrophy.

■ MITOCHONDIAL DISEASES (TABLE 7-3)

Mitochondrial DNA is transmitted exclusively by the mother via the mitochondria found in the egg. Sperm are almost devoid of mitochondria; therefore, sperm does not transmit mitochondrial DNA.

Chronic Progressive External Ophthalmoplegia (CPEO)

This is a disease of progressive limited eye movements, ptosis, retinal pigmentary degeneration, and heart block. Onset can occur in childhood, but often occurs in the second or third decade of life. Patients often present with ptosis and diplopia. The retinal degeneration consists of pigmentary alterations that have a "salt and pepper" appearance. About 40% of affected patients will experience decreased visual acuity or night blindness. Cardiac abnormalities include conduction defects and heart block. Red ragged fibers of skeletal and cardiac muscles are present, and patients are frequently managed with a cardiac pacemaker. Other systemic findings include decreased brain stem ventilatory response to hypoxia and possible sudden death, cerebellar ataxia, deafness, vestibular dysfunction, loss of intelligence, and multiple endocrine abnormalities including diabetes mellitus, growth hormone deficiency, adrenal dysfunction, and hypoparathyroidism. Endocrine dysfunction may be triggered by corticosteroids and hypersensitivity to anesthetic that may even precipitate a fatal event.

The majority of patients with CPEO are sporadic; however, when familial, the disease is transmitted maternally via mitochondrial DNA.

There are many types of CPEO with the most well-known of the syndromes considered to be a subset of CPEO is Kearns-Sayre syndrome. Its unique phenotype notwithstanding, Kearns-Sayre syndrome may be one particular manifestation of a larger group of abnormalities, all caused by deletions of mitochondrial DNA. Deletions lead to similar biochemical abnormalities that are found to produce clinical syndromes that differ. Diagnostic criteria include 2 obligatory features: early-onset CPEO (prior to age 20) and retinal pigmentary degeneration, plus one of the following 3: heart block, CSF protein greater than 100 mg/dL, or cerebellar syndrome.

MELAS Syndrome

(**M**itochondrial myopathy, **E**ncephalopathy, **L**actic acidosis, and **S**troke-like episodes)

MELAS syndrome is characterized by seizures, vomiting, and lactic acidosis occurring during the first years of life. Patients with MELAS syndrome may experience vision loss secondary to cortical blindness; however, they do not develop progressive retinal degeneration. The disorder is secondary to respiratory dysfunction of cortical neurons caused by the mitochondrial dysfunction. Patients experience problems with autoregulation of blood flow at the level of the pial arterioles. Although stroke-like episodes occur, the patient usually recovers. Hemianopsia, cortical visual loss, and intermittent hemiparesis may occur. Unlike other mitochondrial diseases, muscle weakness is not a prominent feature of MELAS syndrome; however, the patient does have ragged red fibers of skeletal and cardiac muscle.

MERRF Syndrome—Fukuhara's Disease

(**M**yoclonus **E**pilepsy with **R**agged, **R**ed **F**ibers)

MERFF syndrome is a generalized seizure disorder with patients presenting in the second decade with myoclonus. Severe visual loss may be secondary to optic atrophy; however, retinal degeneration is not a prominent feature. Over time, patients develop ataxia and muscle weakness.

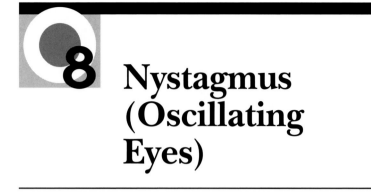

8 Nystagmus (Oscillating Eyes)

Nystagmus is defined as involuntary rhythmic oscillations of the eye. The movements can be described as either pendular or jerk. Pendular nystagmus occurs when the movements have equal velocity in each direction, whereas jerk nystagmus is defined by a fast eye movement in one direction and a slow eye movement in the opposite direction. The direction of jerk nystagmus is determined by the direction of the fast component. **Figure 8-1** depicts a right jerk horizontal nystagmus in primary gaze that increases in right gaze and diminishes in left gaze. Nystagmus can be horizontal (sideways movement), vertical (up and down movement), or rotary (twisting of the eye, or torsion). The oscillations can be described in regard to their amplitude (distance the eye travels) and the frequency (number of oscillations per second).

In most cases, there is a position of gaze where the nystagmus diminishes, referred to as the **null point.** Patients with nystagmus often adopt a compensatory face turn to place the eyes at the null point to enhance visual acuity. **Figure 8-2A** shows a patient with a null point in right gaze. The patient turns his face to the left to place the eyes at the null point in right gaze.

Latent nystagmus is a special form of nystagmus where the nystagmus increases when one eye is covered. Latent nystagmus is often associated with congenital nystagmus and congenital esotropia. Patients with latent nystagmus usually perform poorly on vision testing, as the examiner routinely covers one eye, making the nystagmus worse. To assess the best visual potential in a patient with nystagmus, test vision with both eyes open and allow the patient to adopt a compensatory face turn.

Nystagmus Notation

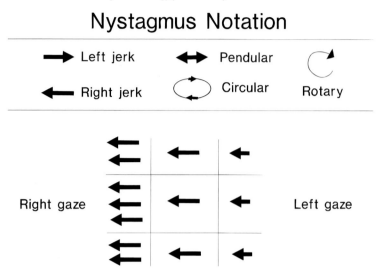

Right gaze   Left gaze

Figure 8-1.
Nystagmus notation. The above schema are useful in describing a patient's nystagmus. Directional arrows are used to indicate the direction of the nystagmus and its basic characteristics. Multiple arrows and the length of the arrow can be used to indicate frequency and amplitude respectively.

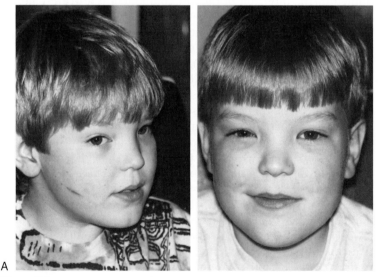

A   B

Figure 8-2.
A, Patient with a face turn to the left, eyes right to damp nystagmus and improve visual acuity. **B,** Same patient after Kestenbaum surgical eye muscle procedure to relocate the null point to the primary position. After surgery, the null point is in primary position and the face turn is improved.

It is helpful to classify nystagmus as either congenital or acquired. It is important to recognize acquired nystagmus, as it maybe a sign of a significant central nervous system disease.

■ CONGENITAL NYSTAGMUS

Congenital nystagmus is nystagmus with onset by 6 to 8 weeks of age. Because of the early onset, infants are able to cortically suppress the motion and do not perceive oscillopsia (ie, perception of cyclic motion associated with nystagmus). Only patients with acquired nystagmus will experience oscillopsia, as they do not have the cortical plasticity to suppress the shaking image. There are 2 basic types of congenital nystagmus: (1) congenital motor nystagmus and (2) sensory nystagmus.

Patients with congenital nystagmus should be referred for full ocular evaluation.

Congenital Motor Nystagmus

Congenital motor nystagmus is bilateral and symmetrical and occurs in the first month of life. It is often inherited as an X-linked recessive trait; however, other modes of inheritance have been documented. By 2 to 4 months of age, the child often establishes a face turn to place the eyes in a position to minimize the nystagmus (null point). Patients with congenital motor nystagmus have relatively good visual potential (usually around 20/50 or better), and the face-turn posturing is used to optimize their vision.

Sensory Nystagmus

Sensory nystagmus is caused by lack of development of the fixation reflex secondary to neonatal blindness. Any disease that results in bilateral blindness, such as congenital cataracts, congenital optic nerve atrophy, and congenital retinal disorders, can cause sensory nystagmus (see Chapter 6). **Table 8-1** lists the more common causes of sensory nystagmus. The pattern of sensory nystagmus is usually indistinguishable from congenital motor nystagmus, except that the nystagmus has a larger amplitude and the eye movements show poor fixation with a "searching" character. The onset of the nystagmus is later than congenital motor nystagmus, usually occurring

Table 8-1.

Causes of Sensory Nystagmus

Diagnosis	Cause of Decreased Vision
Achromatopsia	congenital lack of cones
Albinism	foveal hypoplasia
Aniridia	foveal hypoplasia
Bilateral congenital opacity (eg, corneal, or cataract)	bilateral amblyopia
Infantile retinal dystrophies (eg, Joubert)	retinal degeneration
Leber congenital amaurosis	retinal dysplasia
Optic nerve hypoplasia	optic nerve dysfunction

after 6 to 8 weeks. Patients with sensory nystagmus rarely adopt a compensatory face turn.

■ ACQUIRED NYSTAGMUS

Acquired nystagmus, even if acquired in infancy, may be a sign of a serious neurological condition. Neurologic disease involving the midbrain, cerebellum, vestibular system, and areas throughout the brain stem can cause nystagmus. **Table 8-2** lists types of nystagmus associated with neuroanatomical etiology. In contrast to congenital nystagmus, acquired nystagmus is often associated with the perception of the environment moving, or oscillopsia. Oscillopsia, therefore, is an important indication that the nystagmus is acquired.

Spasmus Nutans

This is an acquired pendular nystagmus that develops between 3 and 18 months of age and is usually asymmetrical and rarely unilateral. The nystagmus appears as shimmering, small-amplitude, pendular eye movements. A distinctive feature of spasmus nutans is the presence of **head nodding.** Children with this disorder nod their heads in a rhythmic manner. The primary form of spasmus nutans is a benign disorder that spontaneously disappears by around 3 to 4 years of age. This is an important type of nystagmus, as several cases of spasmus nutans have been associated with chiasmal or suprachiasmal tumors. Patients with spasmus nutans should have neuroimaging to rule out a central nervous system tumor, even if the nystagmus is the only presenting sign.

Table 8-2.
Types and Characteristics of Nystagmus

Type	Characteristics
See-Saw	Alternating and repetitive elevation and intorsion of one eye with simultaneous depression and extorsion of the fellow eye.
Periodic Alternating (PAN)	Horizontal jerk nystagmus that periodically changes direction every 60 to 120 seconds.
Convergence Retraction	Quick convergence or eye retraction movements on attempted upgaze. Upgaze is usually limited (Parinaud syndrome).
Down-beat	Vertical nystagmus with a fast phase beating downward.
Up-beat	Vertical nystagmus with the fast phase beating upward.
Gaze-evoked	Large amplitude, low-frequency nystagmus in one gaze with higher frequency and smaller amplitude nystagmus in the opposite gaze.
Rebound	Change in direction of gaze-evoked horizontal nystagmus after prolonged eccentric fixation or a horizontal gaze-evoked nystagmus that, upon refixation to primary position, temporally beats in the opposite direction.
Oculopalatal Myoclonus	Fast, vertical, pendular nystagmus, often asymmetric, associated with movements of other muscular structures such as the palate, facial muscles, tongue, pharynx, diaphragm, and extremities.
Opsoclonus	Rapid involuntary multi-vectorial low amplitude chaotic eye movements.
Ocular Flutter	Like opsoclonus, except present only in the horizontal plane.
Spasmus Nutans	High frequency, pendular small amplitude asymmetric or unilateral nystagmus.

9 Abnormal Optic Discs

In this chapter, causes of abnormal appearing optic discs are discussed. They will be classified as congenital or acquired, and are listed in **Table 9-1.**

■ CONGENITAL OPTIC DISC ANOMALIES

Congenital optic disc anomalies are discussed in this section, except for 2 important congenital abnormal optic discs that can cause blindness at birth: **optic nerve hypoplasia** and **optic nerve coloboma,** which are discussed in Chapter 6.

Morning-Glory Disc Anomaly

Morning-Glory disc anomaly is a rare congenital optic disc anomaly that involves the peripapillary retina (area around the optic disc in addition to the optic disc). The optic nerve is large and excavated. The retinal vessels emanate from the mid-periphery of the optic nerve in a straight radial fashion (**Figure 9-1**). There is lack of normal retinal pigment epithelium in the peripapillary area, thus producing scleral show. The retina around the optic disc has multiple radial folds emanating from the optic nerve, thus the term "morning-glory" for its resemblance to the morning glory flower. The Morning-Glory disc anomaly is distinct from optic nerve colobomas; however, their appearance can be similar. Morning-Glory

Table 9-1.
Abnormal Optic Disc Appearance

Congenital
1. Optic Nerve Hypoplasia (Chapter 6)
2. Optic Nerve Coloboma (Chapter 6)
3. Morning-Glory Disc Anomaly (this chapter)
4. Myelinated Retinal Nerve Fibers (this chapter)
5. Pseudopapilledema (this chapter)
6. Grey Pigmented Optic Disc (this chapter)
7. Tilt Myopic Scleral Crescent (this chapter)
8. Optic Nerve Pit (this chapter)
Acquired
1. Papilledema (this chapter)
2. Papillitis (Optic Neuritis) (Chapter 7)
3. Optic Disc Drusen (this chapter)
4. Optic Atrophy (Chapter 7)
5. Glaucoma (Chapter 12)

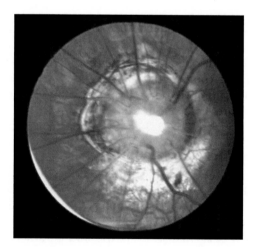

Figure 9-1.
Morning-Glory disc anomaly, black and white photo. Note the enlarged disc with straightened radial retinal vessels emanating from the mid-periphery of the optic nerve. Also note the lack of peripapillary pigmentation and consequent scleral show. The disc has an enlarged appearance.

configuration is distinguished by the pattern of the radial retinal folds coming from the disc and by glial proliferation overlying the peripapillary retina and retinal vessels.

Patients often present with strabismus because of poor vision in the affected eye. Vision is variable (depending on the extent of the macular changes), ranging from 20/50 to legally blind; but fortunately, most cases are unilateral. Bilateral cases do occur; however, visual acuity is usually better than in the unilateral cases. Females tend to be affected more than males, but both sexes are involved. The most important late complication is the high risk for developing a retinal detachment, as almost 40% of affected eyes will develop one. Associated systemic findings include basal encephaloceles and midline facial defects such as hypertelorism, cleft lip, or cleft palate. These systemic findings have also been associated with optic nerve colobomas, and it is possible that optic nerve colobomas have been falsely diagnosed as Morning-Glory disc anomaly (see Chapter 6 for discussion of optic nerve coloboma).

Myelinated Retinal Nerve Fibers

The presence of myelinated retinal nerve fibers is a very dramatic, albeit benign, anomaly. Myelinated retinal nerve fibers are often termed "medullated nerve fibers." Normally, the optic nerve is myelinated up to the point where the optic nerve enters the eye and becomes the optic disc (lamina cribrosa). Myelinated retinal nerve fibers occur when myelinization progresses past the optic disc into the retinal layers. This gives the appearance of a fluffy white material overlying and adjacent to the optic nerve (**Figure 9-2**). The feathery edge and striated appearance occur because the myelin follows the retinal nerve fibers. The blurred disc margins can give the appearance of pseudopapilledema. Occasionally, myelinated nerve fibers have been found to extend into the peripheral retina and macula.

Females are affected more than males, and approximately 80% of cases are unilateral. In the majority of cases, visual acuity is not affected. There is an increased incidence of refractive errors, including unilateral high myopia, and amblyopia may be present. In rare cases, the macula may be involved and macular hypoplasia may result in decreased vision. The condition is stable and does not require treatment other than associated refractive errors and amblyopia.

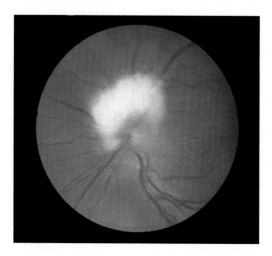

Figure 9-2.
Myelinated optic nerve fibers are the white feathery substance in the inferior peripapillary area of the optic disc.

Pseudopapilledema

The appearance of blurred disc margins, and even a swollen disc, is not always indicative of disc edema. Any process that blurs the disc margins or causes a fullness of the optic nerve may give the appearance of disc edema, and is termed pseudopapilledema. The most common cause of pseudopapilledema is hyperopia associated with a relatively small eye and blurred disc margins. Myelinated nerve fibers are another common cause of blurred disc margins. Some patients have primary blurred disc margins without a specific association or cause (congenital pseudopapilledema) (**Figure 9-3**). **Table 9-2** lists the differential diagnosis of pseudopapilledema.

In contrast to true disc edema, patients with pseudopapilledema have a normal nerve fiber layer and disc color, no vessel engorgement, no peripapillary hemorrhages, and no retinal exudates. Spontaneous retinal venous pulsations are usually present. Vision is normal with most forms of pseudopapilledema.

Congenital Gray Pigmented Optic Disc

The appearance of a congenitally gray optic disc occurs in premature infants with delayed visual maturation, in infants with ocular albinism, and in individuals with isolated chromosomal anomalies

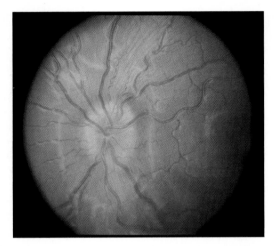

Figure 9-3.
Pseudopapilledema (congenital) showing blurred disc margins, but no retinal vessel engorgement, no nerve fiber edema (hazy appearance), and no flame-shaped hemorrhages.

Table 9-2.
Differential Diagnoses of Pseudopapilledema
(Blurred Disc Margin)

1. Hyperopia
2. Myelinated optic nerve fibers
3. Optic disc drusen
4. Congenital pseudopapilledema
5. Epipapillary hamartomas and tumors

such as partial trisomy 10Q syndrome. In premature infants and neonates, the gray appearance is probably the result of an optical effect, perhaps an overall hypopigmentation of the retina. Over time, the gray discoloration resolves as the retina matures. True pigmentation of the nerve secondary to myelin deposition is rare; however, it may be associated with a chromosomal abnormality of chromosome 17 and Aicardi syndrome. Visual acuity is not affected unless there is associated optic nerve anomaly such as optic nerve hypoplasia.

Congenital Tilted Disc

Congenital tilted disc is characterized by a scleral opening larger than the size of the optic nerve head **(Figure 9-4)**. Typically, there is

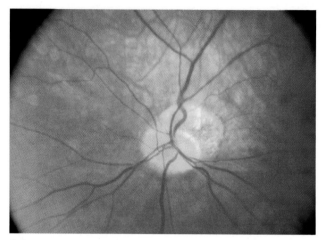

Figure 9-4.
Tilted disc with a crescent of yellow-white scleral show crescent superiorly. This hypopigmented crescent is often seen in children with myopia.

a peripapillary scleral crescent nasal of scleral show, and the vessels emanate in a scattered pattern rather than the normal distribution of nasal and retinal vascular arcades (normal disc—see Chapter 1, Figure 1-8). Some tilted discs are associated with myopia, but visual acuity is generally not affected. In some cases, however, there may be a mild loss of visual acuity that may actually represent a variant of optic nerve hypoplasia. In general, however, there are no associated systemic or neurological diseases.

Optic Nerve Pit

This is a congenital anomaly of the optic nerve consisting of a focal depression within the optic nerve, usually in the temporal aspect of the disc. Optic nerve pits may represent a communication with the subarachnoid space of the optic nerve; however, this theory is still controversial. It is well documented that optic nerve pits are associated with serous retinal detachments in the area of the macula. Laser treatment may improve resolution of these retinal detachments.

■ ACQUIRED OPTIC DISC ABNORMALITIES

Optic Disc Edema

Papilledema is a term often loosely used to imply optic disc swelling or optic disc edema. The term **optic disc edema** should be used to refer to disc edema and swelling caused by a variety of optic nerve and systemic conditions including optic nerve inflammation (**Table 9-3**). Strictly defined, **papilledema** is optic disc edema secondary to increased intracranial pressure. Inflammation of the optic nerve head can produce disc edema, and is termed **papillitis.** Pseudopapilledema is the term for conditions that produce blurred disc margins without associated disc edema (Figure 7-3). Ophthalmoscopically, disc edema is characterized by a full and swollen disc, a feathery blurred disc margin, thickened nerve fiber layer that obliterates underlying peripapillary retinal vessels (inferiorly first, then superiorly), disc hyperemia, small or nonexistent central cup, enlarged veins, and occasional splinter nerve fiber layer hemorrhages (flame-shaped hemorrhages) (**Figure 9-5**). Spontaneous ve-

Table 9-3.
Causes of Optic Disc Edema

1. Papilledema (increased ICP)
   a. Obstructive hydrocephalus
   b. Pseudotumor cerebri (see later in this chapter)
   c. Intracranial hemorrhage (subarachnoid hemorrhage)
2. Papillitis (optic disc inflammation)
   a. Optic neuritis (usually post-viral syndrome)
   b. Toxocara of the disc
   c. Neuroretinitis (chickenpox, mumps, hepatitis B, Cat Scratch disease, Lyme disease, leptospirosis, early neurosyphilis, tuberculosis, sarcoidosis, and toxoplasmosis
3. Malignant Hypertension (ie renal failure)
4. Optic Nerve Venous Outflow Obstruction
   a. Venous sinus thrombosis
   b. Craniosynostosis
   c. Hyperviscosity syndromes

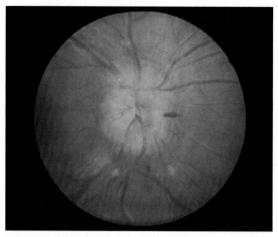

Figure 9-5.
Fully developed papilledema with disc elevation, hyperemia, edematous nerve fiber layer, loss of central cup, and splinter hemorrhages. Note the blurred disc margins and the blurred appearance of the vessels in the mid-periphery of the optic disc.

nous pulsations are absent in papilledema associated with increased intracranial pressure.

Spontaneous Venous Pulsations

Spontaneous venous pulsations are pulsatile collapse and reformation of the retinal veins close to or on the optic disc. The presence of spontaneous venous pulsations over the disc is an important sign, as it indicates that the intracranial pressure is less than 200 mm water. Approximately 20% of the normal population, however, do not have spontaneous venous pulsations and, therefore, the absence of spontaneous venous pulsations does not mean that the intracranial pressure is high.

Differentiating Papilledema, Papillitis, and Pseudopapilledema

This is based on ophthalmoscopic appearance and can be difficult and sometimes impossible to differentiate. **Table 9-4** lists the char-

Table 9-4.
Characteristics of Papilledema, Papillitis, and Pseudopapilledema

	Papilledema	*Papillitis*	*Pseudopapilledema*
Disc Appearance	Blurred margins, elevated disc, loss of cup, dilated vessels, splinter hemorrhages, Obliterated peripapillary vessels, no spontaneous venous pulsations.	Disc appearance similar to papilledema, and vitreous cells with "hazy fundus" view. Macular exudates are common.	Blurred margins, ± elevated disc, no loss of cup (except with drusen), usually no hemorrhage, no dilated vessels, vessels seen clearly. Retinal vessels maybe anomalous, spontaneous venous pulsations usually present.
Symptoms	Headaches, emesis, may have transient visual obscurations.	Acute vision loss with metamorphopsia (distorted vision), may have pain with eye movement.	No symptoms.
Visual Acuity	Usually normal— Late visual loss is associated with optic nerve atrophy.	Usually very poor vision around 20/200 to hand motion; Vision often improves after the acute episode.	Normal; vision is usually 20/20 unless there is a refractive error.

acteristics of papilledema, papillitis, and pseudopapilledema. Both papilledema and papillitis have a similar appearance because both have true optic disc edema. Since papillitis is an inflammatory condition, and inflammation interferes with optic nerve function, papillitis is associated with poor visual acuity and an afferent pupillary defect. In contrast, papilledema usually is associated with excellent visual function. Optic nerves with the appearance of pseudopapilledema are not edematous and do not have signs of true disc edema.

Table 9-5.

Causes of Pseudotumor Cerebri

Endocrine
  Hypothyroidism
  Hyperthyroidism
  Adrenal insufficiency
  Renal insufficiency
  Exogenous growth hormone
Drug
  Corticosteroid use/withdrawal
  Vitamin A
  Tetracycline
  Lithium carbonate
  Nalidixic acid
  Phenytoin
  Indomethacin
  Oral contraceptives
  Amiodarone
  Sulfa
Other
  Sarcoidosis
  Systemic lupus erythematosis
  Pregnancy
  Iron deficiency anemia
  Obesity

Pseudotumor Cerebri

Pseudotumor cerebri (**benign intracranial hypertension**) is a self-limited disorder consisting of increased intracranial pressure of unknown etiology. This diagnosis is made once an intracranial mass lesion and other causes of elevated intracranial pressure are excluded. Typically, intracranial pressure is elevated over 250 mm water and the CSF is normal. The most common symptoms include headaches and transient visual obscurations that last a few seconds. Pseudotumor cerebri may be associated with the use of tetracycline, corticosteroid withdrawal, vitamin A excess, or hyperviscosity syndromes including polycythemia and thrombocytosis. **Table 9-5** lists drugs and endocrine abnormalities associated with pseudotumor cerebri.

In most cases, visual acuity is quite good, in the range of 20/20 to 20/30, even though severe papilledema is present. The typical patient with pseudotumor cerebri is an obese older child or teenager, and the incidence is higher in females. Patients may present with a sixth nerve palsy without other focal signs, as the sixth nerve palsy is secondary to increased intracranial pressure. The treatment of pseudotumor cerebri is to lower the intracranial pressure by serial lumbar punctures or pharmaceutically with carbonic anhydrase inhibitors (acetazolamide or methazolamide). Weight loss is important in obese patients, as well as elimination of any precipitating agents and medication. Some practitioners have recommended urgent therapy with intravenous corticosteroids followed by a slow taper over several months; however, corticosteroids may contribute to the elevation of intracranial pressure. If medical therapy does not improve the condition, then serial lumbar punctures or optic nerve sheath decompression can be performed. A unilateral optic nerve sheath decompression on the more involved side can prevent further visual loss, provide relief from headaches, and may allow resolution of the disc edema bilaterally. These more invasive procedures are usually recommended only after progressive visual field loss occurs despite conservative medical therapy. The natural history of pseudotumor cerebri is spontaneous resolution over approximately 3 months to 1 year. Close ophthalmic follow-up is important to document visual status, as visual loss can occur in a small subset of patients.

Optic Disc Drusen

Optic disc drusen are calcific bodies within the optic disc. Fundus appearance shows blurred optic disc margins and a swelling of the optic disc substance with globular calcific structures on the surface of the optic disc (**Figure 9-6**). They are a result of axonal degeneration and secondary calcification. They first become visible during the teenage years and enlarge over time. Approximately 75% are bilateral and some are inherited as an autosomal dominant trait. Drusen do not produce true disc edema, but do cause optic disc swelling. Visual acuity is usually excellent. Rarely, however, peripheral visual field loss and anterior ischemic optic neuropathy can occur secondary to compression of nerve fibers caused by deep drusen. Optic disc drusen can be identified by B-scan ultrasonography or on CT scan by demonstrating calcium. In young children, the amount of calcium may be small and the scans may be negative. Most optic nerve drusen are idiopathic and not associated with systemic disease; however, they have been reported to occur with hypertensive retinopathy and chronic papilledema.

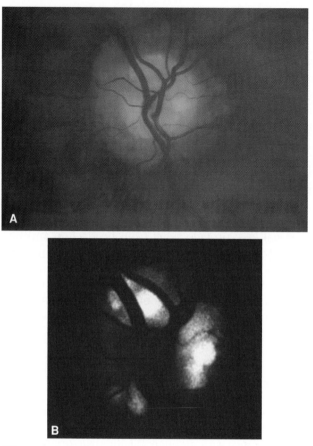

Figure 9-6.
Optic nerve drusen. **A,** Pseudopapilledema appearance with blurred disc margins.
Note the globular calcific structures within the disc substance and note the absence
of a central cup. The retinal vessels tend to be distorted as they leave the optic nerve.
B, Autofluorescence obtained using an exciter filter and barrier filter, showing the
location of the calcific deposits.

Optic Disc Atrophy

Optic disc atrophy is the end stage of optic nerve disease. It can be
caused by diffuse retinal disease or disease of the optic nerve and
chiasm, orbital trauma, or compression from craniosynostosis. The
optic nerve appears pale with decreased capillaries, and there are
diminished nerve fiber layer striations in the peripapillary area (Fig-

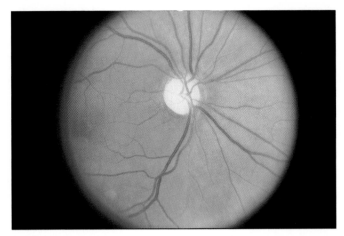

Figure 9-7.
Optic disc atrophy. Optic disc is pale and there is an absence of nerve fibers. This is a traumatic optic disc atrophy from blunt eye trauma.

ure 9-7). The presence of optic atrophy of unknown etiology should prompt a full investigation, including neuroimaging to rule out an orbital lesion compressing the optic nerve or chiasm. See Chapter 7 for discussion of hereditary optic atrophy.

Glaucoma

Glaucoma is optic nerve damage and atrophy caused by increased intraocular pressure. See Chapter 12 for a discussion of glaucoma.

10 Ocular Torticollis

The presence of a face turn or a head tilt is termed torticollis (**Figure 10-1**). The 2 most common causes of torticollis are an ocular problem (ocular torticollis) or a skeletal abnormality of the neck. Other causes include intermittent neck spasms associated with migraine and gastroesophageal reflux (Sandifer syndrome). Ocular torticollis is a compensatory mechanism adopted to obtain the best vision, usually in patients with nystagmus or incomitant strabismus. A simple way to differentiate ocular torticollis from skeletal torticollis is to have patients close their eyes and move the head from side to side with the eyes closed. Skeletal torticollis has restricted neck movement, whereas ocular torticollis should show a relatively free range of motion of the neck. Ocular torticollis can have 3 components: face turn (horizontal head posturing), chin elevation or depression, and head-tilt (tilting to the left or right). Patients with ptosis adopt a chin elevation, whereas patients with incomitant strabismus or nystagmus can adopt any or all 3 components. When examining a patient for ocular torticollis, passively move the head opposite to the face turn, and look for evidence of nystagmus or strabismus.

■ PTOSIS AND OCULAR TORTICOLLIS

Ptosis may cause a chin elevation. The chin elevation compensates for the droopy eyelid, allowing the eye to lower and clear the droopy lid. Both unilateral and bilateral ptosis will induce a chin elevation.

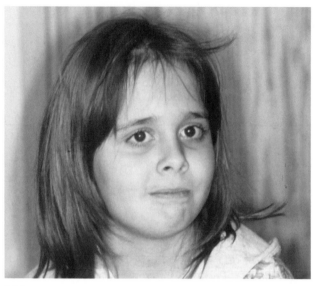

Figure 10-1.
Compensatory face turn to the left. This patient has a face turn to diminish nystagmus. With the eyes in right gaze (at the null point), the nystagmus is minimal and vision is best.

Children with ptosis can have amblyopia even with a chin elevation, so they need prompt referral to an ophthalmologist. See Chapter 17 for more information on ptosis.

■ STRABISMUS AND OCULAR TORTICOLLIS

Patients with incomitant strabismus who have good alignment in an eccentric gaze adopt a compensatory face turn to put the eyes where they are aligned, thereby establishing binocular vision and stereo acuity. Several types of incomitant strabismus can cause ocular torticollis. These include Duane syndrome, Brown syndrome, double elevator palsy, cranial nerve palsies, and restrictive strabismus. Congenital fourth nerve palsy is the most common cause for a head tilt (Figure 4-8), and Duane syndrome is the most common cause for a face turn (Figure 4-12). Eye muscle surgery is often effective in correcting strabismus-related ocular torticollis.

■ NYSTAGMUS AND OCULAR TORTICOLLIS

Patients with congenital nystagmus may show less nystagmus in an eccentric position of gaze. This position of gaze where the nystagmus is least is called the **null point.** Patients with an eccentric null point will adopt a compensatory face posturing in order to place the eyes at the null point to damp the nystagmus and improve vision (**Figure 10-1**). The compensatory face posturing may be a face turn, head tilt, chin elevation or depression, or any combination of these. A patient with a null point to right gaze, for example, adopts a left face turn to move the eyes to the right, placing the eye at the null point. The treatment of nystagmus-related head posturing is based on using eye muscle surgery to move the null point from an eccentric position to primary position. This is called the **Kestenbaum procedure.**

11 Pupil and Iris Abnormalities

■ ABNORMAL PUPILLARY REACTION

Normally, the pupils are round and symmetrical, approximately 3 to 4 mm in diameter. The condition of having pupils of unequal size is called **anisocoria.** Anisocoria of ½ mm is generally accepted as normal, as it occurs in approximately 20% of the normal population. One millimeter or more of anisocoria is abnormal and should prompt further investigation.

When the eyes focus on objects that move from distance to near, a **near reflex** is invoked and the pupil reacts accordingly. This reflex consists of convergence (eyes move in together), miosis (pupillary constriction), and accommodation (increasing lens focus power). These 3 components keep the eyes aligned on an object as it approaches (convergence), increase depth of focus (miosis), and keeps the image in focus (accommodates). Monitoring pupillary reaction during the near reflex may reveal an anisocoria and possibly indicate an abnormality.

■ AFFERENT PUPILLARY ABNORMALITIES

The afferent visual pathway transmits information from the retina through the optic nerves to the lateral geniculate nucleus and on to the occipital cortex. Afferent axons from the retina undergo hem-

141

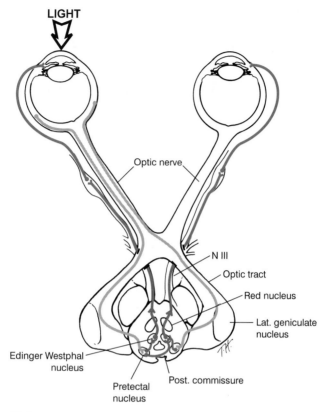

Figure 11-1.
Anatomy of a light reflex pathway with parasympathetic outflow to the iris sphincter. Note that light directed into one eye results in bilateral pupillary constriction. Grey line denotes afferent pathway, red line denotes efferent pathway.

idecussation at the chiasm, with nasal retinal axons coursing to the opposite optic tract and temporal retinal axons coursing to the ipsilateral optic tract (**Figure 11-1**). These afferent fibers synapse with the pretectal nucleus, sending efferent fibers to the ipsilateral and contralateral Edinger-Westphal nucleus. This crossover of the right and left pathways is the reason that both pupils constrict when light is directed into one of the eyes. Ipsilateral pupillary constriction is called the **direct pupillary response,** and contralateral pupillary constriction is called the **consensual pupillary response.** A significant abnormality involving the retina or the optic nerve of one eye can diminish both direct and consensual pupillary responses

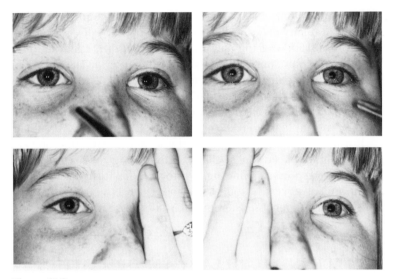

Figure 11-2.
A patient with a right afferent pupillary defect. Light shone on the involved right eye results in minimal constriction of both pupils (top left). When redirected to the uninvolved left eye, both pupils constrict (top right). The same test can be performed with ordinary room light by measuring the pupillary diameter with the uninvolved eye covered (bottom left) and then with the involved eye covered (bottom right). Note that the pupil is larger on the involved right side.

and produces an **afferent pupillary defect (APD),** also called a **Marcus-Gunn pupil.** Patients with an afferent pathway defect of one eye will have symmetrically sized pupils because of the intact consensual pupillary response (**Figure 11-2**).

The **swinging flashlight test** is a method of detecting an afferent pupillary defect and is based on comparing pupillary responses of fellow eyes. An afferent pathway defect of one eye (right eye), results in minimal constriction of both pupils when light is shined into the abnormal right eye (**Figure 11-2, top left**). Light directed into the normal left eye produces strong constriction of both pupils (**Figure 11-2, top right**). This difference in pupillary light reaction can be appreciated by alternating a light source from one eye to the other eye. When the light stimulation moves from the normal eye to the eye with the afferent defect, both pupils will dilate (look at **Figure 11-2**, right photo, first, then compare to the left photo). On a practical note, it is best to perform the swinging flashlight test under dim ambient illumination with a bright, focused light source. Be sure to focus the light only on the eye being tested, as light scatter to the contralateral normal eye will confound the test. An afferent pupillary defect indicates afferent pathway disease anterior to the decussation of the chiasm, such as a large retinal lesion, a lesion of the optic nerve, or a lesion of the anterior chiasm. Small retinal lesions do not cause a clinically significant afferent pupillary defect even though small macular lesions may severely affect vision. Media opacities such as cataracts or corneal opacities will not cause an afferent pupillary defect.

If a pupil of one eye is damaged and not functioning, one can test for light perception in that eye by testing for a **consensual pupillary response.** Shine light into the eye with the damaged pupil and observe the sound eye for a consensual pupillary response. Lack of a consensual pupillary response indicates no light perception.

■ EFFERENT PUPILLARY ABNORMATITIES

Patients with unilateral efferent (motor) pupillary abnormalities have asymmetric pupil size. The efferent motor pathway controls pupillary size by the combined actions of the parasympathetically innervated iris sphincter muscle (pupillary constriction), and the sympathetically innervated iris dilator muscle (pupillary dilatation). Lack of sympathetic innervation (Horner syndrome) results in a constricted pupil, whereas decreased parasympathetic innervation causes a dilated pupil.

Horner Syndrome

Horner syndrome is characterized by a small constricted (miotic) pupil and ipsilateral ptosis (**Figure 11-3**). This syndrome is caused by a lesion in the parasympathetic pathway (**Figure 11-4**). The Horner pupil is small because the sympathetic input to the iris dilator muscle is interrupted. This is best seen in low-light conditions because the normal pupil dilates in the dark, while the Horner pupil remains constricted. Under bright light illumination, both pupils constrict normally. Thus, in Horner syndrome, anisocoria is greater under dark ambient illumination than in bright light. This is an important sign, because it indicates that the anisocoria is secondary to a miotic pupil with lack of sympathetic innervation to the dilator muscle (ie, Horner syndrome), rather than a dilated pupil because

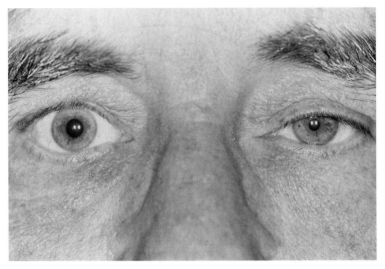

Figure 11-3.
Left Horner syndrome. Note the characteristic ptosis and miosis. The miosis is greater with the room lights down. Note that the lower lid is also slightly ptotic and that the eye appears to be enophthalmic.

of lack of constriction. A mild ptosis is also part of Horner syndrome because sympathetic fibers innervate Müller's muscle, which helps to elevate the upper eyelid. Since nerves for facial perspiration travel with the sympathetic nerves along the external carotid artery, ipsilateral facial anhydrosis can be associated with some cases of Horner syndrome.

Lesions that cause Horner syndrome are localized at the first order neuron (central), second order neuron (pre-ganglion), or third order neuron (post-ganglion) (**Figure 11-4**). First order, or central, lesions include hypothalamic infarcts and tumors. Symptoms are not limited to Horner syndrome because of the proximity of other structures. Second order neuron lesions are often produced by significant pathology in the area of the lung apex or neck. Third order neuron lesions are usually benign and may be caused by aneurysms, trauma, vascular headaches, or inflammatory disorders. Acquired Horner syndrome in children is an important diagnosis, as it may be a sign of an occult tumor such as neuroblastoma.

Congenital Horner Syndrome

This is an uncommon condition consisting of small pupil, ipsilateral ptosis, and ipsilateral decreased pigmentation of the iris (heteroch-

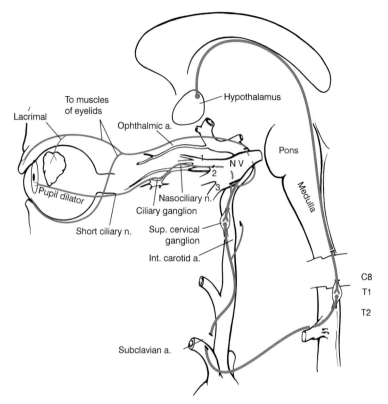

Figure 11-4.
The oculosympathetic pathway. The origin begins in the hypothalamus with connections down through the brainstem to synapse in the upper cervical cord (central or first neuronal pathway). Fibers then travel around the subclavian artery and over the base of the lung to join in the thoracic sympathetic trunk, which then synapses in the superior cervical ganglion (preganglionic or second neuronal pathway). The third order neuron travels with the first branch of the trigeminal nerve and passes through the ciliary ganglion to reach the pupillary dilator muscle.

romia). The decreased pigmentation is usually noted after 2 to 3 years of age when the normal iris undergoes the physiologic process of increased pigmentation. The Horner iris fails to have normal melanocyte development. Birth trauma to the brachial plexus is the most common cause of Horner syndrome, although other causes include vascular occlusion, chest or neck tumors, and pneumothorax.

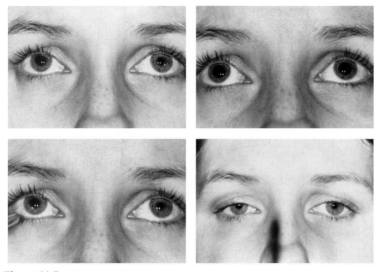

Figure 11-5.
Patient with a right Aide pupil. Note that the pupils are larger under room light (top left) than with the lights off (top right). The pupil constricts purely to light (bottom left) and better to near (bottom right).

Tonic Pupil (Aide Syndrome)

Aide syndrome, or Aide tonic pupil, is characterized by a large pupil with no constriction to light and slow constriction to near stimulus (**Figure 11-5**). This produces anisocoria that is greater in bright light than dark conditions, just the opposite of Horner syndrome. Aide syndrome is caused by an abnormality of the parasympathetic fibers in the ciliary ganglion. It is usually seen in females who are between the ages of 20 and 40, but occasionally can occur in children. The condition is almost always unilateral, and is often associated with decreased deep tendon reflexes in approximately half the cases. Patients may be otherwise completely asymptomatic when the anisocoria is noted on routine examination. Aide tonic pupil is generally felt to be a benign condition; however, 20% will be associated with other disorders such as herpes zoster, neurosyphilis, sarcoidosis, perineal plastic syndrome, diabetes mellitus, and neuropathies such as Charcot-Marie-Tooth disease and Guillain-Barré syndrome.

Argyll Robertson Pupil

This condition is usually bilateral and consists of small, often irregularly shaped pupils that are nonreactive to light, but briskly react to the near response and accommodation. The lesion is believed to be near the Edinger-Westphal nucleus of the third nerve. The lesion occurs from both the ipsilateral and contralateral pretectal areas, thereby sparing the fibers from the near response. The Argyll Robertson pupil is typically associated with neurosyphilis.

■ IRIS ABNORMALITIES

Iris Coloboma

Iris coloboma is caused by a localized absence of a normal iris so that the pupil takes on a keyhole shape (**Figure 11-6**). Typical iris colobomas are caused by an abnormality of closure of the fetal optic fissure. Because the optic fissure closes inferiorly at the 6 o'clock position, typical iris colobomas are located inferiorly. The optic fissure closes first at the equator of the globe, and then progressively closes in an anterior and posterior direction. The 2 most common locations for colobomas are at the anterior extent of the globe (iris

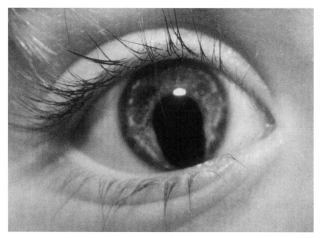

Figure 11-6.
Photograph of a typical iris coloboma with a keyhole pupil located inferiorly, and slightly nasally at approximately 5 o'clock position. The eye is slightly small.

colobomas) and the posterior extent of the globe (optic nerve colobomas). Isolated iris colobomas do not interfere with vision. Colobomas that involve the macula and/or the optic nerve often reduces binocularity. (See Chapter 6 for further discussion of choroidal and optic nerve colobomas.) Isolated iris colobomas are common and usually not associated with a systemic abnormality. Posterior colobomas, however, are more commonly associated with a systemic abnormality and with microphthalmia. Because iris colobomas may be associated with a posterior coloboma or optic nerve coloboma, patients with iris coloboma should be referred for a full ocular examination.

Aniridia

Aniridia, as the name implies, is the absence of an iris (**Figure 11-7**). This is, however, somewhat of a misnomer as there is almost always some amount of iris present. More importantly, aniridia is not confined to the iris but involves the entire eye. It is associated with optic nerve hypoplasia and foveal hypoplasia resulting in poor vision, often 20/200 or worse. Other ocular-associated abnormalities include cataracts, lens subluxation, glaucoma, and corneal opacification occurring later in life. Infants typically present with nystag-

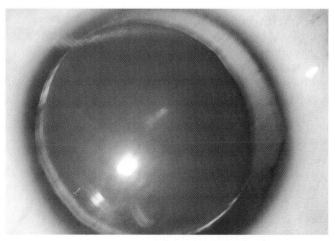

Figure 11-7.
Aniridia. Note the large pupil with minimal iris present. The complete lens is seen because the iris is absent. The lens is slightly subluxed up and to the right.

mus, large pupils, and very poor vision. Patients are often sensitive to light (photophobia). Aniridia can be inherited as an autosomal dominant trait or can be sporadic. Approximately one third of sporadic cases will have an associated Wilms' tumor. It is important to obtain an abdominal ultrasound, and investigate for renal abnormalities and Wilms' tumor in patients with sporadic aniridia. Because there have been a few reported cases of Wilms' tumor in a family with aniridia, it is probably best to work up all aniridic cases for the possibility of Wilms' tumor. The aniridia gene has been localized to chromosome 11p13. Large deletions in this area produce a syndrome with the triad of aniridia, mental retardation, and genitourinary abnormalities (ARG triad). This triad has been linked with a deletion of the short arm of chromosome 11(11p). Aniridia appears to be secondary to a mutation of the PAX 6 gene, a key regulator for eye development. Associated with aniridia and PAX 6 gene mutations are other ocular developmental anomalies such as **autosomal dominant keratitis** and some forms of **Peters anomaly** (congenital corneal opacification, see chapter 15, Figure 15-4 A-C). Dominant keratitis consists of progressive vascularization of the cornea and partial aniridia, with or without nystagmus. The ocular prognosis in aniridia is relatively poor, as foveal hypoplasia usually limits vision to 20/200 or worse, and many patients will develop progressive corneal opacifications, vascularization, glaucoma, and cataracts.

Heterochromia Irides

Heterochromia irides is a difference in iris color. This can be caused by either increased pigmentation in one eye or decreased pigmentation in the other eye. **Table 11-1** lists some of the more common causes of heterochromia irides.

Table 11-1.
Causes of Heterochromia Irides

Increased Iris Pigmentation
1. Congenital pigmented tumors and nevus
2. Oculodermal melanocytosis
3. Iris ectropion
Decreased Iris Pigmentation
1. Congenital Horner syndrome
2. Accidental or surgical trauma
3. Waardenburg syndrome

Rieger Anomaly

Rieger anomaly is an ocular malformation characterized by an abnormal iris that is hypoplastic. Patients may have multiple defects, termed pseudopolycoria. In most cases, the pupil appears irregular. There is also dysgenesis of the anterior segment, including the peripheral aspect of the cornea. Glaucoma occurs in approximately half of patients with Rieger anomaly. **Rieger syndrome** is an autosomal dominant oculoskeletal syndrome consisting of Rieger ocular anomaly with systemic anomalies including teeth abnormalities (microdontia, hypodontia), facial anomalies (maxillary hypoplasia-flattening of the mid-face), deafness, and umbilical hernia. The most important ocular complication of Rieger anomaly or syndrome is the development of glaucoma, which can be difficult to control.

Tearing

■ NASOLACRIMAL DUCT OBSTRUCTION, CONGENITAL GLAUCOMA, AND DRY EYE

Tearing is a common presenting complaint in a pediatric examination. The causes of abnormal tearing (epiphora) is classified according to the age of onset: neonatal onset or acquired tearing. **Table 12-1** lists the most common causes of tearing in childhood.

At birth, there is minimal baseline tear production by the lacrimal gland. Normal tearing develops several days to 2 weeks after birth. Tears are produced in the lacrimal gland and cross the cornea to exit via the superior and inferior puncta. Tears then travel through the canaliculus into the lacrimal sac, to the nasolacrimal duct, and finally through Hasner's valve into the posterior nasal pharynx (**Figure 12-1**). There are 2 physiologic types of tearing: basal tear production that keeps the eye moist during normal conditions, and reflex tearing that occurs in response to ocular irritation or emotion. Epiphora can be caused by an increased production of tears (hypersecretion) or obstruction of the nasolacrimal outflow system.

■ NASOLACRIMAL DUCT OBSTRUCTION

The nasolacrimal drainage system develops from an invagination of surface ectoderm that originates in the nasal-optic fissure. Canali-

Table 12-1.
Pediatric Epiphora

Neonatal Epiphora
1. Nasolacrimal duct (NLD) obstruction (this chapter)
2. Amniotocele (dacryocystocele) (this chapter)
3. Punctal atresia (this chapter)
4. Trichiasis-"lashes rubbing the eye" (epiblepharon or congenital entropion) (Chapter 17)
5. Corneal exposure (craniosynostosis with proptosis, orbital mass such as congenital hemangioma, congenital facial nerve palsy, congenital anesthetic cornea) (this chapter)
6. Congenital glaucoma (this chapter)

Child Onset Epiphora
1. Corneal trauma (foreign body or abrasion) (Chapter 23)
2. Allergic conjunctivitis (Chapter 13)
3. Crocodile tears (this chapter)
4. Dry eyes (this chapter)
5. Trichiasis (Chapter 17)
6. Posterior fossa brain tumor
7. Exposure (acquired proptosis and facial palsy, such as Bell's palsy)

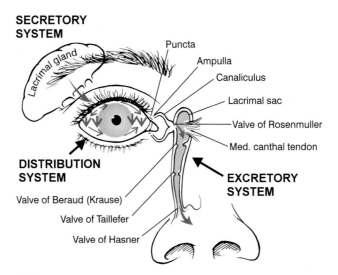

Figure 12-1.
Three integral components of the lacrimal system including secretory system (lacrimal glands), distribution system (eyelid blinking), and excretory system (puncta, canaliculus, nasolacrimal duct). The nasolacrimal duct is the entire structure that connects the canaliculus to the nose (red-colored structure).

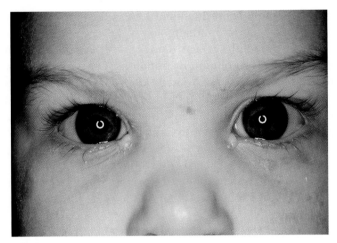

Figure 12-2.
One-year-old with bilateral NLD obstruction. Note the increased tear lake and mucus in the nasal canthal area.

zation of this system first occurs in the central aspect of the nasolacrimal passage and then proceeds both superiorly and inferiorly. Normally, the process of canalization is completed by the end of the ninth month of gestation, but it may fail to completely canalize. If canalization is incomplete, it most often occurs at the distal end of the nasolacrimal duct at Hasner's valve (**Figure 12-1**). This causes tear outflow obstruction at Hasner's valve and is, by far, the most common cause for a nasolacrimal duct obstruction (NLD obstruction). There are other less common anatomic variations within the nasolacrimal system that can cause obstruction of tear outflow, including crowding of the inferior turbinate or a bony obstruction of the nasolacrimal duct.

Infants with a nasolacrimal duct obstruction present with a watery eye and an increased tear lake, mattering of the eyelashes, and mucus in the medial canthal area (**Figure 12-2**). Congenital nasolacrimal duct obstruction is common and occurs in 1% to 5% of the population, with approximately one third being bilateral. If left untreated, almost half of the cases with a nasolacrimal duct blockage spontaneously open by 6 months of age. The incidence of spontaneous resolution after 13 months of age decreases to only 15%.

Management of Nasolacrimal Duct Obstruction

Significant controversy exists about optimal timing for initial nasolacrimal duct probing. Some advocate probing even at a few months of age and suggest that it should be done in the office without anesthesia. Most pediatric ophthalmologist, however, suggest waiting until at least 6 months of age, since almost half the children will have spontaneous resolution by 6 months. Others suggest waiting until 1 or 2 years of age for probing. There is evidence that delaying probing until 1 ½ to 2 years of age lessens the likelihood that a single probing will be successful. This author recommends initial probing be performed between 6 months and 1 year of age. This allows time for most patients to spontaneous resolve, yet will provide the highest rate of probing success. There is one important situation, however, when nasolacrimal duct probing should be performed on an urgent basis, and that is in the case of an amniotocele (discussed later in this chapter).

Medical management during the observational period is a combination of nasolacrimal sac massage and intermittent topical antibiotics. Some suggest massaging inferiorly to push the tears out the nasolacrimal duct, while others suggest massaging superiorly so the material exits the punctum. This author suggests using both methods. The initial massage is directed inferiorly to push the tears in the normal direction out the nasolacrimal duct. Subsequent massage is directed superiorly, so that any tears that did not exit are at least cleared from the punctum. On occasion, inferior pressure itself will open a mild nasolacrimal duct obstruction. The use of topical antibiotic drops or ointments is indicated if there are signs of infection, such as mucopurulent discharge. Antibiotic drops such as polymyxin B/trimethoprim sulfate or sulfacetamide work well, but should only be prescribed when there is evidence of a true infection.

Nasolacrimal Duct Probing

This is a simple but delicate procedure. A small steel wire is passed through the nasolacrimal system, through Hasner's valve, and into the nose. In some cases, the inferior turbinate is infractured to relieve crowding. The success rate for nasolacrimal duct probing is higher than 90% when performed before 1 ½ years of age. In cases where nasolacrimal duct probing fails, intubation with silicone tubes is indicated to establish a patent system (**Figure 12-3**). In general, tubes are only used for patients who have failed the probing procedure.

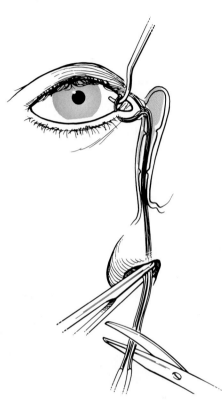

Figure 12-3.
Drawing of silicone stent in the canaliculi and nasolacrimal system. Tubes are left in place for 1 to 3 months to keep the system open.

Amniotocele (Dacryocystocele)

An amniotocele presents as a swelling of the nasolacrimal sac. This is caused by an accumulation of fluid within the sac, as a result of punctal and nasolacrimal duct obstruction. A few days after birth, a bluish swelling appears in the medial canthal area, representing fluid that is sequestered within a distended nasolacrimal sac (**Figure 12-4**). Treatment for a noninfected amniotocele is local massage. If decompression does not occur within a few days, infection (ie, **dacryocystitis**) is almost certain. Because of this, the author suggests probing the nasolacrimal duct to open the obstruction. An infected amniotocele is red, warm, and quite large, approximately 1 cm in diameter (**Figure 12-5**). Once infected, treatment consists

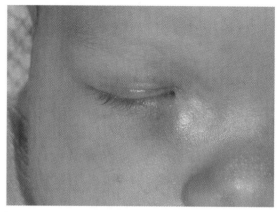

Figure 12-4.
Amniotocele right lacrimal sac in 4-day-old newborn. The amniotocele is the bluish mass inferior to the medial canthus.

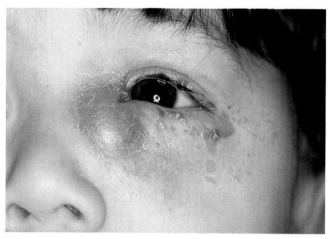

Figure 12-5.
Infected amniotocele: This patient was admitted to the hospital and treated with IV antibiotics. Probing of the nasolacrimal duct opened the obstruction, drained the abscess, and cured the infection.

of intravenous (IV) antibiotics (cephalosporin) and urgent nasolacrimal duct probing to relieve the obstruction and drain the abscess. Some have suggested performing a cutaneous incision into the sac to decompress the abscess; however, this leaves a scar and may produce an external fistula. Nasolacrimal duct probing does not leave a scar, avoids the fistula complication, and has the advantage of directly addressing the primary cause of the abscess by opening the NLD obstruction. If the abscess is not drained, an infected amniotocele can result in cellulitis and even sepsis.

Congenital Nasolacrimal Duct Fistula

In rare instances, the nasolacrimal duct connects to the skin overlying the base of the nose, causing tears to drain down the cheek (congenital NLD fistula). Often, there is a concurrent nasolacrimal duct obstruction associated with the fistula. A nasolacrimal duct fistula is best treated by closing the fistula surgically, opening the NLD obstruction with nasolacrimal probing, and performing intubation using silicone tubes.

Punctal Atresia

Punctal atresia is lack of the eyelid puncta. If only one punctum of the pair is obstructed, normal tear drainage can still occur through the other punctum. In cases where punctal atresia is causing tearing, surgical intervention is indicated to create a new punctal opening.

■ CONGENITAL GLAUCOMA

Tearing is one of the most common presenting signs of congenital glaucoma. Primary congenital glaucoma refers to increased intraocular pressure occurring at birth or shortly thereafter. Normal intraocular pressure in infants is approximately 10 to 15 mm Hg, whereas intraocular pressure in infants with congenital glaucoma is often higher than 30 mm Hg. Congenital glaucoma is very different from adult glaucoma. In adult glaucoma, increased intraocular pressure damages the optic nerve function, but the eye size does not change. In infants, however, increased intraocular pressure results in expansion of eye size in addition to damaging the optic nerve (**Figure 12-6**). The reason the eye enlarges is that, in infants, the eye wall is elastic and stretches. Normal corneas at birth are approximately 10.5 mm in diameter, and corneal diameters greater than 12 mm are considered abnormally large (megalocornea). As the cornea enlarges, breaks of the basement membrane of the corneal endothelium (**Haab's striae**) occur. This results in corneal

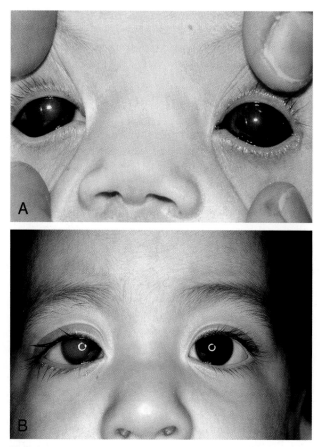

Figure 12-6.
A, Neonate with bilateral severe congenital glaucoma. Note the extremely large corneas and corneal edema that gives the bluish appearance to the eyes. **B,** Congenital glaucoma left eye. Note the white corneal opacity, which is corneal edema secondary to increased intraocular pressure and a break in Descemet membrane (Haab's Striae). The corneal diameter of the left eye is 13.5 mm vs 11.5 mm in the right eye.

edema that reduces vision and can lead to amblyopia. After 3 years of age, the eye wall becomes fairly rigid and ocular enlargement secondary to glaucoma does not occur.

Presenting features of congenital glaucoma include tearing, photophobia, blepharospasm, large cornea, and corneal clouding (edema), with approximately 70% of cases being bilateral. These classic findings of congenital glaucoma are not always present, as

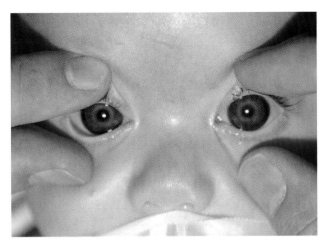

Figure 12-7.
Congenital glaucoma in a 2-month-old infant with bilateral corneal edema and enlarged corneas. The right corneal diameter is 12 mm and the left corneal diameter is 13 mm. This child presented with epiphora and could have been easily misdiagnosed as having a nasolacrimal duct obstruction.

ocular enlargement and corneal edema may be subtle (**Figure 12-7**). In cases that present with tearing, the diagnosis of congenital glaucoma may be misdiagnosed as a nasolacrimal duct obstruction. In contrast to nasolacrimal duct obstruction, however, the tearing associated with congenital glaucoma is caused by corneal edema, which can be seen as a dull red reflex with an ophthalmoscope.

The pathogenesis of congenital glaucoma relates to an abnormal outflow caused by abnormal angle structures, including the trabecular meshwork. Recent studies have identified a congenital glaucoma gene (2p21, 1p36) and juvenile glaucoma gene (1q23-q25). **Juvenile glaucoma** is a type of glaucoma with onset after 2 to 3 years of age. It is difficult to diagnose, as there are virtually no signs or symptoms other than increased intraocular pressure and optic disc cup changes (**Figure 12-8**).

The treatment of congenital glaucoma is based on lowering the intraocular pressure to prevent optic nerve damage, prevent progressive expansion of the eye, and reduce corneal edema. Medications have been used to lower intraocular pressures and can include beta-adrenergic inhibitors (timolol), carbonic-anhydrase inhibitors, which can be administered topically or systemically (Diamox) and, in some cases, adrenergic agonists (apraclonidine). Medical treat-

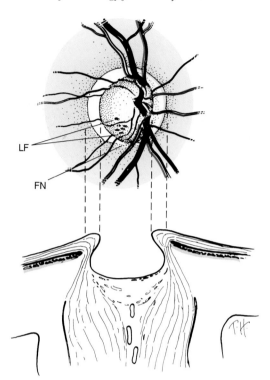

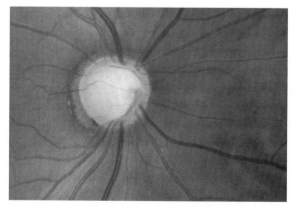

Figure 12-8.
A, Glaucomatous optic nerve (anterior optic nerve head and transverse view, right eye). Note the thinning and undermining of inferior neuroretinal rim and focal notching (FN) of inferior neuroretinal rim, enlarged central cup with visible laminar fenestrae (LF), nasal shift of retinal vessels and peripapillary atrophy. **B,** Glaucomatous optic nerve. Advanced cupping with diffuse thinning and undermining of the neuroretinal rim, nasalization of the retinal vessels, and loss if the normal nerve fiber layer striations (left eye).

ment is not effective in most cases of congenital glaucoma and is, almost always, a surgical disease. Surgery is directed to opening the outflow channels at the trabecular meshwork. The 2 most frequently used procedures are the goniotomy and trabeculotomy ab externum. With a **goniotomy,** a microscopic-sized knife is used to lyse the abnormal trabecular meshwork to open up the angle. With the **trabeculotomy ab externum,** a microscopic probe is placed in Schlemm's canal and then swept through the trabecular meshwork and into the anterior chamber to open up the angle. The success rate of these procedures for congenital glaucoma is approximately 60%-70%. If the first procedure fails, a second goniotomy or trabeculotomy ab externum may be performed. If these procedures are not successful, then a trabeculectomy is usually performed. A **trabeculectomy** is a filtering procedure where aqueous fluid is filtered through a small hole in the eye to the subconjunctival space. Lastly, if these procedures fail, congenital glaucoma can be managed by ciliary body destructive procedures such as cryotherapy and laser surgery. These procedures work by eliminating the ciliary body epithelium that produces aqueous. These are end-stage procedures and have a high failure rate.

The prognosis for congenital glaucoma is fair, with approximately 70% of patients maintaining good, long-term visual acuity. Unfortunately, those who are in the unfavorable outcome group often go on to blindness. The most important cause of visual loss is attributed to optic nerve damage, which is not reversible. Other causes include chronic corneal edema with corneal scarring, refractive errors, and importantly, dense irreversible amblyopia.

Juvenile glaucoma is more amenable to medical treatment. In many cases, however, juvenile glaucoma must also be treated with surgical techniques. Fortunately, juvenile glaucoma is extremely rare.

Other forms of congenital glaucoma, secondary to specific syndromes and ocular anomalies, are listed in **Table 12-2.**

Table 12-2.
Secondary Causes of Congenital Glaucoma

Ocular Anomalies
1. Aniridia
2. Spherophakia
3. Anterior segment dysgenesis (Peters and Rieger anomaly)
4. Posterior pole tumors (retinoblastoma and medulloepithelioma)
Systemic Association
1. Sturge-Weber syndrome
2. Klippel-Trenaunay-Weber syndrome
3. Lowe syndrome (glaucoma and cataracts)
4. Neurofibromatosis I
5. Marfan syndrome
6. Pierre-Robin syndrome
7. Rubinstein-Taybi syndrome
8. Trisomy 13
9. Rubella syndrome
10. Weill-Marchesani syndrome
11. Persistent Hyperplastic Primary Vitreous (PHPV)
12. Retinopathy of Prematurity (ROP)
13. Corticosteroid induced glaucoma

Crocodile Tears

Crocodile tears is a term used to describe tearing secondary to mastication and gustatory stimulation. This occurs because there is an aberrant innervation of the lacrimal gland by the nerve to the salivary glands. The innervation is usually a result of a facial nerve injury causing secondary misdirection of the salivary fibers to the greater superficial petrosal nerve.

■ DRY EYE IN CHILDREN

It may seem paradoxical, but a dry eye often presents with symptoms of tearing. A dry eye, either from corneal exposure or lack of tear production (hyposecretion), causes irritation to the corneal epithelium, stimulating reflex tearing. Exposure caused by poor eyelid closure is often associated with proptosis, lid retraction (shortening of lid skin and cicatricial ectropion), lid defects (lid coloboma), and facial nerve palsy. Exposure can also be caused by lack of a blink response due to an anesthetic cornea.

Table 12-3.
Causes of Dry Eye

- Exposure (proptosis, eyelid retraction, lid coloboma, and poor blink response)
- Hyposecretion (Riley Day syndrome—Familial dysautonomia, hereditary alacrima)
- Conjunctival Scarring (Stevens-Johnson syndrome, alkaline burn, ocular pemphigoid, vitamin A deficiency, trachoma)

Dry eye caused by hyposecretion of tears is rare in children and can be diagnosed by the **Schirmer test.** The Schirmer test is performed by placing a filter paper wick in the temporal fornix of the lower eyelid for 5 minutes to measure the amount of tear production. Normal wetting is a measurement greater than 10 mm, and less than 8 mm indicates hyposecretion. Diffuse conjunctival scarring also produces dry eye syndrome due to loss of mucus-producing goblet cells and closure of accessory lacrimal glands. Conjunctival scarring occurs in diseases such as **Stevens-Johnson syndrome** (see Chapter 13). **Table 12-3** lists causes of pediatric dry eye.

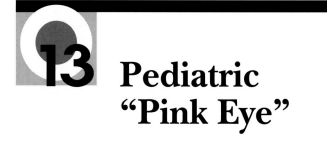

13 Pediatric "Pink Eye"

■ NEONATAL CONJUNCTIVITIS (Ophthalmia Neonatorum)

Neonatal conjunctivitis is a conjunctivitis occurring during the first month of life. Before the use of topical prophylaxis, ophthalmia neonatorum was a devastating disease associated with high morbidity. Routine topical prophylaxis with 1% silver nitrate, 1% tetracycline ointment, or 0.5% erythromycin ointment has dramatically reduced the incidence of ophthalmia neonatorum. Infections can be acquired from vaginal microorganisms during birth or from hand-to-eye contamination from hospital workers. An infection from the birth canal is usually associated with a vaginal delivery, but also can occur after a cesarean delivery if the amniotic membranes rupture prior to delivery.

The most common cause of red, watery eyes in the first few hours of life is chemical conjunctivitis secondary to silver nitrate prophylaxis. Most infants who receive silver nitrate prophylaxis will develop some degree of chemical conjunctivitis. This occurs immediately after silver nitrate is administered, is self-limited, and, in most cases, lasts for less than a day. Infectious causes of neonatal conjunctivitis present later, usually at least 48 hours after birth, and include *Chlamydia trachomatis*, *Neisseria gonorrhoeae*, Group B streptococcus, *Staphylococcus aureus*, *Escherichia coli*, *Haemophilus influenzae*, and herpes simplex virus Type 2. To a large extent, the etiology of the conjunctivitis can be determined by the time of onset of the conjunctivitis (**Table 13-1**).

Table 13-1.
Causes of Neonatal Conjunctivitis

Etiology	Onset and Presentation	Conjunctival Scraping	Treatment
Silver nitrate toxicity	**Within 24 hours** Watery discharge.	Negative Gram/ Negative Giemsa, Few PMN	None needed
Neisseria gonorrhea	**2 to 4 days** Lid swelling, purulent discharge. Corneal involvement can lead to corneal ulcer and perforation.	Gram-negative intracellular diplococci and culture	Topical erythromycin and IV cefotaxime Treat parents even if asymptomatic
Other Bacteria (staphylococci, streptococci)	**4 to 7 days** Purulent discharge, with or without lid swelling.	Gram-positive for specific bacteria and culture	Topical erythromycin or trimethoprim-polymyxin B drops (Polytrim)
Chlamydia	**4 to 10 days** Variable severity of lid swelling and serous or purulent discharge.	Giemsa stain basophilic cytoplasmic inclusion bodies, positive direct immunofluorescent assay, and culture	PO erythromycin, 50 mg/kg/day for 14 days. Treat parents even if asymptomatic.
Haemophilus	**5 to 10 days** Serous or serosanguinous discharge. Hemorrhagic conjunctivitis common. Lid swelling with petechiae and bluish lid skin indicate preseptal cellulitis.	Gram-negative coccobacillus and culture	Topical trimethoprim-Polymyxin B drops (Polytrim) and IV cefotaxime
Herpes Simplex Virus Type 2	**6 days to 2 weeks** Usually unilateral; Serous discharge with keratitis, positive corneal staining.	Gram stain multinucleated giant cells, Papanicolaou stain—intranuclear inclusion bodies and Herpes culture	Topical trifluorothymidine (Viroptic), and IV acyclovir

Differential Diagnosis of Neonatal Conjunctivitis

In addition to neonatal conjunctivitis, other causes of a red, teary eye in a newborn include congenital glaucoma (Chapter 12), dacryocystitis (Chapter 12), and, in rare instances, endophthalmitis. **Endophthalmitis** is a devastating infection within the eye, often resulting in blindness (also see Chapter 14). It is associated with vitreous inflammation that disrupts the red reflex. It is extremely rare, but a neonate can develop endophthalmitis from a blood-borne infection originating from a contaminated indwelling catheter (author's experience). **Congenital glaucoma** is characterized by clear tears, large cornea, and corneal edema. **Dacryocystitis** is an infection of the nasolacrimal sac that causes a swelling in the medial canthal area of the lower lid, and should be distinguished from conjunctivitis.

Evaluation and Treatment of Neonatal Conjunctivitis (Table 13-2)

As for all newborns, the ophthalmic examination should start with the red reflex test. If the pathology is isolated to the conjunctiva and does not involve the cornea or intraocular structures, then the red reflex should be normal. Conditions such as endophthalmitis, congenital glaucoma, and corneal infections have an abnormal red reflex. An urgent consult is indicated if the patient has significant lid swelling, a unilateral conjunctivitis (which may indicate herpes 2 keratitis), shows no improvement over a day or 2, or has an abnormal red reflex. Consider an ophthalmology consultation for any neonate with conjunctivitis.

The initial workup for presumed infectious neonatal conjunctivitis includes conjunctival cultures on chocolate agar, Thayer-Martin agar, and blood agar. Conjunctival scrapings should be obtained and examined by Gram stain, Giemsa stain, and indirect immunofluorescent antibody assay for chlamydia. If a herpes keratitis is suspected (unilateral conjunctivitis with corneal fluorescein staining), a corneal scraping for herpes culture should be obtained. A Venereal Disease Research Laboratories test (VDRL) for a concurrent congenital syphilis infection is advised for venereal neonatal conjunctivitis.

The treatment of a presumed infectious neonatal conjunctivitis prior to receiving laboratory results includes the use of topical erythromycin ointment and IV cefotaxime. Cefotaxime is preferred over

Table 13-2.
Initial Evaluation and Treatment of Presumed Infectious Neonatal Conjunctivitis

Evaluation
1. Red reflex test and ophthalmology consultation.
2. Conjunctival scraping and obtain Gram stain, Giemsa stain, and direct immunofluorescent assay for Chlamydia.
3. Conjunctival culture on blood agar, chocolate agar, and Thayer-Martin agar. Consider viral culture, especially in unilateral cases.

Therapy
Initial therapy prior to laboratory results is erythromycin topical ointment and IV cefotaxime. Consider trifluridine and IV acyclovir if herpes is suspected. Once the offending organism is identified, then specific treatment is given.

ceftriaxone because ceftriaxone binds with albumin and may result in hyperbilirubinemia in neonates. Antibiotic treatment should be given immediately after cultures are taken. Add topical trifluridine (Viroptic) every 2 hours and IV acyclovir if herpes is suspected. Once the laboratory results are known, therapy is tailored to treat the offending organism.

Specific Infectious Causes of Neonatal Conjunctivitis

Gonococcal Conjunctivitis

Gonococcal conjunctivitis occurs approximately 48 hours after birth. It may occur even earlier if rupture of the amniotic membranes occurs several hours prior to delivery. Typically, gonococcal conjunctivitis presents as a bilateral, purulent conjunctivitis with copious discharge and lid edema (**Figure 13-1**). *N gonorrhoeae* is one of the few bacteria that can penetrate intact corneal epithelium causing a corneal ulceration and even corneal perforation. The diagnosis is usually made by identifying Gram-negative intracellular diplococci on conjunctival scrapings and verifying by conjunctival culture. The treatment for gonococcal conjunctivitis is topical erythromycin ointment and IV cefotaxime. If indicated, parents should also be evaluated for possible treatment.

Chlamydial Conjunctivitis

Chlamydial conjunctivitis typically presents bilaterally, with mild to moderate conjunctivitis, around 4 to 10 days after birth. Eyelid

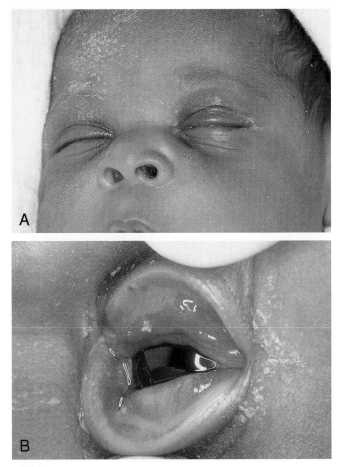

Figure 13-1.
A, Two-day-old infant with culture-positive gonococcal conjunctivitis. Note the bilateral lid swelling (right > left). **B,** With lids everted, a severe conjunctivitis is disclosed.

swelling and a tarsal conjunctival pseudomembrane may be present (**Figure 13-2**). A conjunctival **pseudomembrane** is an accumulation of debris, not a true vascular tissue. The diagnosis of chlamydia is confirmed by conjunctival scrapings identifying cytoplasmic inclusion bodies in corneal epithelial cells (Giemsa stain) or by indirect immunofluorescence assay or culture. The treatment of choice for chlamydial conjunctivitis is topical erythromycin ointment and oral erythromycin 30 to 50 mg/kg per day for at least 2 weeks. Oral

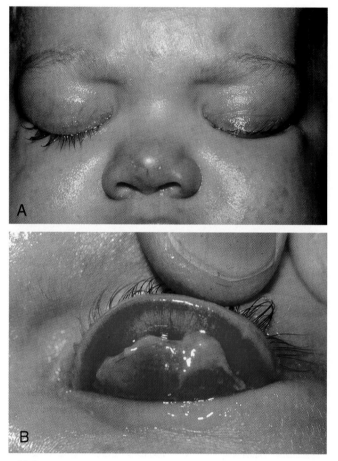

Figure 13-2.
A, Two-week-old infant with severe lid swelling caused by a Chlamydia conjunctivitis.
B, Everting the upper eyelid discloses a severe conjunctivitis, and a conjunctival
pseudomembrane. A pseudomembrane is an accumulation of cellular debris and
fibrin, not a true vascular tissue.

erythromycin is used to remove chlamydia organisms from the naso-
pharynx to decrease the risks of chlamydia pneumonia that presents
between 1 and 3 months of age. Parents should be warned of the
possibility that chlamydial pneumonitis can occur after neonatal
conjunctivitis (**Harrison, et al, 1987**). Parents are the source of the
infection and should be treated with oral erythromycin or tetracycline for 2 to 3 weeks, even if they are asymptomatic.

Herpes Simplex Virus Type 2

Herpes simplex virus type 2 can cause neonatal conjunctivitis usually associated with a keratitis (corneal infection). Herpes keratoconjunctivitis occurs as an isolated eye infection, but may be associated with systemic disease and encephalitis. The onset of herpes keratoconjunctivitis is usually between 1 and 2 weeks postpartum, presenting as a serous discharge with moderate conjunctival injection. In contrast to other infectious causes of neonatal conjunctivitis, herpes keratoconjunctivitis almost always presents as a unilateral infection. Breakdown of the normal epithelial barrier can result in a secondary bacterial corneal ulcer (**Figure 13-3**). Early stages of the keratitis are detected by corneal fluorescein staining showing a geographic or dendritic pattern. The diagnosis is confirmed by viral cultures that may take up to 7 to 10 days to become positive. If herpes neonatal conjunctivitis is suspected, the treatment of choice is topical trifluridine every 2 hours combined with IV acyclovir. Topical antibiotics should be used to prevent a secondary bacterial infection.

Neonatal Conjunctivitis Prophylaxis

There has been some controversy about the best agents to use to prevent neonatal conjunctivitis. Studies have shown that the efficacy of 0.5% erythromycin ointment, 1% tetracycline ointment, and 1% silver nitrate is approximately the same. The use of povidone-iodine 2.5% in a single dose has been advocated for prophylaxsis (**Isenberg and Apt, 1995**). The advantages of povidone include effective coverage of a broad spectrum of bacteria and coverage for viruses such as herpes simplex and human immunodeficiency virus (HIV) with little chemical irritation reaction.

■ PEDIATRIC CONJUNCTIVITIS

"Pink eye," or conjunctivitis, is a nonspecific finding that simply indicates conjunctival inflammation. A variety of disease processes can cause conjunctival inflammation, including an extraocular foreign body, chemical toxicity, trauma, uveitis (Chapter 14), episcleritis (Chapter 14), allergic disease, viral or bacterial infections, and eyelid inflammation (blepharitis). Intraocular processes, including endophthalmitis (infection within the eye) and tumors associated

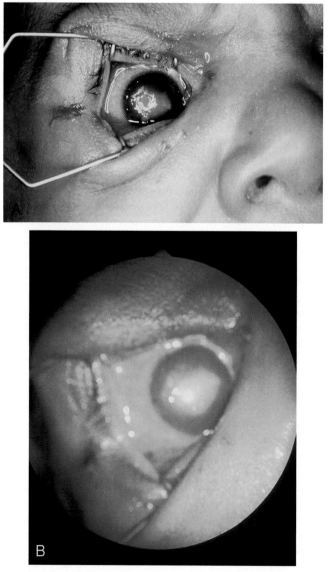

Figure 13-3.
Three-week-old infant with a combined bacterial corneal ulcer and herpes simplex virus type 2 keratitis. **A,** The white corneal lesion represents the area of infection. **B,** Fluorescein staining shows a central epithelial defect.

with necrosis (such as retinoblastoma), can also produce conjunctival inflammation, and may present as conjunctivitis. The vast majority of children who present with pink eye, however, will have a benign, self-limiting conjunctivitis. The most common causes of pediatric conjunctivitis are listed in **Table 13-3.**

Table 13-3.
Common Causes of Pediatric Conjunctivitis

1. Blepharitis
   a. Staphylococcal
   b. Meibomian Gland Dysfunction
2. Allergic conjunctivitis
   a. Seasonal
   b. Vernal
   c. Atopic
3. Bacterial conjunctivitis
   a. *H influenzae*
   b. *S pneumoniae*
   c. *S epidermidis*
   d. *S aureus*
   e. *Corynebacterium*
   f. *Moraxella catarrhalis*
4. Viral conjunctivitis
   a. Adenovirus
   b. Herpes virus
   c. Papovavirus (conjunctival warts)
   d. Poxvirus (molluscum contagiosum)
   e. Picornavirus
   f. Paramyxovirus
5. Trauma (Chapter 23)
   a. Foreign body
   b. Corneal abrasion
   c. Chemical burn
   d. Subconjunctival hemorrhage
   e. Trichiasis
6. Ocular inflammation (Chapter 14)
   a. Juvenile rheumatoid arthritis
   b. Sarcoidosis
   c. Endophthalmitis
   d. Episcleritis
7. Neoplasm
   a. Conjunctival nevus (Figure 13–17)
   b. Lymphangioma
   c. Retinoblastoma

Table 13-4.
Distinguishing Features of Pediatric Conjunctivitis

Feature	Blepharitis	Allergic	Bacterial	Viral
Discharge	Minimal	Watery	Purulent	Watery
Itching vs irritation	Minimal itching (moderate irritation)	Marked itching (minimal irritation)	Minimal itching (marked irritation)	Minimal itching (marked irritation)
Pre-auricular lymphadenopathy	Absent	Absent	Absent	Common
Laboratory	Staphylococcus on culture common	Eosinophils on conjunctival scraping	Bacteria on Gram stain, PMN response	Lymphocytes and monocytes

It is often difficult to determine the etiology of conjunctivitis based on the appearance of the eye. Even so, there are basic distinguishing features of the common causes of pediatric conjunctivitis (**Table 13-4**).

Evaluation and Treatment of Pediatric Conjunctivitis

Initial evaluation and treatment of pediatric pink eye should include a history and an ocular examination using "I-ARM" (inspection, acuity, red reflex, and motility—see Chapter 3). A history of friends or family members with conjunctivitis usually indicates a contagious origin, commonly a viral infection. Itching is an important symptom since it is the hallmark of allergic conjunctivitis. Conjunctivitis associated with **contact lens** use may be secondary to an allergy to contact lens solutions or, even more importantly, a vision-threatening bacterial corneal ulcer. Conjunctivitis associated with contact lens use deserves an immediate ophthalmology referral.

As in the case of neonatal conjunctivitis, the red reflex test should also be performed on older children with conjunctivitis, as an abnormal red reflex may indicate a serious disease process. Benign pediatric conjunctivitis almost never interferes with vision. Conjunctival cultures are not routinely obtained, and patients are treated on the basis on their signs and symptoms. Indications for an ophthalmology referral include decreased visual acuity (worse than 20/40) or an abnormal red reflex. Fluorescein staining of the corneal epithelium is indicated if a corneal abrasion is the suspected cause of the pink eye. Fluorescein staining indicates a defect of the corneal

Table 13-5.
Initial Evaluation and Treatment of Nonspecific Pediatric Pink Eye

1. History (trauma or foreign body, personal contacts, contact lens use, or allergy/itching)
2. I-ARM (inspection, acuity, red reflex, motility)
3. Fluorescein staining to identify abrasion or ulcer
4. No itching—treat with topical antibiotic 3 times a day, (eg polymyxin B-trimethoprim, tobramycin, levofloxacin, or ciprofloxacin)
5. Itching—treat with topical antimicrobial or mast cell stabilizer
6. Refer to an ophthalmologist if a corneal ulcer is suspected, conjunctivitis worsens with treatment, or no improvement over 5 to 7 days.

epithelium most commonly caused by a traumatic abrasion or, less frequently, an infectious process such as a bacterial corneal ulcer or herpes simplex keratitis. Be suspicious of a **unilateral conjunctivitis,** as it may be caused by a foreign body, corneal ulcer, or herpes simplex keratitis. **Table 13-5** lists the initial workup and evaluation of nonspecific pediatric pink eye.

Hemorrhagic Conjunctivitis

An alarming form of pediatric pink eye is conjunctivitis and subconjunctival hemorrhage, or **hemorrhagic conjunctivitis.** The most common causes of hemorrhagic conjunctivitis include *H influenza*, adenovirus, picornavirus, and spontaneous subconjunctival hemorrhage without infection. *H influenza* hemorrhagic conjunctivitis is associated with a purplish discoloration of the eyelids caused by multiple tiny subcutaneous hemorrhages (**Figure 13-4**).

A spontaneous **subconjunctival hemorrhage** is a painless rupture of a small conjunctival vessel, usually for no known reasons. The conjunctiva surrounding the hemorrhage will be normal, and there is no tearing or exudate. The hemorrhage resolves without treatment and a systemic workup is usually not necessary unless the hemorrhage becomes recurrent, or if there is a history of prior bleeding or bruising.

■ BACTERIAL CONJUNCTIVITIS

The conjunctiva is constantly exposed to bacteria, but conjunctival and tear defense mechanisms work to prevent infection. When bac-

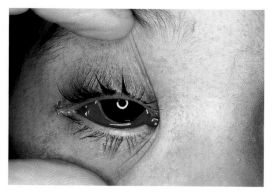

Figure 13-4.
Patient with hemorrhagic conjunctivitis secondary to *Haemophilus influenzae* infection. Patient also has an otitis media. Note the purplish or violaceous hue to the eyelid.

terial infections do occur, they present as watery irritation of the eyes that can progress to a mucopurulent discharge (**Figure 13-5**). Children with a bacterial conjunctivitis often complain that their eyelids stick together in the morning. Most often, one eye is involved; subsequently, the fellow eye becomes involved. The bulbar conjunctiva is diffusely injected and a mucopurulent exudate is present in the inferior conjunctival fornix. The most common bacteria in children include *H influenza, Streptococcus pneumoniae, Mora-*

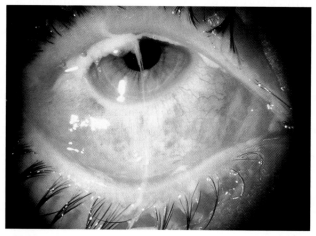

Figure 13-5.
Severe bacterial conjunctivitis with mucopurulent discharge.

Table 13-6.
Causes of Bacterial Conjunctivitis

Acute Conjunctivitis
1. *Staphylococcus aureus*
2. *Haemophilus aegyptius*
3. *Haemophilus influenzae*
4. *Streptococcus pneumoniae*
5. *Streptococcus pyogenes*
6. *Beta streptococcus*
7. *Pseudomonas aeruginosa*
8. *Corynebacteria diphtheriae*
9. *Moraxella catarrhalis*
Chronic Conjunctivitis
1. *Staphylococcus aureus*
2. *Moraxella lacunata*
3. *Proteus*
4. *Klebsiella*
5. *Serratia*
6. *Beta streptococcus*

xella catarrhalis, and staphylococcus. Other organisms that cause conjunctivitis are listed in **Table 13-6** and are categorized as acute or chronic bacterial infections.

In general, cultures and Gram stain are not routinely performed for mild to moderate conjunctivitis, and patients are treated with topical antibiotic drops every 4 to 6 hours. Treatment of presumed bacterial conjunctivitis usually consists of topical trimethoprim sulfate and polymyxin B sulfate (Polytrim solution), or a fluoroquinolone such as ciprofloxacin (Ciloxan), ofloxacin (Ocuflox), or levofloxacin (Quixin). This author prefers a fluoroquinolone because they provide broad-spectrum coverage including *Haemophilus,* and the drops do not sting. Consider an ophthalmology referral for severe conjunctivitis or a chronic conjunctivitis that does not improve after 7 days of treatment.

■ VIRAL CONJUNCTIVITIS

Viral conjunctivitis is usually caused by an adenovirus and is extremely contagious. Patients often present with a history of one eye involvement and subsequent second eye involvement. There is extreme tearing, redness, and the sensation of having a foreign body lodged in the eye. This combination of findings is termed "catarrhal conjunctivitis." In children, the eyelids may be quite swollen and present with reactive ptosis as well as severe conjunctival hyperemia and hemorrhagic conjunctivitis. The cornea may be involved and, in these cases, patients are very light-sensitive (photophobia). Often, there is a history of other family members or friends having pink eye.

Pharyngoconjunctival Fever

Pharyngoconjunctival fever is usually seen in children and consists of an upper respiratory infection (pharyngitis and fever) with bilateral conjunctivitis. It is most commonly associated with adenovirus type 3 and type 7. There is a severe, watery conjunctival discharge; hyperemic conjunctivitis; chemosis (conjunctival edema); preauricular lymph adenopathy; and, quite often, a "foreign body" sensation due to corneal involvement. The disease is highly contagious and lasts approximately 2 to 3 weeks.

Epidemic Keratoconjunctivitis

Epidemic keratoconjunctivitis (EKC) is caused by adenovirus types 8, 19, and 37, and occurs most often in older children and adolescents. In contrast to pharyngoconjunctival fever, EKC is isolated to the eyes. This is a severe bilateral conjunctivitis with conjunctival hyperemia, watery discharge, eyelid swelling, and a reactive ptosis (**Figure 13-6**). Petechial conjunctival hemorrhages are also common. In addition, there may be a pseudomembrane along the conjunctiva, and pre-auricular adenopathy is often present. Usually, one eye is involved first and, several days later, the second eye becomes infected.

Approximately one third of patients develop corneal inflammation (keratitis) with subepithelial infiltrates, 7 to 10 days after onset of the conjunctivitis (**Figure 13-7**). The keratitis is a hypersensitive reaction to the virus, not a true viral infection. Corneal infiltrates cause severe photophobia and irritation.

The treatment of adenovirus conjunctivitis is prevention of further transmission. If a patient presents with possible adenoviral conjunctivitis, be sure to thoroughly wash everything before seeing another patient. A patient with this disease will be contagious for up to 2 weeks and should observe isolation precautions during this

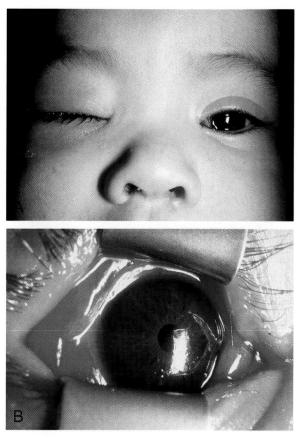

Figure 13-6.
Epidemic keratoconjunctivitis (EKC) bilateral involvement. **A,** Note the severe lid swelling, right eye, and tearing, left eye. There is a wide spectrum of severity; some are mild while others present with a severe conjunctivitis that may have severe lid swelling and the appearance of a preseptal cellulitis. **B,** A lid speculum is placed to open the right eye to show a severe hemorrhagic conjunctivitis.

time. Because of the possibility of corneal involvement, patients with adenoviral conjunctivitis should be referred to an ophthalmologist. Unfortunately, there is no effective antiviral treatment at this time. Cold compresses and topical nonsteroidal anti-inflammatory drops may reduce symptoms. Because of the contagious nature of the adenoviral conjunctivitis, a scraping for viral antigen quick prep is indicated. If positive, patients should not return to school for 1 to 2 weeks. Topical corticosteroids historically have been discouraged

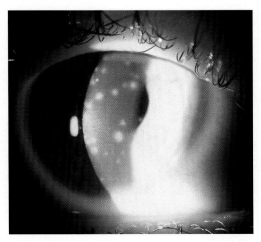

Figure 13-7.
Subepithelial infiltrates of the cornea associated with epidemic keratoconjunctivitis. These infiltrates occur during the second week of the infection and may persist for several months or longer. The infiltrates represent an immune response to the disorder and will resolve spontaneously.

except for the treatment of keratitis. Recent data suggest that topical corticosteroids may reduce the incidence and severity of the post-viral keratitis. If given, topical corticosteroids should be administered only by an ophthalmologist.

Primary Ocular Herpes Simplex Virus Type I

Most normal adults have been exposed to Herpes simplex virus type 1 and, unless immunocompromised, have circulating antibodies to the virus. Only 1% of the population will manifest clinical herpes simplex, as most infections are asymptomatic. Primary ocular herpes represents the first exposure to the herpes simplex type 1 virus. It presents as a skin eruption with multiple vesicular lesions (**Figure 13-8**). Virus can be cultured from vesicle fluid. The use of antiviral medications is controversial, but many feel that systemic or topical acyclovir may speed recovery if given within 1 or 2 days of onset. Topical antibiotics applied to the skin may be useful for preventing secondary bacterial infection. Over several days to 2 weeks, the skin lesions heal, with or without treatment, and usually without significant scarring. The cornea is involved in 10% to 30% of

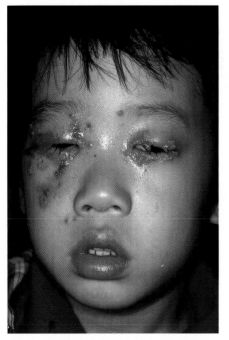

Figure 13-8.
Four-year-old boy with primary herpes cutaneous eruption both eyes. Multiple vesicular lesions around the eyelid and eyelid margins. This resolved after 2 to 3 weeks without significant scarring.

patients with primary ocular herpes simplex type 1. Primary ocular herpes simplex virus rarely causes intraocular inflammation or uveitis.

Recurrent Ocular Herpes Simplex Virus

After initial cutaneous facial infection or infection of the mucous membranes, the herpes virus gains access to the sensory nerve endings and travels up the axons to the trigeminal ganglion. The virus remains sequestered and protected within the ganglion. Recurrent ocular herpes occurs when virus from the ganglion travels down the sensory nerve and infects the cornea or eyelids. The cutaneous eyelid disease consists of a vesicular reaction similar to primary herpes simplex.

The corneal disease from recurrent herpes simplex virus affects the corneal surface epithelium. Active viral replications cause punctate, dendritic, or geographic epithelial defects. The dendritic pattern is a classic sign of herpes simplex keratitis (corneal infection)

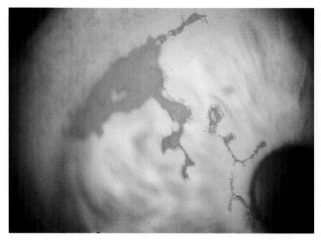

Figure 13-9.
Active herpes keratitis with both dendritic and geographic patterns. Superiorly at the limbus is the confluent area of staining showing a geographic pattern, while the mid-cornea shows the branching, dendritic pattern.

(**Figure 13-9**). Recurrent herpes keratitis is almost always unilateral. In addition, the cornea becomes anesthetized due to sensory nerve damage. With recurrent herpes, the cornea can scar and a secondary inflammatory reaction can occur in response to the viral antigen.

The treatment for acute recurrent herpes keratitis is topical antivirals, usually Viroptic 1% every 2 hours while awake. Systemic treatment with acyclovir has been shown to be effective. There is an ongoing study using daily prophylactic acyclovir to prevent occurrences. Topical corticosteroids are not indicated for active herpes keratitis, as this will decrease the body's immune response.

Herpes Zoster and Varicella Zoster Virus

Chickenpox, or varicella zoster, rarely affects the eye even when vesicular lesions occur on the eyelid or eyelid margin. Some physicians have advocated topical trifluridine (Viroptic) 1% every 2 hours if the conjunctiva becomes involved; however, oral acyclovir early in the course is the preferred treatment. In immunocompromised patients, herpes zoster can present a high risk, and these patients especially should be treated with antivirals. Secondary, or recurrent, herpes zoster ophthalmicus is a disease striking patients over age

50 or immunocompromised children. Herpes zoster ophthalmicus is a severe ocular inflammation and can affect all layers of the eye.

■ BLEPHARITIS

Blepharitis, or eyelid inflammation, is one of the most common causes of pediatric pink eye. The 2 most common types of blepharitis are staphylococcal blepharitis and meibomian gland dysfunction. Both types of blepharitis are treated with lid hygiene (baby shampoo lid scrubs) and topical antibiotics.

Staphylococcal Blepharitis

Children with staphylococcal blepharitis complain of itching and burning and often awaken with their eyelids stuck together with crusting. Their eyes are irritated, but there is not the "true" itching as there is in patients with allergic conjunctivitis. Other signs of staphylococcal blepharitis include crusting and scales at the base of the eyelashes. Scales that encircle an eyelash are called **collarettes.** The eyelid margins are thickened and hyperemic with vascularization of the eyelid margin. Over time, lashes may become misdirected, broken, or absent (**madarosis**). The formation of a stye, or external **hordeolum,** is common. An external hordeolum is an abscess of the gland of Zeis on the anterior eyelid margin (**Figures 13-10 and 13-12**). This is in contrast to a **chalazion,** which is deeper and represents inflammation of the meibomian gland secondary to breakdown of the fatty secretions. Blepharitis may be associated with corneal changes that cause severe photophobia. These corneal deposits represent an immunologic response to the bacterial antigen.

Treatment of staphylococcal blepharitis includes eyelid hygiene and topical antibiotic ointment, usually erythromycin, applied 3 times a day. In severe cases, systemic erythromycin may be indicated. Eyelid hygiene may include baby shampoo lid scrubs, twice a day. Prevention of recurrent blepharitis consists of ongoing lid hygiene. Eyelid cultures are not routinely performed, since most eyelids are normally colonized with staphylococcus organisms.

Phlyctenular Conjunctivitis

Phlyctenular conjunctivitis is a delayed hypersensitivity reaction to bacterial protein, usually associated with staphylococcal blepharitis.

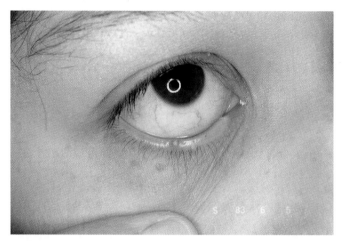

Figure 13-10.
Staphylococcal blepharitis with small external hordeolum.

The lesions are usually located at the 3- and 9-o'clock position around the limbus and are creamy-white or yellowish colored elevated nodules with a surrounding erythematous base (**Figure 13-11**). Treatment consists of treating the blepharitis (lid scrubs and topical antibiotics) and the use of topical corticosteroids. If topical

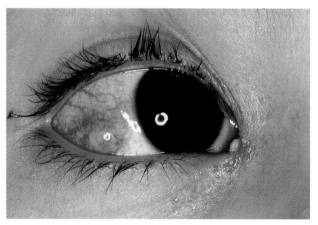

Figure 13-11.
Photograph of phlyctenule in a patient with staphylococcal blepharitis. The phlyctenula is the yellow lesion at the lower lid margin surrounded by erythematous conjunctival reaction.

corticosteroids are recommended, treatment should be monitored by an ophthalmologist. When tuberculosis was prevalent, it was a significant cause of phlyctenulosis. Patients with phlyctenular conjunctivitis, who are at risk for having tuberculosis, should have a tuberculosis workup.

Meibomian Gland Dysfunction—Blepharitis

Meibomian glands are sebaceous glands with orifices at the eyelid margins (**Figure 13-12, top**). Meibomian gland secretions consist of sterol esters and waxes that provide a covering to the tear film, thereby preventing evaporation. Dysfunction or blockage of the meibomian gland orifice by desquamated epithelial cells results in stagnation of the lipids and causes a secondary local inflammation (**Figure 13-12, bottom**). Microbial lipases from *Propionibacterium acnes* and other bacteria contribute to producing irritating fatty acids that increase the inflammatory response.

Meibomian gland dysfunction produces irritation, burning, and redness of the eyelid margins and conjunctiva, causing a blepharoconjunctivitis. The treatment of meibomian gland dysfunction is eyelid hygiene with baby shampoo lid washes and eyelid massage to express the meibomian glands. The use of oral erythromycin may be necessary in severe cases. Controlling meibomian gland dysfunction helps prevent chalazia.

Chalazion

Obstruction of the meibomian gland orifices may result in a **chalazion,** which is a constipated meibomian gland. A chalazion appears as a lump near the eyelid margin, either on the upper or lower lid. Since the chalazion is a swelling of a meibomian gland, the swelling can occur externally as a lump on the skin or internally as a lump underneath the conjunctiva (**Figure 13-13 A through C**). A chalazion is not an infection but, in fact, is a granulomatous inflammation secondary to the irritating lipids within the meibomian gland. Chalazia may resolve spontaneously; however, applying hot soaks several times a day with baby shampoo eyelid washes twice per day helps drain lipid material, decompressing the chalazion. If the chalazion does not resolve over several weeks of treatment, incision and drainage may be necessary.

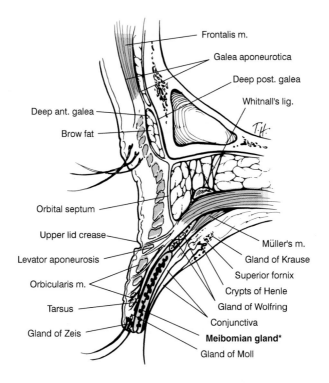

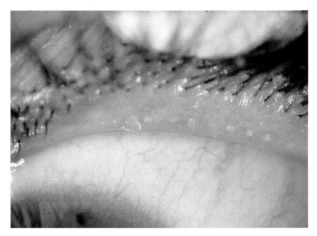

Figure 13-12.
Top, Sagittal section of the upper lid showing various tear-secreting glands. **Bottom,**
Photograph of eyelid margin showing droplets at the orifice of the meibomian
glands.
*Note: the meibomian gland opens at the lid margin.

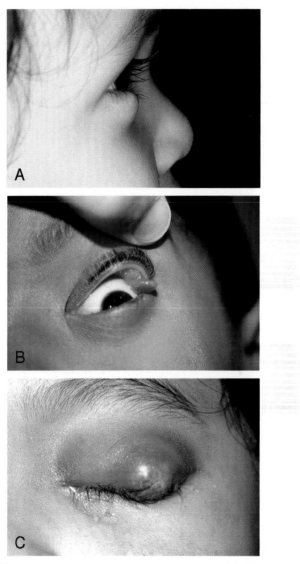

Figure 13-13.
A, Chalazion lower lid. Note that there is a subcutaneous lid mass with some erythema. Over time, the overlying skin can become erythematous and inflamed. **B,** Internal chalazion where the meibomian gland has extended posteriorly under the conjunctiva. This is sometimes called pyogenic granuloma. **C,** Infected chalazion.

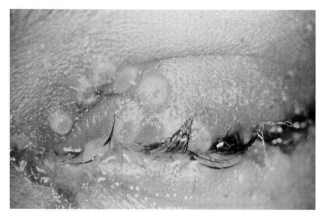

Figure 13-14.
Molluscum Contagiosum.

External Hordeolum

Infections of the accessory glands (Zeis and Moll) of the eyelids cause small styles called **external hordeolum (Figure 13-10).** They are best treated with erythromycin ophthalmic ointment and not soaks. They can be prevented by daily eyelid washes with dilute baby shampoo.

Molluscum Contagiosum

Molluscum contagiosum is a viral disease of the skin, often occurring on the eyelids, caused by a DNA virus of the pox virus group. The lesions are small, round, discrete bumps with a central pit (**Figure 13-14**). They are presumed to be contagious, transmitted by direct touch. When present on the eyelid margin, they can cause a conjunctival reaction and a follicular conjunctivitis. These lesions can be treated by excising the central core, or rarely, through the use of cryotherapy or application of chemical caustics such as trichloroacetic acid or aqueous phenol.

■ ALLERGIC AND INFLAMMATORY PEDIATRIC CONJUNCTIVITIS

Seasonal Allergic Conjunctivitis

Seasonal allergic (hay fever) conjunctivitis is very common and affects approximately 10% of the general population. The hallmark of this allergy is itching and tearing, with the eye being relatively quiet compared to the severity of the symptoms. Seasonal allergic rhinitis often accompanies seasonal allergic conjunctivitis. Seasonal allergic conjunctivitis is a type 1 hypersensitivity reaction, and conjunctival scrapings or biopsy reveals mast cells and eosinophils. Serum quantitative IgE are usually elevated, and skin tests may be positive for environmental allergen. Allergic conjunctivitis is most common in the spring when pollen levels are high; however, a significant number of cases occur during the winter when the forced air heating is turned on and filters have not been cleaned or replaced.

A laboratory workup is usually not necessary, as a diagnosis can be made through clinical signs and symptoms. Family history may be positive for allergies, atopic disease, or asthma. For chronic, recurrent conjunctivitis, therapy consists of removal of environmental allergens and the use of topical mast cell stabilizing agents such as cromolyn sodium, lodoxamide, and pemirolast. Mast cell stabilizers prevent the release of histamine and require 2 to 3 days of continued use to reduce symptoms. This is because mast cell stabilizers stop the release of histamines, but do not inhibit activity of circulating histamines, and time is required for circulating histamines to dissipate. Topical antihistamines, such as olopatadine (Patanol) and levocabastine (Livostin), provide immediate relief because they directly block histamine receptors. Topical histamines are used for episodic allergic conjunctivitis and are added to mast cell stabilizers for breakthrough symptoms for patients with chronic allergic conjunctivitis. The combined use of a mast cell stabilizer along with an antihistamine works well for severe allergic conjunctivitis. Oral systemic antihistamines such as loratadine (Claritin) or cetirizine (Zyrtec), can be used alone or in combination with topical medication to treat allergic conjunctivitis. Topical corticosteroids are reserved for severe allergic conjunctivitis such as vernal conjunctivitis, and are only used for short courses of a few days. If corticosteroids are used, an ophthalmologist should monitor the patient for the potential side effects of glaucoma and cataracts.

Vernal Conjunctivitis

Vernal conjunctivitis is a severe allergic condition presenting with severe itching, tearing, mucus production, and giant papillae of the

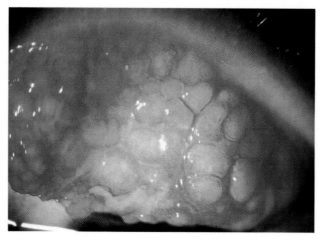

Figure 13-15.
Vernal Conjunctivitis. An everted upper eyelid discloses a giant papillary conjunctival reaction. Patients present with severe itching, burning, and mucous discharge. Eversion of the upper lids shows the classic giant papillary reaction.

upper tarsal conjunctiva (**Figure 13-15**). It most commonly affects young boys of the Mediterranean and Central and South America region. Patients often have reactive ptosis and squint in bright light due to secondary keratitis caused by the giant papillae scraping the cornea. There may be papillae around the limbus (junction of the sclera and cornea) with characteristic white centers (Trantas dots) that represent an accumulation of inflammatory cells (predominantly eosinophils). Conjunctival scrapings of the papillae show many eosinophils.

Treatment is based on avoiding allergens and using topical antihistamines along with topical mast cell stabilizers. It is critical to use mast cell stabilizers 3 to 4 times every day, without exception, and use topical antihistamines intermittently to control vernal conjunctivitis. In some instances, severe episodes of inflammation can only be controlled with intermittent short courses of topical corticosteroids. Topical corticosteroids should be administered and supervised by an ophthalmologist to monitor intraocular pressure (to rule out glaucoma) and to monitor the lens status (to rule out cataracts). Long-term corticosteroid use should be avoided. The prognosis is fair because uncontrolled patients may sustain permanent vision loss as a result of corneal scarring.

Giant Papillary Conjunctivitis

Giant papillary conjunctivitis is secondary to soft contact lens use. Like vernal conjunctivitis, there are large papillae underneath the superior tarsal conjunctiva. The reaction is due to a sensitization of the conjunctiva to allergic materials present on the surface of the contact lens or in contact lens solutions. Recommended treatment is the use of topical mast cell stabilizers such as nedocromil (Alocril), pemirolast (Alamast), cromolyn (Crolom); discontinuing contact lens wear; or changing to a regimen of frequent contact lens replacement. Prognosis is good.

Atopic Conjunctivitis

Atopic conjunctivitis is a form of allergic conjunctivitis associated with atopic dermatitis (eczema). Serum IgE concentrations are often elevated, resulting from what appears to be a deficiency in cellular immunity (deficiency of T-suppressor cells). Patients with atopic dermatitis often have associated conjunctivitis with itching, burning, and mucus discharge. Symptomatic treatment of eye complaints includes using cold compresses, topical vasoconstrictors, topical antihistamines, and topical mast cell stabilizers. Topical corticosteroids should be used for only short periods of time while being monitored by an ophthalmologist.

■ CONJUNCTIVITIS ASSOCIATED WITH SYSTEMIC DISEASE

Stevens-Johnson Syndrome (Erythema Multiforme Major)

Stevens-Johnson syndrome is most likely a type 3 hypersensitivity reaction. It may be associated with mycoplasmal pneumonia, herpes simplex virus, and drugs such as sulfonamides, tetracycline, and penicillin. Patients present with fever, malaise, headache, loss of appetite, and nausea. There is a generalized erythematous papular rash. The skin is very friable and traction on the skin can produce tears. Mucous membranes including the nose, mouth, vagina, anus, and conjunctiva are most severely affected. Eye involvement consists of conjunctival injection and the formation of bullae that can rupture and lead to secondary scarring. Conjunctival scarring can distort the eyelids and turn the lashes towards the cornea, causing corneal damage. Therapy remains controversial. This author has found fewer ocular complications if topical corticosteroids are administered early, before advanced disease leads to conjunctival scarring. A topical corticosteroid/antibiotic combination, used every to 2 to 4 hours, may prevent the severe ocular sequelae. Once conjunctival scarring occurs, however, there is no effective treatment. It is this author's suggestion that patients with Stevens-Johnson syndrome should have an immediate ophthalmology consultation, with topical corticosteroids being started promptly. In addition to topical corticosteroids, a topical antibiotic should be prescribed to prevent secondary bacterial infection. This treatment is controversial, as there are no controlled studies that establish a specific treatment protocol.

Kawasaki Disease

Kawasaki disease is a systemic vasculitis occurring in children under 8 years of age. It has an onset of fever, present for more than 5 days, along with 4 out of the following 5 criteria: non-purulent conjunctivitis, oral mucus membrane injection and/or swelling, erythema and edema of the hands and feet, polymorphous rash, and cervical lymphadenopathy. The vasculitis may involve the coronary arteries and cause a coronary aneurysm or a thrombosis that may lead to sudden death. The cause of Kawasaki disease is unknown.

Toxic Epidermal Necrolysis (Lyell Syndrome)

Toxic epidermal necrolysis is a generalized peeling of the epidermis in large geographic areas of the skin and mucous membranes and, in children, is actually the result of medication. The ocular manifestations are similar to Stevens-Johnson syndrome, with acute conjunctivitis and secondary scarring being the most common presenting features. It is important that children with this syndrome be referred to an ophthalmologist for evaluation and treatment, with close follow-up during the acute periods.

Graft-Versus-Host Disease

Approximately 40% of patients who receive a bone marrow transplant will have graft-versus-host disease. Donor T-lymphocytes attack the recipient cells, primarily affecting the skin, liver, intestine, oral mucosa, conjunctiva, lacrimal gland, vaginal mucosa, and esophageal mucosa. The ocular effects of graft-versus-host disease consist of conjunctivitis, dry eye, corneal epithelial erosions, and corneal ulcerations. Treatment with topical artificial tears, short courses of topical corticosteroids and, in severe cases, cyclosporine may improve symptoms. These patients should be referred to an ophthalmologist for careful follow-up.

■ CONJUNCTIVAL NEVI

These are congenital or acquired lesions of the conjunctiva usually located near the corneal limbus, and may be darkly pigmented or appear as pink or inflamed conjunctiva (**Figure 13-16**). Nevi come from melanocytes but have varying amounts of pigmentation with 30% having minimal pigmentation. Most common types include junctional, compound, and subepithelial nevi. All have low malignant potential, and usually become noticeable in the first decade of life through puberty. Treatment is controversial, but growth or

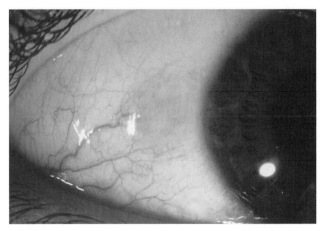

Figure 13-16.
Lightly pigmented compound conjunctival nevi.

change in pigmentation of the nevus may be an indication for surgical removal. Malignant **melanoma** is very rare in children, but has been reported to occur.

■ BIBLIOGRAPHY

1. Harrison JR, English MG, Lee CK, Alexander ER. Chlamydia trachomatis infant pneumonitis: comparison with matched controls and other infant pneumonitis. *N Engl J Med.* 1978;298:702–708
2. Isenberg SJ, Apt L, Wood M. A controlled trial of povidone–iodine as prophylaxis against ophthalmia neonatorum. *N Engl J Med.* 1995; 332:562–566

14 Ocular Inflammation and Uveitis

This chapter covers ocular inflammation including uveitis, episcleritis and scleritis, endophthalmitis, acute retinal necrosis syndrome, and ocular manifestations of acquired immunodeficiency syndrome (AIDS).

■ UVEITIS

Uveitis is a term for intraocular inflammation involving the uveal tract (iris, ciliary body, and choroid). Ophthalmologists classify uveitis according to the location: either anterior uveitis—affecting anterior chamber and iris; intermediate uveitis—affecting the ciliary body area and anterior vitreous; posterior uveitis—affecting the choroid and retina; or panuveitis—affecting the entire uveal tract. Normally, the vitreous and the aqueous fluid are devoid of cells. In patients with uveitis, leukocytes circulate in the aqueous and also can be found in the vitreous. In addition, the protein content of the aqueous humor increases with inflammation. Clinically, the ophthalmologist uses a slit-lamp to identify **cells and flare** (representing protein) circulating in the anterior chamber. Cells can only be seen by high-powered magnification, and flare is the light scatter in the protein-laden aqueous humor. White cells can precipitate on the back of the cornea, and are termed **keratic precipitates (KP)** (**Figure 14-1**). The term **iritis** refers to anterior inflammation, and **iridocyclitis** describes intermediate intraocular inflammation. Ophthalmologists often send patients with uveitis to the pediatri-

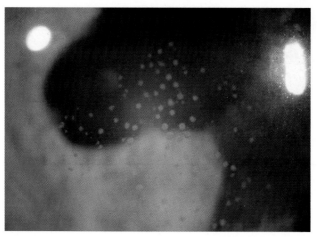

Figure 14-1.
A photograph of a patient with chronic uveitis and keratic precipitates on the posterior surface of the cornea. Note the multiple white circular lesions.

cian for evaluation of systemic disease. **Table 14-1** lists the more common diseases associated with pediatric uveitis.

■ JUVENILE RHEUMATOID ARTHRITIS

Juvenile rheumatoid arthritis (JRA) represents approximately 70% of all pediatric arthritis and can be divided into 3 types.

• Still's Disease
• Polyarticular JRA
• Pauciarticular JRA

Still's Disease

Still's disease (systemic JRA) accounts for approximately 20% of all JRA cases; however, it is rarely associated with uveitis. Patients with this form of JRA present with fever, salmon-colored rash, lymphadenopathy, and hepatosplenomegaly. Less than 6% will develop uveitis.

Polyarticular Juvenile Rheumatoid Arthritis

Polyarticular JRA involves more than 4 joints. This accounts for approximately 40% of all patients with JRA. Most patients are fe-

Table 14-1.
Common Diseases Associated With Pediatric Uveitis

Disease	Uveitis	Lab Test
1. Juvenile Rheumatoid Arthritis (JRA)	Anterior uveitis	Antinuclear antibodies (ANA) Erythrocyte Sedimentation Rate (ESR)
2. Sarcoidosis	Panuveitis	Angiotensin-converting enzyme (ACE) Chest x-ray Gallium scan Biopsy of suspicious nodules
3. Seronegative spondyloarthropathies	Anterior uveitis	HLA-B27
4. Inflammatory bowel disease	Anterior uveitis	HLA-B27
5. Behçet syndrome	Anterior/posterior uveitis	HLA-B5 (subset BW 5 1) in 50% of Mediterranean or Japanese patients Skin abrasion test
6. Syphilis	Anterior/posterior uveitis	VDRL/RPR; FTA-ABS
7. Toxoplasmosis	Posterior uveitis	Toxoplasma ELISA Titer
8. Toxocara	Posterior uveitis	Toxocara ELISA Titer
9. Acute Retinal Necrosis syndrome	Posterior uveitis	Herpes Zoster Virus Titer, or Herpes Simplex Virus Titer

males, and approximately 30% will be negative for the rheumatoid factor. Uveitis may occur, although uncommon, and is present in about 15% of patients with polyarticular JRA.

Pauciarticular Juvenile Rheumatoid Arthritis

Pauciarticular JRA involves 4 joints or fewer, and 2 forms of this type of JRA have been described. Pauciarticular type 1 (early onset) is predominantly seen in girls younger than 5 years of age and is associated with a high incidence of uveitis (25% of patients). Most patients are antinuclear antibody positive (ANA+). Pauciarticular type 2 (late onset) is usually seen in older boys and is often associated with recurrent anterior uveitis. Approximately 75% will test positive for HLA-B27. Many of the boys with late onset pauciarticular JRA will develop ankylosing spondylitis.

The ocular inflammation associated with JRA does not parallel the joint inflammation. The uveitis seen in patients with JRA usually occurs within 7 years of the onset of the arthritis; however, late onset uveitis may occur up to 20 years after JRA is diagnosed. Since uveitis associated with JRA is asymptomatic until severe ocular damage occurs, children with JRA should be screened early for uveitis. Patients with JRA who have the highest risk of developing uveitis are female, have early-onset pauciarticular JRA, and are ANA+. The early detection of ocular inflammation is critical to decreasing the visual loss that can occur with JRA uveitis. **Table 14-2** lists a recommended screening schedule for ocular examinations.

Complications of JRA uveitis include keratic precipitates (white cells on the posterior surface of the cornea), posterior synechiae (iris adherence to the cornea), cataracts, glaucoma, cyclitic membrane (scarring in the area of the ciliary body), and blindness. Treatment is based on reducing ocular inflammation to prevent these ophthalmologic complications. Topical corticosteroids are used to reduce anterior chamber inflammation, and may be required as frequently as a drop every hour in severe cases. Corticosteroids should be quickly tapered when inflammation is controlled, as corticosteroids can cause cataracts and glaucoma. The use of topical mydriatics to keep the pupil mobile and avoid pupillary scarring to the lens (posterior synechiae) is also advocated. Most patients with JRA uveitis are treated with chronic topical corticosteroids and many experience serious side effects (cataracts and glaucoma). Systemic methotrexate may be used in those children with severe uveitis to reduce the topical corticosteroid dose necessary to control inflammation.

Table 14-2.
Screening Schedule for Ocular Examinations in Patients With Juvenile Rheumatoid Arthritis

Juvenile Rheumatoid Arthritis Type	*Frequency of Ocular Examinations*
Systemic onset (Still's Disease)	Annually
Polyarticular onset	Semiannually
Pauciarticular onset or ANA+	Every 3 months

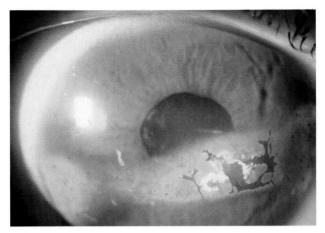

Figure 14-2.
Band keratopathy in a child with juvenile rheumatoid arthritis. Note the white band opacity extending horizontally across the cornea. Band keratopathy represents calcium deposits within the corneal epithelium.

Another complication of JRA is **band keratopathy,** representing calcium deposits within the surface corneal epithelium (**Figure 14-2**). Once severe pathology occurs, such as glaucoma, cataracts, and band keratopathy, the prognosis for good vision is poor (**Figure 14-3**). Approximately one third of cases with glaucoma progress to no light perception vision.

■ SPONDYLOARTHROPATHIES ASSOCIATED WITH UVEITIS (HLA-B27 Related Uveitis)

Next to JRA, spondyloarthropathies associated with uveitis is the most common cause of anterior uveitis in children. The majority of these patients will have an HLA-B27 haplotype, but are negative for rheumatoid factor. Juvenile spondyloarthropathy-related uveitis is divided into the following 4 types:

• Juvenile Ankylosing Spondylitis
• Juvenile Reiter Syndrome
• Juvenile Psoriatic Arthritis
• Juvenile Bowel-Associated Arthritis

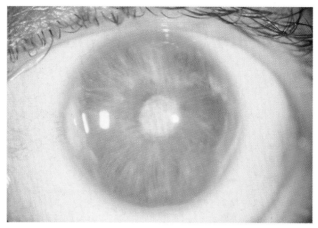

Figure 14-3.
Patient with advanced uveitis associated with juvenile rheumatoid arthritis. Note the peripheral band keratopathy at the 3- and 9-o'clock position, the white pupil indicating a dense cataract, and a relatively small cornea indicating end-stage severe ocular disease (pre-phthisis bulbi).

Juvenile Ankylosing Spondylitis

Juvenile ankylosing spondylitis primarily affects older boys, with the mean age being 11 years. Typically, the arthritis presents with lower limb involvement rather than lower back pain, which is more commonly seen in older patients. The anterior uveitis may be quite severe, and may result in a hypopyon (layered white cells in the anterior chamber) (**Figure 14-4**). More than 90% of patients with juvenile ankylosing spondylitis will be HLA-B27 positive.

Juvenile Reiter Syndrome

Juvenile Reiter syndrome is a rare entity consisting of the classic triad of arthritis, urethritis, and conjunctivitis (really uveitis). Children typically develop this syndrome after an episode of salmonella or shigella enterocolitis.

Juvenile Psoriatic Arthritis

Juvenile psoriatic arthritis is associated with skin changes, nail pitting, and joint involvement. It is seen more frequently in girls and may be associated with a chronic anterior uveitis.

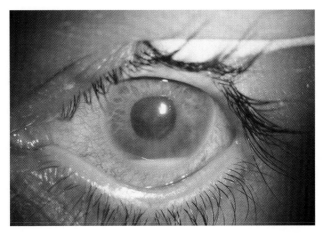

Figure 14-4.
Patient with HLA-B27 positive uveitis associated with ankylosing spondylitis. Note the white hypopyon inferiorly. The hypopyon represents layered white cells within the anterior chamber.

Juvenile Inflammatory Bowel Disease

Juvenile inflammatory bowel disease is an enteropathic arthropathy and is associated with rheumatological manifestations such as ulcerative colitis and Crohn's disease. Patients with inflammatory bowel disease and HLA-B27 haplotype have a higher incidence of sacroiliac joint disease and uveitis. Uveitis is a common ocular complication and occurs in approximately 11% of patients diagnosed with HLA-B27-positive inflammatory bowel disease. Other ocular manifestations include conjunctivitis, corneal infiltrates, episcleritis, scleritis, and optic neuritis. The ocular inflammation tends to parallel the intestinal inflammation. Some have suggested that a colectomy, resulting in improvement of the ulcerative colitis, also improves the ocular disease.

As with JRA-related uveitis, patients should be treated with topical corticosteroids and mydriatics based on the degree of inflammation. Uveitis associated with spondyloarthropathies runs a course of recurrent bouts of acute inflammation. If treated early, the prognosis is usually quite favorable.

■ SARCOIDOSIS

Sarcoidosis is a granulomatous inflammatory disease most commonly seen in adults between the ages of 20 and 50 years but, occasionally, is also seen in children. There are 2 distinct groups of pediatric sarcoidosis patients—one group with early onset of 5 years and younger, and the second group with later onset of 8 to 15 years of age. Pulmonary involvement is seen in almost 100% of patients in the older age group, even though the patients may not have symptoms. Lymphadenopathy, hepatosplenomegaly, and ocular involvement are common findings. Arthritis in this group is rare, and black children are affected approximately 3 times more often than white children. In contrast to the older group, the younger children with this disorder are predominantly white and exhibit the triad of arthritis, erythema nodosum, and uveitis.

Pediatric sarcoidosis often affects the eyes in both the younger and older pediatric groups, with approximately 50% to 80% of children affected. The most common ocular inflammation is an anterior uveitis that classically presents with large keratic precipitates (mutton-fat) and granulomatous nodules on the iris. In some cases, the posterior segment will be involved as well, causing choroiditis, vitritis, and even papillitis (**Figure 14-5**). Inflammatory granulomas can occur in the conjunctiva and even in the orbit, sometimes causing proptosis. In contrast to adults, children rarely have lacrimal gland involvement or retinal periphlebitis (versus inflammation).

The workup of suspected sarcoidosis in children should consist of a test for angiotensin-converting enzyme (ACE), chest radiography,

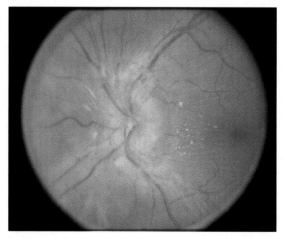

Figure 14-5.
Patient with sarcoidosis and inflammatory papillitis. Note the blurred disc margins and the hard exudates in the peripapillary region.

and possibly gallium scanning. Angiotensin-converting enzyme levels in children tend to be higher than in adults; therefore, it is important to use age-matched normal levels for comparison. Juvenile rheumatoid arthritis and Lyme disease can present similar to sarcoidosis, making it very important to rule them out before treatment is started. The diagnosis can be confirmed by a biopsy of the skin, lymph node, and conjunctival nodule. Blind biopsy of the conjunctiva is usually not productive.

Treatment of systemic sarcoidosis consists of using systemic corticosteroids to treat the systemic inflammation. Ocular inflammation is also controlled through the use of corticosteroids. These are given topically or orally, along with a mydriatic agent, to keep the pupil mobile. Because of the high incidence of ocular involvement, children with sarcoidosis should have regular ocular examinations.

Ocular Toxocariasis

The dog roundworm, *Toxocara canis*, may be found in the dirt of parks and playgrounds and is present in up to 80% of puppies. This is the most common nematode that causes ocular infections in the United States. In the dog, *T canis* has a complete life cycle. In humans, however, the cycle is incomplete. Typically, a child ingests soil that contains toxocara ova. The ova hatch in the small intestines and the larvae pass through the intestinal wall to spread to various organs including the liver, lung, brain, and eye. This dissemination of the larvae is called visceral larva migrans (VLM).

Visceral larva migrans (VLM) presents as a cough, fever, malaise, loss of appetite, and, in some cases, seizures. The peripheral blood has generalized leukocytosis with prominent eosinophilia. The VLM syndrome most commonly occurs in children between 6 months and 3 years of age, often with a history of pica and in proximity to puppies. Ocular infestation involves the choroid and retina, and may result in severe inflammation with secondary scarring and even blindness. The larvae incite a granulomatous response that will not interfere with the vision if it is confined to the periphery. Toxocara granulomas within the foveal area, however, can result in decreased vision and even legal blindness (**Figure 14-6**). In some cases, severe inflammatory reaction occurs, resulting in endophthalmitis and possible loss of the eye.

Toxocara ocular disease is one of the causes of leukocoria in infants and children. The diagnosis is made by the characteristic

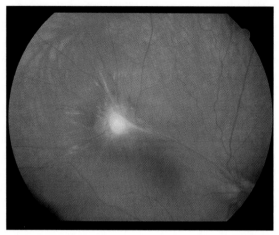

Figure 14-6.
Toxocara granuloma with traction on the optic disc.

retinal lesions seen on ophthalmoscopy and by ocular ultrasound, in addition to obtaining serum ELISA titers for antibodies to toxocara. Treatment is observation for small peripheral lesions; however, larger lesions close to the macula and cases with severe inflammation (endophthalmitis) should be treated with systemic or periocular corticosteroids. If a worm has been identified within the retina, anthelminthics should be avoided. If anthelminthics are used, however, corticosteroids should also be prescribed since larval death will cause severe intraocular inflammation. The use of laser to kill the larvae has been advocated by some, but this also leads to severe intraocular inflammation.

Congenital Toxoplasmosis
(see Chapter 6)

Lyme Disease

Lyme disease is caused by the spirochete, *Borrelia burgdorferi.* It is transmitted to humans by the bite of a deer tick commonly found in New England, Middle Atlantic, and upper-Midwest States. Three stages of Lyme disease have been described, and all 3 stages may affect the eye.

Early Localized Disease

This first stage occurs within 1 month after the tick bite and consists of headaches, stiff neck, malaise, fever, lymphadenopathy, and a migratory erythematous skin rash termed erythema migrans. Ocular involvement is usually a conjunctivitis.

Early Disseminated Disease

This second stage occurs approximately 1 to 4 months after infection and results in secondary erythema migrans skin lesions, and neurologic, musculoskeletal, cardiac, and ocular disease. Neurologic disease occurs in approximately 40% of patients and can take the form of encephalitis, meningitis, or Bell's palsy (facial nerve palsy). Almost 10% of the patients will develop cardiac involvement disease. Ocular manifestations of Lyme disease include keratitis, uveitis, and optic neuritis. Treatment therapies include ceftriaxone IM, penicillin, or doxycycline for children younger than 8 years of age.

Late Disease

The final stage has its onset months after the initial infection. Complications consist of chronic neurological disease and arthritis. Ocular findings include uveitis. Laboratory workup includes ELISA titers for the antibody to *B. burgdorferi*; however, not all patients with Lyme disease will have elevated titers. Because of the similarity to syphilis, patients with Lyme may have a false positive syphilis serology. Treatment consists of tetracycline, erythromycin, or penicillin. Patients with encephalitis or meningitis should be treated with ceftriaxone IM, penicillin, or doxycycline for children younger than 8 years of age.

■ EPISCLERITIS AND SCLERITIS

Episcleritis is an inflammatory condition of the scleral surface. It occurs in adolescents and young adults as a unilateral or, more often, bilateral conjunctivitis. Patients present with localized injection of the conjunctiva and deeper episcleral tissue, with the injection usually localized over the rectus muscle insertion. There is often pain on eye movement, distinguishing episcleritis from allergic or infectious conjunctivitis where there is no pain on eye movement. The area of inflammation is tender to palpation. Another distinguishing characteristic is the localized nature of the conjunctival

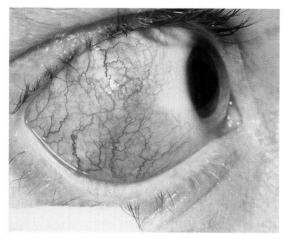

Figure 14-7.
Episcleritis with conjunctival injection localized around the lateral rectus muscle. Note that the conjunctiva close to the cornea (perilimbal conjunctiva) is clear and the sclera is white. This localized pattern of inflammation is distinct from the generalized pattern of inflammation associated with an infectious conjunctivitis.

injection (**Fig. 14.7**). In contrast to allergic conjunctivitis, episcleritis is not associated with itching; but it is associated with some tearing, discomfort, and tenderness to the touch. Although often recurrent, episcleritis is a self-limiting disorder usually not associated with systemic disease. In contrast, true inflammation of the sclera (**scleritis**) is usually seen in adult patients, and is often associated with rheumatoid arthritis. Patients with a localized conjunctival inflammation and tenderness should be referred for a full ophthalmic evaluation. The treatment of episcleritis is usually topical nonsteroidal anti-inflammatory agents or topical corticosteroids. Systemic anti-inflammatory agents such as ibuprofen and indomethacin may be required.

■ ENDOPHTHALMITIS

Endophthalmitis is an intraocular infection that may be caused by a bacteria or fungus. This is a devastating ocular condition with an extremely poor prognosis, even when treated with high-dose antibiotics and vitrectomy to remove the infection. Damage to intraocular structures occurs, not only from the toxins released by the microorganism, but also from the inflammatory response produced by the host. The retina and anterior segment structures may be directly injured. Scarring, secondary to inflammation, can cause a secondary retinal detachment.

Endophthalmitis can be divided into 2 basic causes:

1. Exogenous endophthalmitis is caused by direct penetration of a microorganism into the eye, such as in the case of traumatic endophthalmitis. Features include
   - Bacterial corneal ulcer that penetrates the anterior chamber
   - Ruptured globe with contamination of the intraocular structures
   - Postoperative endophthalmitis after intraocular surgery
2. Endogenous endophthalmitis is caused by hematogenous spread of an infectious agent into the eye. This disease is
   - Rare
   - Associated with an indwelling catheter and colonization by the infecting organism

Characteristics of endophthalmitis include pain, decreased vision, and a severely inflamed eye with conjunctival injection. There are usually an associated hypopyon (white cells layered out in the anterior chamber) and white cells in the vitreous cavity, producing a dull red reflex (**Figure 14-8**).

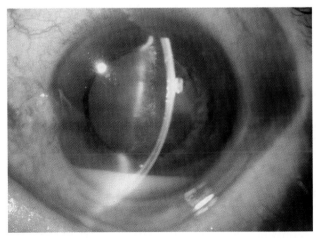

Figure 14-8.
Endogenous endophthalmitis with diffuse injection of the conjunctiva, a hypopyon (which is the white layered material in the anterior chamber), and vitreous cells evidenced by the whitish appearance in the pupil.

Traumatic endophthalmitis occurs in approximately 3% to 8% of patients with penetrating ocular injuries. *Bacillus cereus* accounts for almost one fourth of traumatic endophthalmitis cases and is commonly found in soil. Therefore, soil-contaminated penetrating ocular injuries are usually associated with bacillus endophthalmitis. Fungal endophthalmitis (eg, *Candida albicans*) should be suspected if plant or organic intraocular debris is present. *Streptococcus epidermidis*, streptococcus, and *Staphylococcus aureus* are also common causes of traumatic bacterial endophthalmitis.

Endogenous endophthalmitis occurs from infections arising at sites distant from the eye and is spread by hematologic dissemination. Patients who are immunosuppressed, chronically ill, or who have indwelling catheters are predisposed to developing endogenous endophthalmitis. Common organisms responsible for endogenous endophthalmitis include *Staphylococcus* spp. (associated with endocarditis), *S. aureus* (associated with a cutaneous infection), and *B. cereus* (associated with intravenous drug use). *Neisseria meningitidis* and *Hemophilus influenzae*, *Escherichia coli*, and *Klebsiella* spp. can also cause endophthalmitis. Endogenous fungal endophthalmitis is most commonly caused by Candida and Aspergillus fungi. Fungal endophthalmitis typically presents with a quiet eye and focal, or multifocal, chorioretinal lesions. Candida infections are usually seen in patients who are immunosuppressed, on hyperalimentation, or who have chronic indwelling catheters.

The treatment of endophthalmitis consists of intravenous systemic antimicrobials along with topical, subconjunctival, and intraocular antimicrobials. Topical and intraocular corticosteroids are often administered to limit the host-mediated intraocular inflammation, thus reducing intraocular tissue damage.

The prognosis of patients with endophthalmitis depends on the causative organism; however, the prognosis is generally poor, and the majority of patients end up legally blind in the involved eye. Traumatic endophthalmitis caused by *B. cereus* has an especially poor prognosis.

■ ACUTE RETINAL NECROSIS SYNDROME

Acute retinal necrosis syndrome (ARNS) is caused by a viral infection of the retina. Herpes simplex virus, herpes zoster virus, and cytomegalovirus (CMV) have been implicated as infectious causes. Patients present with symptoms of photophobia, pain, and de-

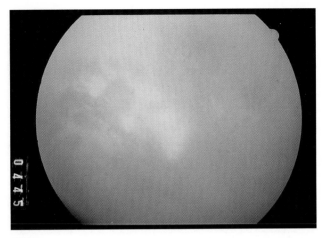

Figure 14-9.
Fundus photograph of a patient with acute retinal necrosis. Note the white retinal lesions representing areas of retinal necrosis. Also note that fundus details are not well seen because of vitreous cells and flare that produce an opacity.

creased vision. Acute retinal necrosis syndrome can occur in either sex and in any age group, but most commonly occurs in the third and fifth decade of life. Acute retinal necrosis syndrome presenting in children may indicate an immunocompromised host. Retinal inflammation causes a severe uveitis with retinal necrosis (**Figure 14-9**). Over time, the areas of necrotic retina form chorioretinal scars (**Figure 14-10**).

Acute retinal necrosis syndrome is diagnosed by the appearance of the retinal lesions. Antibody titers to herpes simplex or herpes zoster virus may support the diagnosis, but these titers may not be elevated with isolated ocular involvement. Intravenous acyclovir is the treatment of choice to diminish the retinitis. Because acyclovir does not affect the uveitis, corticosteroids are often prescribed 2 days after initiation of acyclovir. Visual prognosis is relatively poor, with 75% of patients developing a retinal detachment.

■ OPHTHALMIC MANIFESTATIONS OF AIDS

In contrast to adults, children with AIDS rarely have eye involvement. In a study of 125 patients, 9 children had CMV retinitis, 2 children had HIV cotton-wool spots retinitis, 1 had herpes zoster retinitis, and 1 had toxoplasmosis retinitis. Of these findings, cyto-

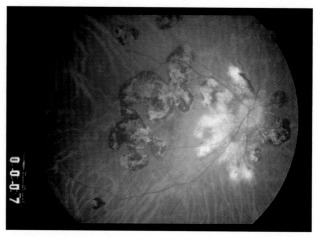

Figure 14-10.
Fundus photograph of end-stage scars in a patient with ARN. Note the hyperpigmented and hypopigmented areas in the macular area and surrounding the optic nerve.

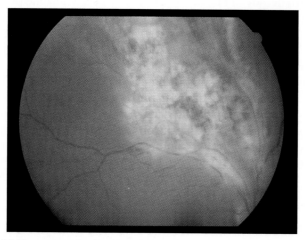

Figure 14-11.
Fundus photograph of cytomegalovirus retinitis. Note the areas of intraretinal hemorrhage associated with white areas of edematous retina. The retinitis follows retinal vessels and produces severe retinal necrosis.

megalovirus retinitis is the most vision threatening. Cytomegalovirus retinal lesions are characterized by areas of intraretinal hemorrhages and are located along vascular arcades in conjunction with white, edematous retina (**Figure 14-11**).

The treatment of CMV retinitis in patients with AIDS consists of antiviral agents (ganciclovir or foscarnet) and/or the use of colony-stimulating factors. In addition, CMV retinitis can be treated with an intravitreal ganciclovir implant. This is a polymer implant that slowly releases ganciclovir into the vitreous cavity. Relapses of CMV retinitis are common in patients with AIDS, and patients must be followed closely for recurrence.

15 Corneal Abnormalities

■ ABNORMAL CORNEAL SIZE

Microcornea

Microcornea is defined as a corneal diameter of less than 10 mm. Isolated presence of microcornea, without other ocular problems, is consistent with normal visual acuity. Isolated microcornea can be unilateral or bilateral, and sporadic, inherited as an autosomal dominant or recessive trait. Microcornea can be associated with other ocular abnormalities, most commonly coloboma of the optic nerve or choroid, and congenital cataracts, including persistent hyperplastic primary vitreous (PHPV). Systemic syndromes associated with microcornea include Ehlers-Danlos syndrome, Weill-Marchesani syndrome, Rieger anamoly, Fetal Alcohol syndrome, Congenital Rubella syndrome, and Trisomy 13-15 syndrome. Microcornea should be distinguished from nanophthalmos. **Nanophthalmos** is an otherwise normal eye that is small, including the cornea. A small eye is termed **microphthalmia.**

Megalocornea

Megalocornea is defined as a cornea larger than 13 mm in diameter. Isolated, or primary, megalocorneais consistent with excellent visual acuity and an otherwise normal eye. Primary megalocornea is usually bilateral and is most commonly seen as an X-linked recessive trait in males. It is important to rule out congenital glaucoma in any child with a large cornea, as increased pressure in children under 2 to 3 years of age can result in corneal enlargement. Megalocornea is also associated with systemic syndromes such as Down syndrome, Marfan syndrome, and Apert syndrome.

■ CLOUDY CORNEA

A cloudy cornea is distinct from leukocoria, which is a white pupil and is discussed in Chapter 22. With a cloudy cornea, structures within the eye cannot be seen clearly. Note that with leukocoria, the iris and pupil are clearly visualized; but a cloudy cornea blocks the view of iris structures. **Tables 15-1 and 15-2** list the common causes of a cloudy cornea at birth, in early infancy, and in childhood.

Congenital and Neonatal Onset of Cloudy Cornea

Corneal Dystrophy

There are 2 important corneal dystrophies that cause clouding of the cornea at birth or in early infancy: Congenital Hereditary Endothelial Dystrophy (CHED) and Posterior Polymorphous Dystrophy (PPMD). These are disorders of the corneal endothelium. The corneal endothelium actively pumps water out of the cornea, keeping the cornea clear. Dysfunction of the endothelium results in edema of the cornea and corneal clouding.

Congenital Hereditary Endothelial Dystrophy
Congenital hereditary endothelial dystrophy (CHED) is inherited as autosomal dominant or autosomal recessive. The autosomal recessive form is more common and presents at birth or in the neonatal period with bilateral corneal opacities. The opacities can cause decreased visual acuity in the neonatal period and, therefore, may cause bilateral amblyopia and nystagmus. The cornea has an opaque, ground-glass appearance secondary to corneal edema (**Figure 15-1**). CHED appears similar to cloudy corneas secondary to congenital glaucoma; however, in congenital glaucoma, the intraocular pressure is high and corneal diameters are large. In CHED, the cause of the corneal edema is abnormal corneal endothelium

Table 15-1.
Cloudy Cornea: Congenital and Neonatal Onset

1. Birth trauma (forceps injury) *Chapter 23*	Unilateral, central, stromal and/or epithelial opacity due to breaks in Descemet's membrane. Usually resolves, though amblyopia may result from slow resolution.
2. Congenital glaucoma *Chapter 12*	Unilateral or bilateral epithelial and stromal opacity later. Increased corneal diameter with high intraocular pressure.
Infectious Keratopathy	
3. Herpes 2 keratitis *Chapter 13*	Unilateral localized cloudy corneal lesion (ulcer), positive fluorescein corneal staining. Viral culture for herpes.
4. *Neisseria Gonorrhoeae* *Chapter 13*	Severe neonatal purulent conjunctivitis with punctate epithelial fluorescein staining that can lead to corneal ulcer.
Metabolic Disease	
5. Mucopolysaccharidoses (Hurler syndrome, Scheie syndrome) *Chapter 24*	Bilateral, diffuse opacities by 6 to 12 months. Progressive, corneal opacity but does well with corneal transplant.
6. Mucolipidosis IV *Chapter 24*	Bilateral corneal clouding in first year of life. Conjunctival biopsy shows typical inclusion cells.
7. Cystinosis *Chapter 24*	Bilateral cystine corneal deposits. Widespread systemic crystal deposition. Renal involvement in infantile form (Fanconi syndrome).
Corneal Dystrophy	
8. Congenital Hereditary Endothelial Dystrophy (CHED) *This chapter*	Bilateral, diffuse corneal thickening. Autosomal recessive form is stationary, while autosomal dominant form is progressive.
9. Congenital Hereditary Stromal Dystrophy (CHSD) *This chapter*	Bilateral, central, flaky, corneal clouding. Autosomal dominant non progressive.
Corneal Dysgenesis	
10. Sclerocornea *This chapter*	Bilateral or unilateral peripheral opacity. Associated with other abnormalities (Goldenhar syndrome).
11. Peters anomaly *This chapter*	Central corneal opacity with defects in posterior stroma, Descemet's membrane and endothelium. Eighty percent are bilateral.
12. Limbal dermoid *This chapter*	Unilateral, temporal opacity. Increasing size or post-excision scarring may cause astigmatism and amblyopia.

Table 15-2.
Cloudy Cornea: Late Infancy and Childhood

Metabolic Disease	
1. Mucopolysaccharidoses *Chapter 24*	Bilateral, diffuse opacities. Types I and VI present in early childhood.
2. Tyrosinemia *Chapter 24*	Corneal epithelial deposits start in infancy. Blood and urine positive for tyrosine.
Trauma	
3. Corneal blood staining *Chapter 23*	Unilateral diffuse brown staining following hyphema. Slow resolution can result in amblyopia.
Infectious Keratitis	
4. Congenital syphilis Late interstitial keratitis *This chapter*	Bilateral with corneal edema and vascularization in acute stage (salmon patch). In quiescent stage, "ghost vessels" in stroma.
5. Rubella keratitis *Chapter 22*	Microcornea, central epithelial and stromal opacities, and cataract. May cause infantile glaucoma.
6. Measles keratitis *This chapter*	Corneal epithelium involved, positive punctate fluorescein staining pattern. Keratitis occurs 1 to 2 days prior to skin rash.
7. Herpes type 1 keratitis *Chapter 13*	Unilateral recurrent keratitis with mild conjunctivitis and faint clouding of the cornea. Positive fluorescein staining often in a dendritic pattern.
8. Infectious Keratitis; Bacterial and Fungal, and Protozoan (Corneal ulcer) *This chapter*	Usually unilateral localized white corneal lesion associated with conjunctival inflammation. Positive fluorescein staining. Often a history of extended wear contact lens use, or corneal trauma.
Dry Eye and Exposure	
9. Dry eye syndromes *Chapter 12*	Lid retraction, facial nerve palsy, anesthetic cornea, tear hyposecretion.
10. Familial dysautonomia (Riley-Day syndrome) *Chapter 12*	Autosomal recessive, corneal opacity secondary to reduced lacrimation or decreased corneal sensation.
11. Anesthetic cornea (neurotrophic ulcer) *This chapter*	Decreased corneal sensation, lack of sensory innervation, isolated congenital trigeminal anesthesia, fifth cranial nerve damage, chronic topical anesthetic cornea, chemical burns.

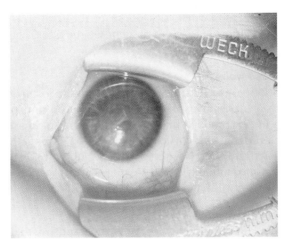

Figure 15-1.
Congenital hereditary endothelial dystrophy (CHED). A baby with a cloudy and thickened, but normal-sized, cornea. The patient had a bilateral disease with nystagmus because of decreased vision since birth.

resulting in abnormal hydration of the cornea. Treatment for this disorder is **corneal transplantation;** however, the prognosis of corneal transplantation in infancy is guarded. Children with autosomal dominant CHED develop corneal clouding later (at a few years of age), do not develop nystagmus, and have a better visual prognosis.

Posterior Polymorphous Dystrophy

Posterior polymorphous dystrophy (PPMD) results in bilateral cloudy corneas at birth or in early infancy. Corneal clouding is quite mild and usually does not interfere with visual acuity. Since the corneal opacity is very mild, treatment is usually not necessary. In rare cases, however, the opacity will progress and corneal transplantation may be indicated. In most cases, PPMD is an isolated corneal problem, but some cases have been associated with glaucoma.

Corneal Dysgenesis (Anterior Segment Dysgenesis)

In contrast to the corneal dystrophies (which are progressive), corneal dysgenesis syndromes are usually static. These diseases represent embryologic dysgenesis, probably related to abnormal neural crest cell migration. In addition to corneal changes, the iris and lens may also be abnormal. Dysgenesis of the cornea, iris, and/or lens is termed anterior segment dysgenesis (see also Chapter 11 — Rieger anomaly and Aniridia).

Posterior Embryotoxon

Posterior embryotoxon is, perhaps, the mildest form of anterior segment dysgenesis. It is an anteriorly displaced and prominent Schwalbe's line. Schwalbe's line is the anatomical landmark separating the sclera from the cornea (**Figure 15-2**). This is present in 15% of normal children. Isolated posterior embryotoxon is a benign condition. Approximately 90% of patients with Alagille syndrome (see Chapter 24) will have posterior embryotoxon.

Axenfeld-Rieger Syndrome

This is a peripheral anomaly of the cornea and iris that includes posterior embryotoxon (anteriorly displaced Schwalbe's line) and prominent iris processes attached to Schwalbe's line and peripheral cornea. Many consider Axenfeld syndrome to be a mild form of Rieger anomaly (see Chapter 11). More than 50% of patients with Axenfeld syndrome will have glaucoma.

Sclerocornea

Sclerocornea is a very white cornea and almost has the appearance of sclera (**Figure 15-3**). This disease may be unilateral or bilateral and is nonprogressive. Patients with bilateral sclerocornea often have bilateral amblyopia and nystagmus. Unilateral sclerocornea is often associated with unilateral dense amblyopia. Sclerocornea is not inherited and has no known causes. Treatment is corneal transplantation if the disease is bilateral. In unilateral cases, however, many pediatric ophthalmologists do not suggest surgery. The prog-

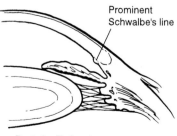

Prominent
Schwalbe's line

Posterior Embryotoxon

Figure 15-2.
Diagram of posterior embryotoxon.

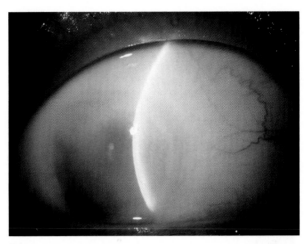

Figure 15-3.
Sclerocornea. A 20-year-old man born with sclerocornea with extension of the opaque scleral tissues onto the cornea and absence of the usual limbal change in contour. The other eye has minimal sclerocornea with good visual acuity.

nosis of corneal transplantation is very poor in infants because of low survival rates for corneal grafts and because of the unilateral dense amblyopia.

Peters Anomaly

Peters anomaly is a central corneal opacity of unknown etiology (**Figure 15-4**). It is usually not inherited; however, there are some families who show a high incidence of Peters anomaly. Some cases have been associated with maternal drug use. The cause of this corneal opacity is the congenital absence of both Descemet's membrane and the corneal endothelium (**Figure 15-5**). This anomaly probably represents abnormal migration of neural crest cells. Associated systemic anomalies have been described including cardiac defects, cleft lip, cleft palate, craniofacial dysplasia, and skeletal changes. In most cases, however, the Peters anomaly is isolated to the eye. Treatment of Peters anomaly depends on the severity of the opacity. If the opacity is bilateral and blocks the visual axis, nystagmus and dense bilateral amblyopia are common. Under these conditions, corneal transplantation is advised. The prognosis for corneal transplantation is guarded because of the complications of graft rejection and dense amblyopia. Because of the poor results

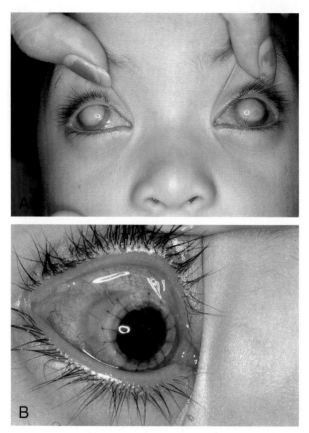

Figure 15-4.
A, Bilateral Peters anomaly showing central corneal opacity. This patient also had glaucoma. Note that the corneas are large. **B,** Eye from Figure 15-4A after corneal transplantation, showing the clear corneal graft. Unfortunately, a massive graft rejection occurred 6 months after surgery.

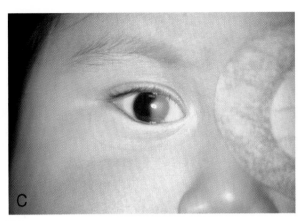

Figure 15-4.
(continued) **C,** Unilateral Peters anomaly that splits the pupil. This patient was treated conservatively with pupillary dilatation to expand the involved pupil and improve vision, and part-time occlusion of the fellow eye to manage the amblyopia. This opacity improved over several years.

with corneal transplantation, patients with unilateral Peters anomaly are often treated conservatively without surgery. In some cases, Peters anomaly is associated with lens subluxation and lens adherence to the cornea (**Figure 15-6**).

Limbal Dermoids
Limbal dermoids are choristomas and represent abnormal surface ectodermal tissue on the surface of the cornea. These are white or

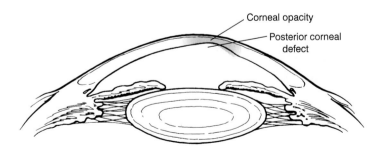

Figure 15-5.
Drawing of a corneal opacity. Peters anomaly is a defect in the posterior cornea with overlying corneal scarring.

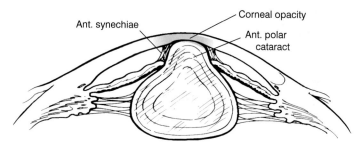

Ant. synechiae

Corneal opacity

Ant. polar cataract

Peters Anomaly

Figure 15-6.
Drawing of lens adherence to cornea. Peters anomaly comes in various forms, all having a central corneal scar with a posterior defect and central iris adhesions.

yellowish masses at the periphery of the cornea (limbus) and are usually unilateral (**Figure 15-7**). The limbal mass can cause irritation secondary to interference with blinking and tear coverage of the cornea. Corneal dermoids can also induce astigmatism, cause decreased visual acuity, and require surgical excision. In some cases, a corneal graft is required to replace corneal tissue. Close examination of the dermoid often shows the presence of hair and hair follicles. The tissue limbal dermoid cysts may be isolated or occur in association with Goldenhar syndrome (see Chapter 24).

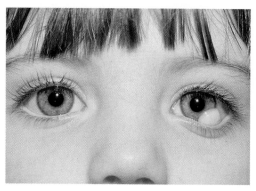

Figure 15-7.
Limbal dermoids. A young child with a dermoid tumor at the corneal limbus. It was removed with a shave keratectomy.

Acquired Cloudy Cornea in Childhood

There are numerous causes of an acquired cloudy cornea, and the more important causes are listed in **Table 15-2.** The following are topics not covered in other chapters.

Congenital Syphilis

Syphilis is acquired in utero at any stage of pregnancy. At birth, there may be a generalized skin rash, jaundice, hepatosplenomegaly, rhinitis, and anorexia. The eyes appear normal. The first ocular complication includes a retinochoroiditis, occurring in the first few months to a year of life. By age 2 years, patients often show signs of neurosyphilis and central nervous system involvement. The classical Hutchinson's teeth occur as notched teeth and are late manifestations. The corneal involvement usually occurs late, between 5 and 20 years of age, as **interstitial keratitis.** This is an inflammation of the deep corneal stroma that leads to corneal opacity. The cornea can become quite vascularized, and the vascular pattern can produce what is termed as a corneal salmon patch. Treatment for ocular manifestations consists of using topical corticosteroids and cycloplegics along with systemic treatment for the neurosyphilis. The systemic treatment of the neurosyphilis alone does not treat the interstitial keratitis, as it is an inflammatory reaction and not necessarily caused by active infection.

Measles

Measles is caused by an RNA paramyxovirus and presents with an acute cough and conjunctivitis. In addition, patients have a keratitis with superficial punctate epithelial fluorescein staining. There are characteristic Koplik's spots on the conjunctiva and caruncle. In most cases, the eye involvement is relatively mild; however, in chronically ill or malnourished children, the keratitis can be quite severe. In developing countries, measles is a self-limiting disease, but can be devastating and sometimes life-threatening in underdeveloped countries where there are large numbers of malnourished children. The more severe systemic complications of measles include pneumonia and acute encephalitis. Rarely seen is the occurrence of subacute sclerosing panencephalitis (SSPE). The treatment for the keratitis in uncomplicated measles is symptomatic relief with artificial tears. If there is a keratitis demonstrated by fluorescein staining of the cornea, then topical antibiotics should be used to prevent secondary bacterial infection. Topical corticosteroids-antibiotic combination can be used to reduce inflammation in severe cases.

Corneal Ulcers

Corneal ulcers are caused by a breakdown of the corneal epithelium with resultant necrosis of the corneal stroma. Corneal ulcers can be noninfectious (trophic ulcer), and caused by chronic corneal diseases such as vasculitis, severe corneal exposure, lack of sensory innervation (neurotrophic ulcer), or lack of vascular supply to peripheral cornea (lye burn). Infections cause corneal ulcerations when the infection violates the corneal epithelium and invades the corneal stroma. Clinically, the corneal ulcer presents as a white lesion in the cornea (**Figure 15-8** and see Chapter 13, Figure 3). There is usually positive fluorescein staining in the area of the ulcer indicating the absence of corneal epithelium. If the lesion is in the visual axis, vision will be severely affected. Infectious corneal ulcers are difficult to treat, as the cornea is avascular and therefore immu-

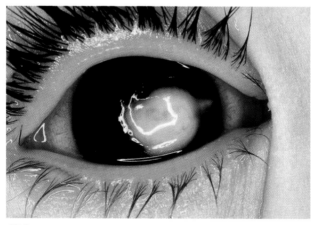

Figure 15-8.
Bacterial corneal ulcer is the white lesion in the central area of the cornea.

nocompromised. In many cases, weeks of high-dose antimicrobial therapy are necessary to eradicate the offending organism. One of the major problems is secondary corneal scarring that occurs after the infection is cured. Corneal scarring may interfere with vision necessitating corneal transplantation. The presence of a white corneal lesion and an inflamed eye should prompt immediate referral to an ophthalmologist. Infectious corneal ulcers can be caused by bacteria, fungus, virus, and even protozoa.

Bacterial Ulcer

Bacterial corneal ulcers are quite rare in children, because the intact corneal epithelium prevents penetration of bacteria within the corneal stroma. A breakdown of the corneal epithelium, however, will provide a portal of entry for bacteria. Eyelid abnormalities (entropion with eyelash rubbing of the cornea), dry eyes, corneal exposure, and corneal trauma break down the corneal epithelium and increase the risk of bacterial infection. The use of extended-wear contact lenses is another risk factor for developing bacterial keratitis. A history of conjunctivitis associated with contact lens use should prompt immediate referral, as this may represent a bacterial keratitis.

Bacterial species that cause corneal ulcers include pseudomonas, staphylococcus, Moraxella, *Streptococcus pneumoniae*, bacillus, and even acid-fast bacilli. Treatment of bacterial keratitis includes the use of a topical antibiotic every half-hour to every hour once cultures and Gram stain of the ulcer have been obtained. Intravenous antibiotics are not used because of insufficient drug delivery to the avascular cornea. Early diagnosis and treatment are critical. Once the central visual axis is involved, visual acuity is often lost as a result of secondary scarring after the bacterial infection has resolved. Patients are often admitted to the hospital for treatment of large bacterial ulcers that threaten the visual axis.

Fungal Ulcer

Fungal infection of the cornea is very rare, occurring much less frequently than bacterial corneal ulcers. Fungal keratitis occurs more often in temperate climates and in the tropics, often associated with vegetation foreign bodies and corneal trauma (**Figure 15-9**). Candida and Aspergillus are 2 of the most common causes of fungal keratitis. Treatment consists of topical and systemic antifungal agents.

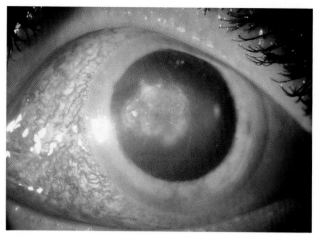

Figure 15-9.
Fungal ulcer. A 29-year-old outdoor laborer, 1 week after being struck in the eye with a branch. He was treated with topical antibiotic steroid ointment with worsening of the condition. Culture grew Aspergillus.

Protozoan Corneal Ulcer

Corneal ulcers can be caused by Acanthamoeba, a protozoan found in contaminated water and contaminated homemade contact lens solution. Acanthamoeba keratitis presents with severe pain and foreign body sensation appearing to be out of proportion to the ocular inflammation. Treatment includes debridement and topical treatment with antimicrobial agents. Diamidines, aminoglycoside, and imidazole compounds can be used in conjunction to eradicate the infestation. In addition, polymeric biguanides used in swimming pools can be diluted and used for acanthamoeba keratitis. In many cases, corneal transplantation is required.

Neurotrophic Ulcer

Denervation of the corneal sensory nerves from the trigeminal ganglion results in corneal disease. Sensory deprivation results in decreased cellular metabolism and decreased mitotic rate. Over time, usually several weeks, lack of sensory innervation to the cornea leads to decreased corneal clarity, corneal epithelial defects, and, eventually, corneal vascularization and opacification (**Figure 15-10**). Causes of decreased innervation are listed in **Table 15-3**.

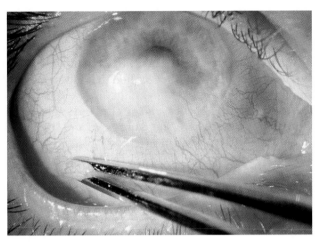

Figure 15-10.
Anesthetic cornea. A teenager with congenital absence of fifth cranial nerve function demonstrating severe changes of neurotrophic keratopathy. The patient did not feel the forceps moving the conjunctiva.

Table 15-3.
Causes of Neurotrophic Ulcer

Congenital Onset:
1. Congenital trigeminal anesthesia
2. Familial dysautonomia
Acquired Onset:
1. Fifth trigeminal nerve damage
2. Closed head trauma
3. Intracranial tumors
4. Intracranial aneurysm
5. Neurosurgery
Corneal Disease:
1. Herpes Simplex keratitis
2. Herpes Zoster keratitis
3. Chronic contact lens wear
Chronic Topical Anesthetic Abuse:
1. Timolol (topical glaucoma medications)
2. Chemical burns

Treatment of neurotrophic ulcers includes the use of artificial tears and topical lubricants. Patients should be warned not to use topical anesthetic drops, as this is an important cause of a neurotrophic ulcer. In severe cases of neurotrophic ulcer, a conjunctival graft is placed over the cornea, even though it blocks vision. A **tarsorrhaphy,** a procedure where the eyelids are sutured together, can be used to protect the cornea and preserve the globe. Unfortunately, in severe cases where the damage to the sensory nerve is permanent, the neurotrophic ulcer can progress to ulceration and perforation, with loss of the globe.

■ KERATOCONUS

Keratoconus is a noninflammatory, self-limiting ectasia of the central portion of the cornea. It is characterized by progressive thinning and steepening of the central cornea. Keratoconus occurs in about .15% to .6% of the general population; however, data on prevalence of keratoconus vary greatly. Onset of keratoconus occurs during the teenage years—mean age of onset is age 16 years, but onset has been reported to occur at ages as young as 6 years. Keratoconus shows no gender predilection and is bilateral in more than 90% of cases. Often, patients with keratoconus have had several spectacle prescriptions in a short period of time, and none has provided satisfactory vision correction. Refractions are often variable and inconsistent. Patients with keratoconus often report monocular diplopia or polyopia and complain of distortion rather than blur at both distance and near vision. Some report halos around lights and photophobia. During the active stage, change may be rapid; although unusual, contact lenses may have to be refit as often as every 3 to 4 months. In general, the disease develops asymmetrically.

Atopic disease (eg, hay fever, atopic dermatitis, asthma) has been suggested as an etiologic component of keratoconus. Patients with keratoconus are chronic eye rubbers, and it is theorized that rubbing indents the cornea, and may make the cornea yield at its weakest point, the center. Hormonal influence has been addressed as a possible cause, a supposition supported by the initial onset around puberty and tendency to progress during pregnancy or to exacerbate during menopause. Systemic conditions linked to keratoconus include Down syndrome, Ehlers-Danlos syndrome, Crouzon syndrome (craniofacial dysostosis), and Marfan syndrome. To date, no single, clear-cut cause of keratoconus has been found. Treatment consists of providing a hard contact lens to establish a smooth surface to the cornea. If the contact lens fails and the cornea becomes thin and distorted causing decreased visual acuity, a corneal transplant may be necessary. It is rare that a child would have severe keratoconus that would require a corneal transplant.

16 Eyelid and Orbital Masses

A mass, or tumor, behind the eye will push the eye forward causing proptosis (exophthalmos), an important sign that an orbital mass is present. Proptosis often presents with one eye appearing larger than the other eye, as the proptotic eye pushes the eyelids apart, causing a wider lid fissure (**Figure 16-1**). Anterior orbital masses and eyelid masses cause narrowing of the lid fissure (**Figure 16-2**). An acquired lid or orbital mass requires immediate evaluation, with orbital imaging to rule out severe orbital disease such as Rhabdomyosarcoma. **Table 16-1** presents the differential diagnosis of pediatric proptosis.

■ CAPILLARY HEMANGIOMA

The most common vascular ocular tumor seen in children is the capillary hemangioma. This is a hamartoma, as it is made up of tissue normally found in the eyelid. During the first few weeks of life, the lesion will be small. Over the next few months, it progressively increases in size. The tumor generally shows spontaneous regression by 4 to 7 years of age. If the tumor is superficial, it has a red or strawberry appearance (**Figure 16-2A**—nose and right brow). Deeper tumors will have a bluish appearance or no significant cutaneous color change (**Figure 16-2**—left upper lid). The diagnosis can often be facilitated by everting the eyelid to visualize the vascularity of the hemangioma (**Figure 16-3**).

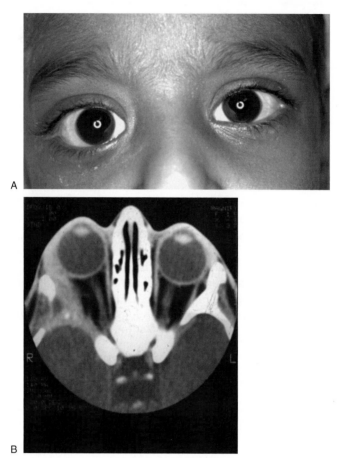

Figure 16-1.
A, Four-year-old boy with Hand-Shuller-Christians disease and proptosis of the right eye caused by a posterior orbital mass. Note that the lid fissure is wider on the right.
B, Axial CT scan of the patient in Figure 16-1A, demonstrating right lateral orbital lesion with destruction of the lateral orbital wall. Note that the right eye is proptotic and forward as compared to the left eye. From Johnson T, et al: Clinicopathological correlation. *Saudi Bul Ophthalmol* 1988;3:31.

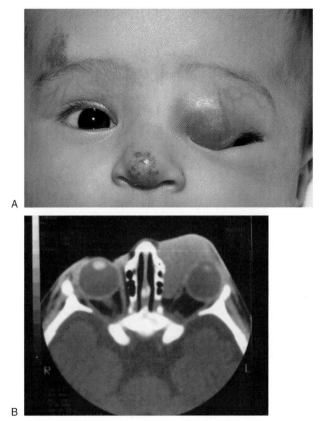

Figure 16-2.
A, Infant with large hemangioma involving the left upper lid and orbit, tip of the nose, and superior aspect of right eyebrow. Note that the mass is causing severe ptosis and obstructing the visual axis. **B,** Contrast enhanced CT scan of the child pictured in Figure 16-2A, showing large anterior orbital mass involving the right upper lid and medial orbit.

Table 16-1.
Differential Diagnosis of Pediatric Proptosis

Disease	History and Symptoms	Findings	Treatment
Orbital Cellulitis	Pain, fever, eyelid swelling, associated sinus disease, tooth extraction, trauma.	Proptosis, poor ocular motility, possible decrease in vision, Marcus Gunn pupil. Orbital imaging shows inflammation, possible abscess.	IV antibiotics, possible surgical abscess drainage.
Infantile Hemangioma	Congenital mass increasing within the first year of life, then stabilizes, then regresses by 4 to 7 years of age.	Possible association with a red, strawberry birthmark or a bluish discoloration of the skin. Posterior lesions cause proptosis. Ptosis may cause amblyopia.	Observation, unless amblyopia is present, then intralesional corticosteroid injections are indicated.
Lymphangioma	May go unnoticed until acute intralesional hemorrhage occurs during the first decade of life; may increase in size with upper respiratory tract infections.	Acute proptosis with ecchymosis, multi-lobulated lesion on CT scan, blood chocolate cysts, severe hemorrhage can lead to optic nerve compression.	Avoid head trauma, curtail activity. Surgical decompression if optic nerve is compromised or amblyopia present.
Plexiform Neurofibroma	Neurofibromatosis, painless lid mass.	Café-au-lait spots, S-shaped lid deformity; "bag-of-worms" on palpations. If sphenoid wing is involved, there is pulsatile exophthalmos.	Observation, unless proptosis is severe; then surgical debulking.
Optic Nerve Glioma	First decade, painless proptosis, slow growth; often associated with NF1.	CT scan shows optic nerve tumor. Optic atrophy late in the disease, firm to retropulsion, poor visual acuity, Marcus Gunn pupil.	Observation; if chiasm threatened, radiation and/or neurosurgery.

Table 16-1.
(continued)

Disease	History and Symptoms	Findings	Treatment
Rhabdomyosarcoma	Rapid onset, painless proptosis, any age (7 to 8 years median).	Tumor usually in orbit with inferior globe displacement, lid edema and erythema common.	Biopsy urgent, radiation and chemotherapy; good prognosis if tumor is confined to orbit.
Metastatic Neuroblastoma	Young child with rapid onset of proptosis, eyelid ecchymosis.	Horner syndrome. Abdominal mass on MRI, increased urine VMA, diaphoresis, tachycardia, orbital bony distruction on CT.	Urgent biopsy, irradiation and chemotherapy, poor prognosis.
Orbital Pseudotumor	Rapid onset of proptosis, pain on eye movements, malaise, fever, often bilateral.	Lid swelling, edema, possible proptosis, possible iritis, diffuse inflammatory mass on CT.	Oral corticosteroids.
Langerhans Cell Histiocytosis	Palpable tender mass, skin rash, runny nose, fever.	CT scan shows mass with lytic bone lesions, palpable lymph nodes.	Excision, radiation, chemotherapy.
Dermoid Cysts	Slow growth with onset of diplopia.	CT scan shows cysts attached to bone with bone scalloping.	Surgical excision.
Chorioma (Leukemia)	Rapid growth, fever.	CT scan shows diffuse orbital mass, peripheral blood may show increased white count and cell atypia consistent with leukemia.	Pediatric oncology and chemotherapy.

Capillary hemangiomas are benign tumors, but amblyopia may occur if the mass closes the eyelid compromising the visual axis. Even small amounts of ptosis can cause significant amblyopia. Therefore, any child with ptosis from a lid mass should be referred for ophthalmic evaluation. If the visual axis is clear, treatment is often deferred, as the lesions will regress spontaneously. If amblyopia is present, then treatment includes systemic interferon, sys-

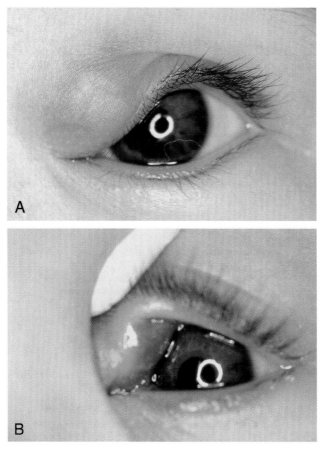

Figure 16-3.
A, Eyelid mass of nasal aspect of the left upper lid. Note that the skin does not have the typical red, strawberry appearance. **B,** Eversion of the upper eyelid discloses the hemangioma seen through the conjunctiva.

temic corticosteroids, or intralesional corticosteroid injection. In this author's experience, corticosteroid injection is the most effective treatment for large hemangiomas that block the visual axis. There have been a few isolated reports of visual loss secondary to retrograde embolization of the central retinal artery during intralesional corticosteroid injection. This complication can be reduced and, perhaps, avoided if the volume of injection is 2 mL or less and minimal pressure is used during the injection. Corticosteroid injections are most effective when done early in infants younger than 8 months of age. Repeat corticosteroid injections can be given; however, long-term local corticosteroid injections can cause adrenal axis depression and increase growth. Some advocate systemic corticosteroids, however, this author has found that systemic corticosteroids can cause significant side effects and do not deliver a large enough dose to significantly shrink most tumors. Surgical excision is reserved for small, localized lesions. It usually is avoided in larger lesions because of the risk of considerable bleeding and because the infiltrative nature of the lesion requires removal of large amounts of skin.

■ LYMPHANGIOMAS

Lymphangiomas are benign, vascular hamartomas that usually appear in childhood. Lymphangiomas may appear superficially, involving the conjunctiva, or may be located deep in the orbit. They tend to increase in size when the child has a viral cold or flu. These tumors have a tendency to spontaneously hemorrhage and develop spontaneous hematomas. Most often, the first sign of a lymphangioma is the rapid onset of proptosis secondary to acute bleeding within the tumor (**Figure 16-4**). The hemorrhage can form a hema-

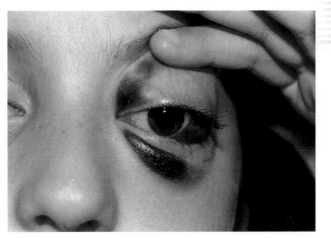

Figure 16-4.
Ten-year-old girl with acute proptosis and ecchymosis, left eye. Patient has a left orbital lymphangioma of the upper and lower lid that had an episode of acute hemorrhage. This was the first presenting sign of the lid angioma.

toma, or chocolate cyst, which is the accumulation of clotted blood. With very large hemorrhages, compression of the optic nerve may necessitate urgent surgical decompression.

There is no good treatment for lymphangiomas. Surgical excision of the lymphangioma is difficult because of the diffuse infiltrative nature of the tumor and its tendency to hemorrhage. Conservative management consists of preventing inadvertent trauma and limiting the child's activity.

■ DERMOID CYST

Dermoid cysts are benign choristomas (tissues not normally found at the involved site). Dermoid cysts arise from bony suture sites, most commonly seen at the anterior lateral orbit (**Figure 16-5**) or just superior to the nasolacrimal sac. Dermoid cysts may also be found deep in the orbit and may displace the eye (**Figures 16-6 A and B**). Dermoid cysts are lined with stratified squamous epithelium and are filled with keratin and adnexal structures such as hair shafts, sweat glands, and meibomian glands. Traumatic rupture of a dermoid cyst may produce severe inflammation and secondary scarring. Because of this, most ophthalmologists suggest early removal, shortly after 6 months of age. Complete excision of the dermoid cyst results in an excellent prognosis.

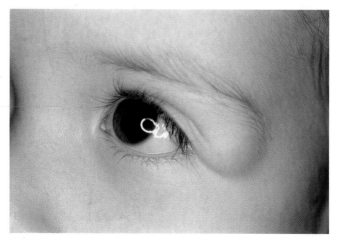

Figure 16-5.
A 6-month-old infant with a superior temporal dermoid cyst, left eye. Note the distortion of the eyebrow and lateral aspect of the upper lid.

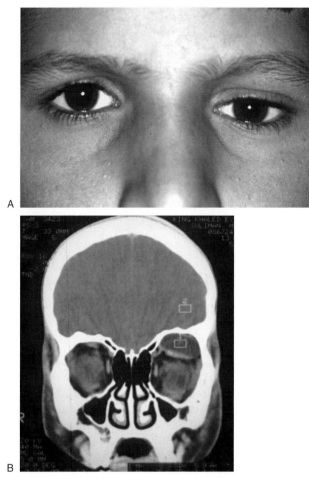

Figure 16-6.
A, Thirteen-year-old boy with downward displacement of the left eye secondary to a deep orbital dermoid cyst. **B,** Coronal CT scan of the patient in Figure 16-6A, showing the superior orbital dermoid cyst and expansion of the left orbit.

■ DERMOLIPOMA

Dermolipoma is a gelatinous mass located in the lateral canthus area (**Figure 16-7**). These masses are choristomas that contain fatty tissues with dermal appendages. Generally, no treatment is needed. Surgical excision is indicated only when the mass presents a signifi-

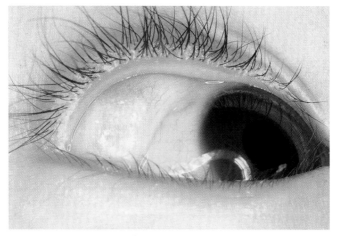

Figure 16-7.
Dermolipoma of the left eye. Note the fatty mass in the lateral canthal area.

cant cosmetic problem. Surgical removal can cause local scarring and limited ocular motility.

■ OPTIC NERVE TUMORS

Optic nerve gliomas are relatively rare in children. Seventy percent of children with optic nerve gliomas will have neurofibromatosis type 1. Most cases are unilateral; however, bilateral cases occur, and are almost always pathognomonic of neurofibromatosis. The tumors may occur anywhere along the course of the optic nerve, chiasm, or optic tracts. Unfortunately, there is no good treatment at this time, and the management remains controversial. Patients with good vision and lesions isolated to the optic nerve (not threatening the chiasm) are usually observed. Tumors that show rapid growth or involve the optic chiasm may require neurosurgical intervention. Radiation therapy has also been used for non-resectable tumors.

■ FIBRO-OSSEOUS TUMORS

Tumors involving fibrous connective tissue from bone and cartilage can occur in the orbit. Patients present with proptosis, and computed tomography (CT) is critical to making the appropriate diagnosis. Of these lesions, **fibrous dysplasia** is one of the more common. This is a hamartoma that involves the bony structure of the orbit. Children present with facial asymmetry, proptosis, and globe displacement. The frontal bone is most commonly affected and results in downward ocular displacement. Malignant transformation is uncommon; however, it has been reported. Computed tomography scan shows characteristic translucent zones within the bone, as well as large sclerotic areas (**Figure 16-8**).

Management includes observation unless there is optic nerve compression or severe proptosis. In those cases, surgery may be indicated.

Ewing's sarcoma is a primary tumor of the bone in childhood that rarely involves the orbit. Most orbital cases are metastatic from distant sites. Ophthalmic symptoms include proptosis, pain, restriction of ocular motility and, occasionally, visual loss. Treatment includes surgical extirpation, radiotherapy, and chemotherapy.

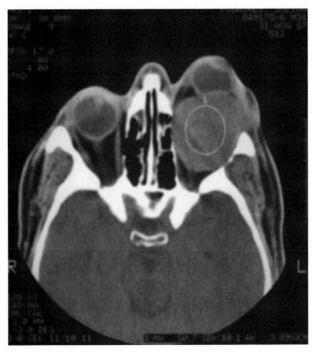

Figure 16-8.
Axial CT scan of a young boy with mono-ostotic fibrous dysplasia with characteristic ground-glass appearance of the bone.

■ LANGERHANS CELL HISTIOCYTOSIS

Abnormal proliferation of histiocytes is termed Langerhans cell histiocytosis. It consists of previously described conditions, eosinophilic granulomas, Hand-Schüller-Christian disease, and Letterer-Siwe disease. Eosinophilic granulomas are most common in children and result in a solitary osseous lesion in the orbit. The lesion causes bony erosion and soft tissue expansion, with the frontal and zygomatic bones most frequently involved. Hand-Schüller-Christian disease has the classic triad of diabetes insipidus, bilateral proptosis, and bony punched-out lesions of the cranial bones (**Figure 16-1**). This disease almost always affects infants and young children and may have a cutaneous component, with orbital involvement rarely being present. Letterer-Siwe disease carries the worst prognosis and is associated with hepatosplenomegaly, lymphadenopathy, jaundice, anemia, respiratory insufficiency, osseous defects, and thrombocytopenia. This disease has a very high mortality rate.

■ RHABDOMYOSARCOMAS

Rhabdomyosarcoma is a malignant tumor that arises from undifferentiated mesenchymal tissues of the orbit that are precursors to striated muscle. This is the most common malignant orbital neoplasm in children. Most children present with a rapid onset of painless proptosis or an acquired lid mass. Tumors most commonly occur between the ages of 6 and 10 years; however, these tumors can present at virtually any age, even infancy. This is a potentially lethal tumor but, if it is confined to the orbit at the time of presentation, there is a 90% survival rate at 3 years. Once the tumor spreads beyond the orbit, the survival rate diminishes significantly. Therefore, it is important to obtain an urgent ophthalmic consultation for any child with an acquired proptosis, in order to rule out rhabdomyosarcoma. At one time, the treatment of this tumor was surgical exenteration of the orbit, which resulted in a poor survival rate. Recently, with the use of radiation therapy combined with chemotherapy, survival rates have improved dramatically. A biopsy may be necessary if orbital imaging does not make the definitive diagnosis.

Of the 3 types of rhabdomyosarcoma tumors (embryonal, alveolar, and pleomorphic), the embryonal tumors most commonly occur within the orbit. Histopathology reveals fascicles of spindle cells with small hyperchromatic nuclei. Electron microscopy often shows cross-striations consistent with striated muscle.

■ METASTATIC TUMORS OF THE ORBIT

The most common metastatic tumors of the orbit include lymphoid tumors and neuroblastoma. Other less common metastatic tumors of childhood include Ewing's sarcoma of orbital bone (can present as primary or metastatic) and Wilms tumor.

Leukemia and Lymphoid Tumors of the Orbit

Orbital tumors known as granulocytic sarcoma, or **chorioma,** may occur with leukemia, especially acute myeloblastic leukemia. An orbital mass with proptosis may precede blood or bone marrow findings. Biopsies of these lesions may be misread as lymphoma, a very unusual orbital childhood tumor.

Neuroblastoma

Neuroblastoma of the orbit is the most common metastatic tumor of the orbit. The primary lesion arises from the abdomen or sympathetic tissue within the mediastinal, cervical, and pelvic regions (**Figure 16-9**). Patients usually present around 2 years of age with rapid onset of painless proptosis often associated with eyelid ecchymosis. The ecchymosis comes from hemorrhage within the tumor resulting from tissue necrosis as the tumor outgrows its vascular supply. Approximately 20% of patients with neuroblastoma develop orbital metastasis.

Tumors within the orbit can cause lytic bony lesions and bone erosion. Other ocular findings of neuroblastoma include Horner syndrome and opsoclonus-myoclonus (dancing eyes, dancing feet syndrome). Urine vanillylmandelic acid (VMA) and homovanillic acid (HVA) are often elevated in patients with neuroblastoma.

■ PRESEPTAL AND ORBITAL CELLULITIS

Cellulitis of the orbit can be divided into **preseptal cellulitis** (periorbital cellulitis) and **orbital cellulitis.**

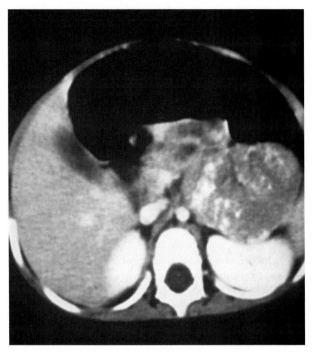

Figure 16-9.
Abdominal CT scan demonstrates primary abdominal neuroblastoma originating in the adrenal gland.

Preseptal Cellulitis

Preseptal cellulitis is an infection of tissues anterior to the orbital septum, which is the connective tissue boundary between the eyelids and the posterior orbit. Preseptal cellulitis, therefore, involves the tissues of the eyelids (**Figure 16-10**), but does not involve the posterior orbit. It is often associated with upper respiratory tract infections, local trauma, bacteremia, or sinusitis. Signs include erythema of the upper or lower lid, swelling of the lid, and tenderness. Since the infection only involves the anterior tissue, the eye motility is normal, there is no proptosis, and vision is good. The most common bacterial pathogens include *Haemophilus influenzae*, *Staphylococcus aureus*, Group A streptococcus, and *Streptococcus pneumoniae*. Children under 4 years of age are particularly susceptible to *H influenzae* infection; however, the incidence has decreased significantly since the advent of vaccination of *H influenzae*. The treatment for infants

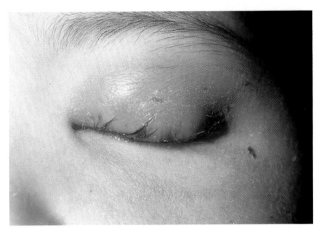

Figure 16-10.
Left preseptal cellulitis with swelling and erythema of the upper lid. The eye has full range of motion, no proptosis, and excellent vision.

with preseptal cellulitis may require admission to the hospital for intravenous antibiotics, but most pediatricians first prescribe cephalexin or amoxicillin/clavulanate as outpatient treatment to cover *S aureus* and Group A streptococcus. If admitted to the hospital, cefuroxime, a cephalosporin effective against *H influenzae, S aureus, and streptococci*, is used most often. For older children with milder preseptal cellulitis, oral cephalosporin can be given on an outpatient basis as long as there is close follow-up.

Orbital Cellulitis

Orbital cellulitis is an extremely dangerous condition and may be vision and/or life threatening. Orbital cellulitis can result in severe complications such as vision loss, meningitis, cavernous sinus thrombosis, brain abscess, and even death. The clinical characteristics of orbital cellulitis include erythema and swelling of the eyelids, proptosis, limitation of eye movement, and, in advanced cases, decreased vision (**Figure 16-11**). Orbital cellulitis is most commonly associated with sinusitis, but it can also occur secondary to an orbital fracture, infection of the skin, or lacrimal sac infection (**Figure 16-12**). Systemic effects of orbital cellulitis may be minimal, or patients may only have a mild increase in peripheral white counts and no fever. If orbital cellulitis is suspected, an immediate ophthalmic consultation along with a CT scan of the orbits is advised.

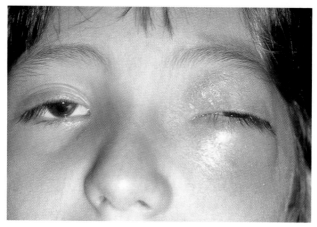

Figure 16-11.
Left orbital cellulitis in a 10-year-old child with a history of sinusitis. Note the swelling and true proptosis. The patient has limited eye movements, exotropia, and poor vision.

Other causes of orbital inflammation include pseudotumor of the orbit (discussed later in this chapter), ruptured dermoid cyst, and orbital neoplasms such as rhabdomyosarcoma. The most common organisms responsible for orbital cellulitis are similar to those of preseptal cellulitis, with the addition of anaerobes and Gram-negative organisms. Often, more than a single organism may be present. Blood cultures and cultures of the conjunctiva may identify the bacterial cause. Initial therapy is always broad-spectrum antibiotic coverage. Treatment of orbital cellulitis is admission to the hospital for intravenous antibiotics, usually cefuroxime. (**Figure 16-12**).

If sinusitis is present, an otolaryngology consultation is imperative to help manage the orbital cellulitis. In many cases, sinus surgery is indicated. A recent study comparing sinus drainage with no sinus drainage in subperiosteal abscesses showed that both groups had equal morbidity and mortality; however, the sinus drainage group improved more rapidly. Should abscesses not respond to antibiotics, or if the clinical course is worsening, then prompt surgical drainage is indicated.

Fungal Orbital Cellulitis

A fungal orbital cellulitis can occur, especially in immunocompromised patients. **Aspergillus** is a ubiquitous fungus that is usually

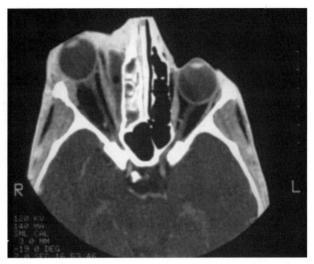

Figure 16-12.
Axial CT scan in a patient with a right orbital cellulitis and ethmoid sinusitis. Note there is a subperiosteal abscess, thickening of the eyelids, and proptosis of the right side.

considered harmless. Aspergillus cellulitis consists of a chronic fibrosing granulomatous infection that does not respond to standard antibiotic therapy. In these cases, culture and biopsy should be taken. Treatment includes surgical debridement and IV amphotericin B.

Mucormycosis

Mucormycosis is another fungal organism that can cause orbital cellulitis. This occurs in debilitated individuals, usually older patients in diabetic ketoacidosis, or immunocompromised patients. The infection starts within the paranasal sinuses and spreads into the orbit. The fungus causes vascular occlusion, leading to infarction and necrosis of the tissue. The disease is often fatal, and management includes local and systemic treatment with amphotericin B in addition to surgical excision of necrotic tissue. Hyperbaric oxygen therapy may be helpful.

■ ORBITAL PSEUDOTUMOR (IDIOPATHIC ORBITAL INFLAMMATORY DISEASE)

By definition, orbital pseudotumor is orbital inflammation having no known cause or underlying disease. Orbital inflammation can

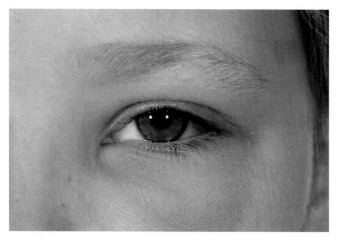

Figure 16-13.
Two-year-old child with pseudotumor involving the left lower lid. Note the erythema and swelling of the lid.

be associated with Wegener's Granulomatosis, Polyarteritis Nodosa, Sarcoidosis, and Systemic Lupus Erythematosus. These systemic diseases should be considered in those patients with noninfectious orbital inflammation. Orbital pseudotumor may affect any part of the orbit and, in children, 45% may be bilateral. The pseudotumor may be anterior to the orbital septum and involve the eyelids, or be posterior and cause proptosis. When anterior, the inflammation presents similar to a preseptal cellulitis with erythema and swelling of the involved eyelid (**Figure 16-13**). In addition to these most common signs, ocular pain and pain with eye movement appear more commonly and are more striking than in infectious cellulitis. Inflammation deep in the orbit will result in proptosis and, in some cases, limited ocular motility.

Tolosa-Hunt Syndrome

Tolosa-Hunt syndrome is a variant of a pseudotumor that affects the superior orbital fissure and cavernous sinus. It is described as a painful, external ophthalmoplegia. Patients present with pain behind the eye and limited motility, secondary to impairment of the third, fourth, and sixth cranial nerves. Affected patients also may have hypoesthesia of skin around the eye and decreased vision if the optic nerve is involved. In addition to the eye involvement, children may present with systemic symptoms such as headaches, fever, vomiting, pharyngitis, anorexia, abdominal pain, and lethargy. Pseudotumor tends to be recurrent and may alternate from one eye to the other. A biopsy may be necessary to establish a diagnosis and rule out a neoplasm. Histology shows nonspecific pleomorphic infiltrate of inflammatory cells including lymphocytes, plasma cells, macrophages, and eosinophils. The eosinophils are more commonly found in children. After the diagnosis is made and neoplasms have been ruled out, treatment is started with oral corticosteroids. Initial doses are 1 mg/kg per day of oral prednisone. After 10 to 14 days, the dose can be tapered over a 3-week period. In difficult cases that do not respond to the corticosteroids, immunosuppressive agents may be used.

■ Viral Papilloma

Viral papilloma are caused by human papilloma virus and may appear anywhere on the conjunctival surface. Papilloma may be difficult to see unless magnification is used for the examination. Papilloma may protrude from the lid margins **(Figures 16-14 A and B)**.

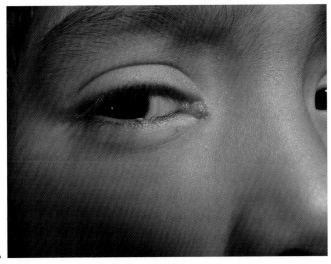

A

Figure 16-14.
Papilloma of the lower eyelid and medial canthus area. **A,** Photo shows lesion in the medial canthus.

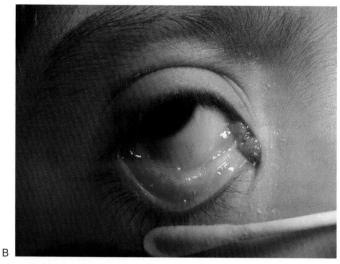

B

Figure 16-14.
(continued) **B,** Photo shows eversion of the eyelid and discloses that the lower eyelid conjunctiva is involved.

"Kissing" lesions may appear where the lids are in apposition. A vascular core serves to differentiate these lesions from nevi with which they may be confused clinically.

Treatment for papilloma is observation and cryotherapy. Surgical excision is likely to be followed by recurrence of the nevi. Cryotherapy should be done with care to avoid freezing the globe, skin, and tarsal plate.

17 Eyelid Disorders

The most common pediatric eyelid malformations are ptosis and epiblepharon (**Tables 17-1**), with less common malformations including entropion, ectropion, colobomas, cryptophthalmos, euryblepharon, and blepharophimosis (**Table 17-2**).

■ CONGENITAL PTOSIS

Congenital ptosis is a condition resulting in droopy eyelids at birth (**Figure 17-1**). This can be unilateral or bilateral. The most common type of ptosis is associated with a deficiency and fibrosis of the striated levator muscle. The levator muscle is the main elevator of the eyelid, with Müller's muscle contributing less significantly. It is thought to be a localized developmental muscle dysgenesis of unknown cause. Some patients may show improvement during the first year or 2 of life but, generally, the disorder remains static throughout life if not repaired. Most cases are sporadic; however, familial inheritance cases have been reported.

Congenital ptosis also can occur as part of blepharophimosis syndrome (discussed later in this chapter), Marcus Gunn jaw winking syndrome, congenital third nerve palsy (see Chapter 4, figure 13), syndromes involving congenital fibrosis of the extraocular muscles, or can occur secondary to trauma at birth. **Marcus Gunn jaw winking syndrome** is a rare syndrome caused by aberrant innervation of the levator muscle of the eyelid from the third branch of the trigeminal nerve. This results in ptosis and eyelid movement

253

Table 17-1.
Common Eyelid Disorders

- **Ptosis**—eyelid drooping
- **Epiblepharon**—eyelashes scratching the eye secondary to a redundant skin fold inducing a vertical orientation of the eyelashes

Table 17-2.
Less Common Eyelid Disorders

- **Blepharophimosis Syndrome**—Autosomal dominant. Most common findings are ptosis, blepharophimosis, epicanthus inversus, and telecanthus.
- **Coloboma**—An embryologic cleft found in the upper or lower eyelid. They can be unilateral or bilateral.
- **Cryptophthalmos**—Failure of eyelid formation. This can involve all of the eyelid or just portions.
- **Ectropion**—Out-turning of the eyelid secondary to insufficient skin.
- **Entropion**—In-turning of the eyelid. The eyelashes scratch the eye.
- **Euryblepharon**—A combination of horizontal eyelid laxity and vertically shortened skin, giving an appearance similar to ectropion.

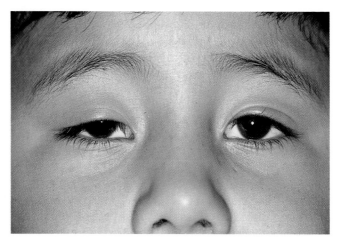

Figure 17-1.
Patient with bilateral upper eyelid ptosis, right greater than left. Note absent lid crease on the right and brow lift as patient attempts to open the eyes.

(winking) synchronized with mouth movement, crying, eating, and sucking. Children with congenital ptosis should be referred for ophthalmologic evaluation. Since ptosis can cause amblyopia, by either blocking the visual axis or inducing astigmatism, the vision of the eye and the refractive error have to be determined. If the vision is affected, then appropriate amblyopia therapy must be started. This can consist of patching the good eye and prescribing glasses. If the eyelid is so droopy that the lid interferes with vision, then early ptosis surgery is indicated. If the vision is not affected, then the child needs to be monitored closely until the ptosis is repaired, generally until the child is 3 to 5 years of age. Amblyopia may still develop as the patient grows while the ptosis is still present. Ptosis can also cause abnormal head positions (chin elevation) from the patient trying to see better, indicating that the ptosis is significant.

There are several different operations that can repair congenital ptosis. The most important factor in determining which operation is necessary is levator function. For a patient with excellent levator function and less than 3 mm of ptosis, surgery to the levator muscle or Müller's muscle can correct the ptosis. For a patient with moderate or excellent levator function and ptosis greater than 3 mm, levator muscle resection is indicated. In a patient with poor levator function, frontalis muscle suspension surgery is indicated. This is an operation whereby suture materials, such as fascia lata or silicone, suspend the eyelid to the frontalis muscle above the eyebrows. There are some surgeons who may still advocate levator surgery even in the face of poor levator function.

■ EPIBLEPHARON AND ENTROPION

Epiblepharon is a condition whereby a horizontal redundant skin fold under the eyelid induces a vertical orientation of the eyelashes, often resulting in the eyelashes touching the cornea (**Figure 17-2**). When eyelashes touch the cornea, this is termed **trichiasis.** Entropion is a true eyelid margin rotation, often causing trichiasis (**Figure 17-3**). Congenital entropion can occur in conjunction with congenital epiblepharon. The causes of congenital epiblepharon or entropion include improper development of the lower eyelid retractors with possible dehiscence near the tarsal plate, microphthalmos, and enophthalmos.

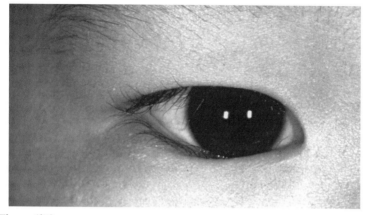

Figure 17-2.
Epiblepharon characterized by redundant pretarsal skin pressing the lashes against the cornea. The tarsal plate is in an upright position.

Epiblepharon tends to get better by itself as the patient grows, whereas entropion does not. The treatment of epiblepharon depends on the presence of corneal damage caused by lashes scratching the cornea. If there is no corneal damage, treatment consists of observation and possible use of artificial tears and ointments. If, however, there is chronic corneal damage with tearing, eye redness, and the patient rubbing his eyes, then conservative treatment with

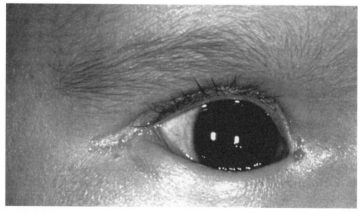

Figure 17-3.
Congenital entropion demonstrating in-turning of the lower lid margin. The tarsal plate is not in an upright position.

drops and ointments may be tried, but surgical correction is often necessary. Since epiblepharon resolves spontaneously with growth of the orbit, it is best to delay performing surgery if possible. Furthermore, if surgery is indicated, then minimal to no skin should be taken so that ectropion does not occur as the patient ages.

The treatment of congenital entropion is surgical. The entropion does not resolve as the patient gets older and, therefore, surgical correction is warranted. Surgery can be delayed as long as the corneal findings are not severe.

■ ECTROPION

Ectropion is a condition that results with the eyelids turning out (**Figure 17-4**). Childhood ectropion is rare, with the most common causes being congenital or cicatricial. Congenital ectropion is due to insufficient eyelid skin, causing the eyelid margin to pull out away from the eyeball. Cicatricial ectropion is secondary to scarring and/or loss of the skin after trauma, radiation, or prior surgery.

Treatment of ectropion consists of release of the traction by placement of a skin graft, flap, or skin and muscle flap. Since congenital ectropion occurs with many other findings (ie, euryblepharon, eyelid tumors, blepharophimosis syndrome, etc), other surgery often needs to be performed at the same time.

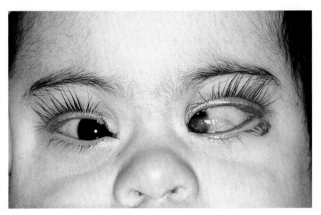

Figure 17-4.
Patient with esotropia and congenital ectropion of all 4 eyelids. This resulted in corneal ulcerations of the left eye.

■ EYELID COLOBOMAS

A coloboma is an embryologic cleft with abnormal closure (**Figure 17-5**). Eyelid colobomas occur from delayed or incomplete union of the mesodermal sheaths of the frontonasal and maxillary processes. They are often associated with other ocular, periorbital, or facial defects. Eyelid colobomas can occur in either the upper eyelid or lower eyelid. Upper eyelid colobomas are often full thickness and triangular in shape (occasionally quadrilateral or irregular). They are most often found medially, and the size ranges from a tiny indentation to the full length of the eyelid. They can be unilateral or bilateral. They often cause corneal exposure problems, especially if the defect is greater than one third the width of the eyelid.

In contrast, lower eyelid colobomas are usually partial thickness (with some remnants of orbicularis, tarsal remnants, cilia, or granular structures) and rounded. They are found most often laterally, and the length ranges from a tiny indentation to the full length of the eyelid. These also are found unilaterally or bilaterally. Lower eyelid colobomas can also cause corneal exposure problems and often cause trichiasis.

Treatment of eyelid colobomas depends on the status of the cornea. If there is minimal corneal exposure, medical treatment with drops or ointments is indicated, with elective surgery during the first 4 years of life. If moderate damage is present, medical treat-

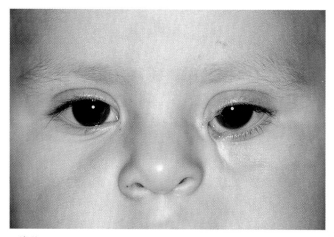

Figure 17-5.
Patient with left lower lid coloboma and associated left upper lid ptosis.

ment with drops and ointments is indicated with possible use of soft contact lenses and close follow-up. If the eye responds to treatment, then elective surgery can be performed during the first 4 years of life. If the corneal problems persist, reconstructive surgery should be done sooner. Finally, if severe corneal damage is present, the previously described temporizing measures should take place until surgery can be performed. Since surgery is easier to perform when the patient is older, due to increased laxity of the surrounding tissues, surgery should be delayed until it is either necessary or there is enough laxity of the surrounding tissues.

■ BLEPHAROPHIMOSIS SYNDROME

Blepharophimosis syndrome is an autosomal dominant syndrome with near 100% penetrance. It is found in males more often than females. The most common findings with blepharophimosis syndrome include ptosis, blepharophimosis, epicanthus inversus (abnormal slant of epicanthus), and telecanthus (wide intercanthal distance and normal interpupillary distance) (**Figure 17-6**). Other findings can include ectropion, trichiasis, punctal or canalicular malformations, broad and flat nasal bridge, bone deficiency at the supraorbital rim, strabismus, nystagmus, and optic disc colobomas.

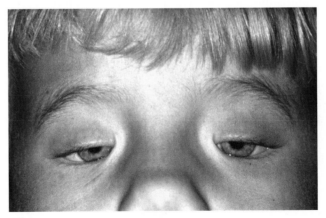

Figure 17-6.
Patient with blepharophimosis syndrome. Note the ptosis, phimosis, telecanthus, and epicanthus inversus.

Treatment of the blepharophimosis syndrome depends on the specific problems. The ptosis is repaired as described earlier in this section. The blepharophimosis, epicanthus inversus, and telecanthus can be repaired if the parents so desire.

■ EURYBLEPHARON

Euryblepharon is a type of ectropion associated with excess horizontal eyelid length and decreased vertical eyelid skin (**Figure 17-7**). As a result, the eyelids are pulled away from the eyeball and give an appearance of ectropion. It is most apparent in the lower eyelids; however, the upper eyelids can be involved. The cause of congenital euryblepharon is not known. It may be associated with other eyelid anomalies, including ptosis and telecanthus. Associated findings of nystagmus and esotropia have also been reported. It may be inherited, and an autosomal dominant variety has been reported.

Treatment of euryblepharon consists of reformation of the lateral canthal angle, removal of excess horizontal eyelid tissue, and replacing the deficient eyelid skin with either skin grafts or flaps. Timing of the surgery will depend on the status of the cornea as described in the eyelid coloboma portion of this chapter.

■ CRYPTOPHTHALMOS

Cryptophthalmos is a condition that results in failure of eyelid formation (**Figure 17-8**) and is often bilateral and symmetric. Autosomal recessive and autosomal dominant inheritance have been

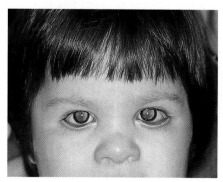

Figure 17-7.
Patient with congenital euryblepharon.

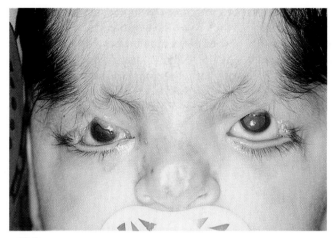

Figure 17-8.
Patient with bilateral cryptophthalmos and upper eyelid colobomas. Note the fusion of the upper eyelid skin to the eyeball.

reported. The globe is often abnormal, resulting in poor visual prognosis. Cryptophthalmos is divided into 3 types: the complete variety, the incomplete variety, and the symblepharon variety. In the complete variety, the eyelids do not form and the eyelid skin grows continuously from the forehead to the cheek, covering the underlying globe. The globe is usually abnormal. The incomplete variety presents with facial skin fusing to the medial aspect of the globe, with no eyelid structures in that area. The lateral eyelid is present and normal. The congenital symblepharon variety presents with fusion of the upper eyelid skin to the superior portion of the globe. The eyelid in this area is absent. There may be a small amount of normal eyelid laterally.

Cryptophthalmos is associated with many other congenital anomalies, including mental retardation, nasal anomalies, ear anomalies, cleft lip and palate, irregular dentition, genitourinary abnormalities, cardiac malformations, meningoencephalocele, abnormal hairline, umbilical hernia, anal atresia, ankyloglossia and laryngeal atresia, and syndactyly.

Syndromes associated with cryptophthalmos include: Fraser syndrome, cryptophthalmos-syndactyly syndrome, malformative syndrome with cryptophthalmos, and cryptophthalmos syndrome.

Treatment of cryptophthalmos is aimed at reconstructing the eyelids and allowing for visual development. The eyelids can be reconstructed with oral mucous membrane grafts in combination with local myocutaneous or eyelid-sharing grafts. The underlying globe must also be reconstructed and may require mucous membrane grafts to the globe as well as corneal surgery in an attempt to allow the formation of vision. Visual prognosis for complete cryptophthalmos is poor.

18 Sublux Lens
(Ectopia Lentis)

Displacement of the crystalline lens from its normal position is termed ectopia lentis or sublux lens. The most common cause of bilateral sublux lens is Marfan syndrome, while the most common cause of a unilateral sublux lens is trauma. The various causes of lens subluxation are listed in **Table 18-1.**

The laboratory assessment of a patient with ectopia lentis depends on the history and physical examination. If a clearly identifiable cause for the subluxation is found, a full laboratory work-up is not needed. **Table 18-2** lists the clinical evaluation of subluxed lens.

Table 18-1.
Causes of Sublux Lens

A. Systemic Associations (bilateral subluxation)
   1. Marfan syndrome (by far, most common)
   2. Weill-Marchesani syndrome
   3. Homocystinuria
   4. Hyperlysinemia
   5. Sulfite oxidase deficiency
B. Isolated Ocular Causes
   1. Trauma (unilateral)
   2. Aniridia (usually unilateral)
   3. Ectopia lentis et pupillae (bilateral)
   4. Autosomal dominant inheritance (bilateral)
   5. Anterior uveal coloboma (usually unilateral)
   6. Idiopathic (unilateral or bilateral)

Table 18-2.
Clinical Evaluation of Sublux Lens

A. History
1. History of trauma, systemic illness, mental retardation, seizures, etc
2. Family history of cardiovascular disease, sudden death in adolescence or early adulthood, skeletal abnormalities
B. Complete Eye Examination
C. General Appearance
1. Height
2. Length of arms versus torso
3. Length of fingers
4. Joint flexibility
D. Laboratory Tests
1. Cardiology consultation and cardiac ultrasound to rule out Marfan syndrome
2. X-rays for possible brachydactyly associated with Weill-Marchesani syndrome
3. Urine for sodium nitroprusside (rule out homocystinuria)

■ SYSTEMIC ASSOCIATIONS

Marfan Syndrome

Marfan syndrome is the most common cause of sublux lenses. It is a connective tissue disorder inherited as autosomal dominant. Recent research has shown that Marfan syndrome is caused by an incorrect expression of a gene product for the 350 kd glycoprotein called fibrillin, which makes up the extracellular microfibril network.

Ocular Findings of Marfan Syndrome

Ocular manifestations of Marfan syndrome include lens subluxation in approximately 80% of patients. The lens is usually displaced up and out; however, it may occur in any direction. Complete dislocation of the lens rarely occurs (**Figure 18-1**). Other ocular findings include hypoplastic iris with pupillary miosis (difficulty dilating), lenticular myopia (axial length usually normal), flat corneal curvature, and possibly a slightly increased incidence of spontaneous retinal detachment.

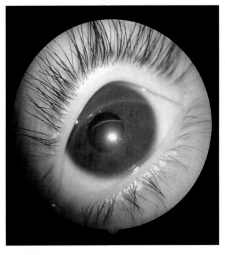

Figure 18-1.
Photograph of a subluxed lens associated with Marfan syndrome. Classically, the lens is displaced up and out (superior-temporally), but in this case, the lens is down and in (inferior-nasally).

Systemic Findings of Marfan Syndrome

Systemic findings are consistent with the abnormal microfibrillar network and include aortic arch dilatation, dissecting aortic aneurysms, femoral hernias, and arachnodactyly (long, thin fingers). Cardiovascular complications cause 90% of the early mortality associated with Marfan syndrome. Echocardiography reveals dilation of the aortic root that is characteristic of this syndrome. Arachnodactyly is the most common skeletal feature in Marfan syndrome, and is present in 88% of patients. Patients tend to be very tall, and their upper body segment is much shorter by comparison to their arms and legs. Scoliosis may occur, generally worsening during the adolescent growth spurt, and can be a deforming complication. Pectus excavatum and joint laxity are also present.

Useful clinical clues to the diagnosis can be elicited via the thumb sign and wrist sign. The thumb sign is considered positive when the thumb projects beyond the ulnar border when making a fist (thumb wrapped under the fingers). The wrist sign is considered positive when the distal phalanges of the first and fifth digit overlap when wrapped around the opposite wrist.

Management of Marfan Syndrome

A patient suspected of having Marfan syndrome must have a cardiologic and ophthalmologic examination and be closely followed with yearly examinations. The ocular examination should include a cycloplegic refraction (with drops), intraocular pressure measurement, and a dilated fundus examination.

Ocular Treatment for Ectopia Lentis in Marfan Syndrome

A mild subluxation with most of the pupil covered by the lens is compatible with excellent visual acuity and does not necessarily need treatment. However, if the edge of the lens bisects the visual axis, this often results in image distortion and amblyopia. In these patients, a trial of pupillary dilatation should be initiated. The patient should be tested with phakic (having the natural lens) correction and aphakic (without the natural lens) correction to find the best vision. Part-time occlusion therapy along with pupillary dilatation may be enough to improve visual acuity. The author's experience, however, is that a subluxed lens that bisects the pupil often results in significant image distortion, even when the pupil is dilated. In these cases, surgical removal of the lens is indicated to clear the visual axis. Removal of the lens should be performed using a microscopic vitrectomy technique. One can approach the subluxated lens from an anterior limbal (corneal) or posterior (pars plana) approach. The efficacy and safety of the anterior limbal versus posterior pars plana approach has been found to be approximately the same, perhaps with a slightly increased risk for retinal detachment using the pars plana approach. Recently published results have shown that lensectomy for subluxated lenses can be performed safely, and visual outcomes are good.

Early studies showed poor results with lensectomy for Marfan syndrome. In one study, visual acuity was unaltered in 14% of patients undergoing lens extraction, and it worsened in 18% (**Cross, 1973**). Complications included retinal detachment, and vitreous loss occurred in 50% of cases. More recent studies with vitrectomy instrumentation have shown that lensectomy can be safely performed of patients with a variety of causes of sublux lens (and specifically Marfan syndrome) without increased risks compared to standard cataract surgery (**Behki et al, 1990**). The safety and surgical outcome of anterior (limbal) approach versus posterior (pars plana) approach have been shown to be the same (**Hakin, 1992**).

The following are indications for lens extraction of a subluxated lens:

1. Lens positioning such that the lens edge bisects the pupil, making optical correction of either the aphakic or phakic part of the lens impossible
2. Displacement of the lens anteriorly, causing secondary glaucoma

Weill-Marchesani Syndrome (spherophakia/ brachymorphia)

Weill-Marchesani syndrome is usually inherited as an autosomal recessive trait and consists of both ocular and skeletal abnormalities (**Table 18-3**). The skeletal abnormalities are the reverse of Marfan syndrome, as patients with Weill-Marchesani syndrome show brachymorphia, short stubby fingers, and are of relatively short stature with hypoflexibility of the joints.

Ocular manifestations include microspherophakia (small round lens) and subluxation in virtually all patients. Subluxation is progressive, with the lens eventually becoming completely dislocated. Dislocation into the anterior chamber is common. Secondary pupillary block glaucoma is an important consideration in Weill-Marchesani syndrome. Some authors have suggested a prophylactic laser peripheral iridotomy (surgical opening in the iris) in all patients with Weill-Marchesani syndrome, as a preventive measure against developing pupillary block glaucoma because it is very diffi-

Table 18.3.
Findings in Weill-Marchesani Syndrome

Systemic	*Ocular Findings*
Brachycephaly	Ectopia lentis (down and anterior)
Short build (Pyknic)	Spherophakic lens
Broad thorax	Lenticular myopia
Brachydactyly	Relatively short axial length
Roentgenologic brachymetacarpia	Pupillary block glaucoma
Hypoextendable joints	Shallow anterior chamber
Inheritance variable	Angle abnormalities

From Wright KW, Chrousos GA. Weill-Marchesani syndrome with bilateral angle-closure glaucoma. *J Pediatr Ophthalmol Strabismus.* 1985; 22:129–132

cult to treat once pupillary block occurs. In addition, patients should be kept on miotics to keep the pupil small and prevent anterior dislocation of the lens. The risk of glaucoma is extremely high, with approximately 80% of patients developing angle-closure glaucoma (**Wright, 1985**).

Homocystinuria

Homocystinuria is caused by a deficiency of the enzyme cystathionine synthase resulting in abnormal methionine metabolism. Laboratory screening tests for homocystinuria include urine for amino acids (homocystine) and blood levels, which show elevated homocystine and methionine. Sodium nitroprusside urine test screens for homocystinuria. Homocystinuria is rare, occurring in approximately 1 out of every 200,000 births.

Ocular manifestations include ectopia lentis, myopia, secondary glaucoma (rarely), and possible retinal detachment. The zonules are weak, and lens accommodation is poor. In contrast to Marfan syndrome, approximately one third of patients with homocystinuria eventually develop complete lens dislocation either into the vitreous or anterior chamber. Subluxation in homocystinuria is bilateral and occurs in almost all patients. Systemic findings include cerebral vascular thrombosis, myocardial infarction, pulmonary embolism, and intermittent claudication, all which contribute to death at an early age. Patients with homocystinuria are at an increased anesthesia risk because of the possibility of thromboembolic disease.

Skeletal abnormalities are very mild in comparison to Marfan syndrome; however, pectus excavatum, joint laxity, hernias, and scoliosis can occur. Some infants with homocystinuria will show developmental delay and failure to thrive.

Sulfite Oxidase Deficiency

This is an extremely rare disorder associated with increased sulfite in the urine. Systemic findings include hemiplegia, progressive choreoathetoid movements, seizures, and decreased mentation. There is cortical atrophy, most prominent in the parietal and frontal lobes. Over time, there is progressive subluxation and dislocation of the lens.

■ ISOLATED OCULAR CAUSES

Ectopia Lentis et Pupillae

This is an ocular anomaly that consists of lens subluxation and corectopia (displaced pupil). The pupil is often misshapen, either oval or slitlike, and is difficult to dilate. Persistent pupillary membranes, with or without lenticular adhesions, may occur. Ectopia lentis et pupillae is frequently bilateral and is often associated with myopia, glaucoma, and retinal detachment.

■ BIBLIOGRAPHY

1. Behki R, Noel LP, Clarke WN. Limbal lensectomy in the management of ectopia lentis in children. *Arch Ophthalmol.* 1990;108:809–811
2. Cross HE, Jensen AD. Ocular manifestations in the Marfan syndrome and homocystinuria. *Am J Ophthalmol.* 1973;75:405–420
3. Hakin KN, Jacobs M, Roger P, Taylor D, Cooling RJ. Management of the subluxed crystalline lens. *Ophthalmology.* 1992;99:542–545
4. Wright KW, Chrousos GA. Weill-Marchesani syndrome with bilateral angle-closure glaucoma. *J Pediatr Ophthalmol Strabismus.* July-August 1985; 22:129–132

19 Retinopathy of Prematurity

I n the late 1940s and early 1950s, retinopathy of prematurity (ROP), or retrolental fibroplasia (RLF) as it was previously called, was the most common cause of blindness in children (**Figure 19-1**). Preterm neonates born during this period were treated in incubators with almost 100% oxygen. Once high-oxygen concentrations

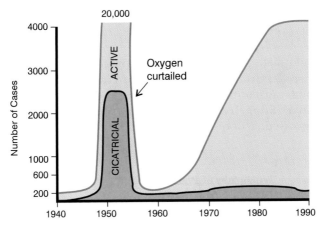

Figure 19-1.
Graph showing incidence of ROP over time from the 1940s to the 1990s. Note that around 1955 the incidence of cicatricial and active ROP dropped significantly, because this is the point in time when oxygen use was curtailed. In the late 1960s through the 1990s, survival of very low birth weight infants increased along with the incidence of active ROP (red area). Note that the incidence of severe cicatricial ROP remained relatively low during this period.

271

were curtailed, a dramatic decrease in the incidence of severe ROP occurred. The use of oxygen monitoring by arterial blood gas and pulse oximeters has greatly improved survival rate and reduced the morbidity of preterm infants. Because of the increased survival of low birth-weight neonates, the potential for increased incidence of ROP is possible.

■ ETIOLOGY AND PATHOPHYSIOLOGY

The exact cause of ROP remains controversial; however, it is clear that hyperoxia plays a major role in the development of ROP (**Table 19-1**). In utero, fetuses are normally in a state of relative hypoxia. Preterm neonates do not have fully vascularized peripheral retina. Hyperoxia in the immature areas of the retina stimulate **Vascular Endothelial Growth Factor (VEGF),** which, in turn, stimulates normal vascularization of the peripheral retina (**Figure 19-2**). Preterm birth exposes neonates to higher oxygen levels than those present in the intrauterine environment, and these higher levels down-regulate normal VEGF production. This causes vaso-obliteration of immature retina vessels and stops the normal process of peripheral vascularization. Over time, the avascular peripheral retina becomes ischemic and retinal hypoxia stimulates a secondary overproduction of VEGF. While physiologic levels of VEGF stimulate vessel growth at the junction between the vascular and avascular retina, abnormally high levels of VEGF stimulate the growth of abnormal new vessels. New vessels form arteriovenous **shunts** that develop into vascular tufts on the surface of the retina called retinal **neovascularization** that hemorrhage, leak protein, and invoke retinal fibrosis. Retinal fibrosis causes retinal traction that can progress

Table 19-1.
Pathogenesis of Retinopathy of Prematurity

---

1. Premature birth with avascular peripheral retina.
⇩
2. Hyperoxia after birth down-regulates VEGF and causes vaso-obliteration.
⇩
3. Avascular retina becomes hypoxic causing overproduction of VEGF.
⇩
4. Overproduction of VEGF stimulates shunts and neovascularization (ROP).

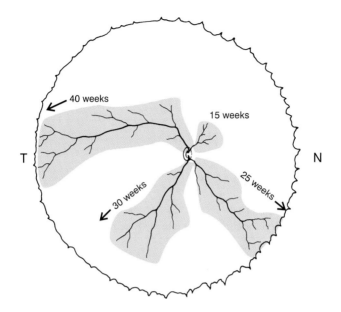

Figure 19-2.
Diagram showing the vascularization pattern of the fetal retina. Retinal vessels grow out of the optic nerve toward the peripheral retina. Because the distance from the optic nerve to the nasal retinal periphery is shortest, the nasal retina becomes vascularized first. Even a full-term infant will have a narrow skirt of avascular retina in the temporal periphery (T: temporal retina; N: nasal retina).

to retinal detachment and blindness. Regression of ROP occurs when low physiologic levels of VEGF stimulate normal vascularization of the avascular peripheral retina.

Almost all cases of ROP are associated with hyperoxia. Providing a stable, controlled, low-oxygen environment while maintaining adequate O_2 saturation for the preterm neonate is one of the most important challenges in the neonatal intensive care unit.

■ RISK FACTORS OF RETINOPATHY OF PREMATURITY

The most significant risk factors for developing ROP are low birth weight and hyperoxia (**Table 19-2**). The lower the birth weight, the

Table 19-2.
Incidence of Retinopathy of Prematurity Versus Birth Weight

Birth Weight (g)	Any ROP	Stage 3	Pre-threshold	Threshold
<750	90%	37%	39%	15%
750–999	78%	22%	21%	7%
1000–1250	47%	8%	7%	2%
Total Group	66%	18%	18%	6%

Modified from Palmer et al, 1991

Table 19-3.
Retinopathy of Prematurity Risk Factors

Birth weight
Hyperoxia
Respiratory distress syndrome
Intracranial hemorrhage
Gestational age
Blood transfusions

higher the risk of ROP. Almost 50% of neonates who weigh between 1,000 and 1,250 g show some sign of ROP; however, only 6% will develop severe vision-threatening ROP (ie, threshold disease). Because neonates who weigh more than 1,500 g almost never develop vision-threatening ROP, screenings should be done in all neonates whose birth weight is less than 1,500 g. Infants receiving high doses of oxygen may sustain severe ROP even if their birth weight was greater than 1,500 g. This author performed observational research in an underdeveloped country, examining several childran with bilateral stage 5 cicatricial ROP (total retinal detachment), who had birth weights over 1,500 g. These children had not been monitored and had received uncurtailed oxygen for prolonged periods of time.

Other than hyperoxia and low birth weight, other risk factors include gestational age, respiratory distress syndrome, infections, intracranial hemorrhage and blood transfusions (**Table 19-3**). Blood transfusions increase ROP risk because adult hemoglobin disassociates oxygen more easily than fetal hemoglobin, providing increased retinal oxygen dose.

■ CLASSIFICATION OF RETINOPATHY OF PREMATURITY

The international classification of ROP uses 3 parameters: (1) zone of the disease (how posterior is the ROP), (2) clock hours of involvement (circumferential extent of ROP), and (3) stage (degree of abnormal vasculature). In general, ROP is more severe in the superior temporal periphery because this is the last area to be vascularized and has the widest avascular zone.

Normal immature retina is not truly ROP, but represents avascular peripheral retina. Immature retina must be watched closely through serial retinal examinations. Immature retina in Zone III usually has a good prognosis.

Zones of Retinopathy of Prematurity

Figure 19-3 shows the various zones of ROP. **Zone I** is the most posterior zone, demarcated by a circle centered on the optic nerve

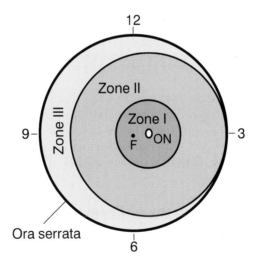

Figure 19-3.
International classification of ROP "zones." Zone I is the circumferential area around the optic nerve with a radius twice the distance from the optic nerve to the fovea (dark red area). Zone II has a diameter from the optic nerve to the nasal retina (pink zone). Zone III is the temporal crescent of retina not covered by Zone I or Zone II (light pink area).

Table 19-4.
Stages of Retinopathy of Prematurity

Stage	Retinal Findings
Immature Retina	Normal vascularized retina with arborization of vessels, no demarcation line between the normal retina and the peripheral avascular zone.
ACTIVE ROP	
Stage 1	A sharp demarcation line between the vascular and avascular zone, which represents an arteriolar-venous shunt. The peripheral vessels line up in a straight parallel configuration (broom bristles), and feed into a flat shunt.
Stage 2	Straightened peripheral vessels inserting into an elevated shunt.
Stage 3	Shunt with neovascularization extending off the surface of the retina into the vitreous.
Stage 3-Plus Disease (Pre-threshold Disease)	Stage 3 with tortuous and dilated posterior retinal vessels.
CICATRICIAL ROP	
Stage 4	Subtotal retinal detachment. A. Extrafoveal. B. Retinal detachment including fovea.
Stage 5	Total retinal detachment—funnel configuration.

that extends twice the distance from the disc to the fovea. **Zone II** is a circle centered on the optic nerve, with the radius being the distance from the optic nerve to the nasal ora serrata. **Zone III** is the temporal crescent of peripheral retina not included in Zones I and II. Therefore, if ROP is present nasally, it has to be in Zone I or II.

Stages of Retinopathy of Prematurity

The stages of ROP denote the severity of the vascular shunt and neovascularization. There are 5 stages: 3 active stages and 2 cicatricial stages (**Table 19-4**).

Active Retinopathy of Prematurity

The three active stages represent the severity of the retinal shunt vessels and the conditions of normal immature retina and Plus

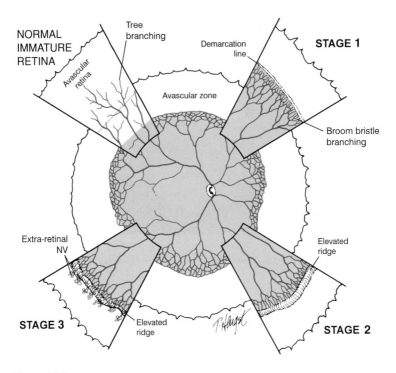

NORMAL IMMATURE RETINA

Tree branching

Avascular retina

Avascular zone

Demarcation line

STAGE 1

Broom bristle branching

Extra-retinal NV

Elevated ridge

STAGE 3

Elevated ridge

STAGE 2

Figure 19-4.
Diagram of the vascular pattern associated with normal immature retina, and stage 1 to stage 3 ROP. The upper left is a diagram of normal immature retina showing the typical tree branching vascular pattern. Upper right shows stage 1 ROP with straightening of the peripheral vessels to insert at the shunt-demarcation line. There is the distinctive broom bristle branching pattern with the vessel ends lining up along the shunt. Lower right stage 2 ROP shows an elevated ridge, which represents an enlarged shunt. Lower left stage 3 ROP shows extraretinal extension of neovascularization (NV) in addition to a shunt.

disease (**Figure 19-4**). Stages 1 and 2 indicate a vascular shunt within the retina, with stage 1 being flat and stage 2 being an elevated ridge. Stage 3 represents neovascularization on the surface of the retina and is a sign of severe disease requiring close follow-up and possible need for treatment. **Plus disease** is tortuosity and dilation of retinal vessels close to the optic disc (**Figure 19-5**). This is a sign of severe disease and may coexist with stage 2 or stage 3 ROP. Stage 3 ROP with Plus disease (pre-threshold disease) indicates significant risk of vision loss and must be followed closely, at least every week, as laser or cryotherapy may be needed.

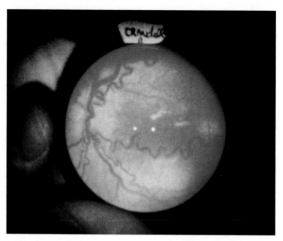

Figure 19-5.
Photograph of Plus disease showing tortuous and dilated retinal arcades emanating from the optic nerve.

Cicatricial Retinopathy of Prematurity

Cicatricial ROP is a type of regression that presents as scarring secondary to severe active retinopathy of prematurity, usually stage 3, Zone I or II. The degree and severity of cicatricial ROP depends on the severity of the active disease, and is quite variable. The hallmark of cicatricial ROP is retinal fibrosis, scarring, and secondary scar contraction that causes retinal traction. In the mild form, cicatricial ROP produces peripheral retinal traction that pulls the retinal vascular arcades temporally, straightening the vessels. More severe temporal traction will drag the macula temporally, which may or may not interfere with vision. The dragged macula causes the eye to turn out to view (fixate) and gives the false appearance of an exotropia. This is called a **positive angle kappa.** Severe fibrosis and traction can lead to retinal detachment, which may be partial (stage 4) or total (stage 5). Circumferential traction causes a funnel retinal detachment as seen in **Figure 19-6**.

Retinopathy of Prematurity Screening

The most important aspects of managing ROP are prevention and early detection. Careful curtailment of oxygen is important to

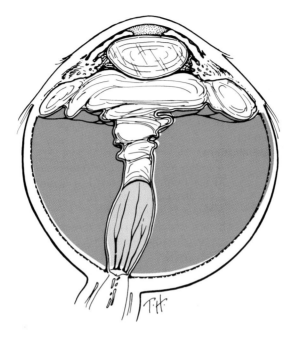

Figure 19-6.
Stage 5 ROP with total retinal detachment. The red area in the cutaway of the closed funnel detachment shows retinal vessels inside the funnel. Note that the retrolental membrane is pushing the lens and iris diaphragm anteriorly. There is a high incidence of angle closure glaucoma in these patients.

prevent vaso-obiliteration and eventual ROP (as discussed earlier in this chapter under Etiology and Pathophysiology). Screening examinations are important to monitor the development of ROP. The multicenter trial investigating cryotherapy for ROP has shown a 50% reduction in vision-threatening sequelae to retinopathy of prematurity when treatment is applied in the active stage before development of retinal detachment. The initial neonatal nursery examination should be performed at 4 to 6 weeks after birth for infants under 1,500 grams, because this is when ROP first becomes evident. Prior to the eye examination in the neonatal intensive care unit, the baby's pupils are dilated with cyclopentolate/phenylephrine combination drops. Drops should be instilled twice at 5-minute intervals. The dilated retinal examination includes scleral depression to visualize the peripheral retina. The insertion of an eyelid speculum is required to do this testing. It is important to remember

Table 19-5.
Screening Protocol for Preterm Infants

A. First Screening
According to guidelines published by the AAP, AAPOS, and AAO:
- Preterm infants ≤1,500 g
- Gestational age ≤28 weeks
- Preterm infants >1,500 g with unstable course (high risk)
- First examination by 4 to 6 weeks chronological age, 31 to 33 weeks post-conception

B. Follow-up Examinations

Zone I	*Immature Retina or any ROP (pre-threshold).* Repeat examination every 1 week until normal vascularization to Zone II.
Zone II	*Immature Retina (No ROP).* Repeat examination every 2 weeks until normal vascularization to Zone III.
Zone III	*With stage 1 or 2.* Repeat examination every 2 to 4 weeks to monitor for progression.
Pre-threshold	(Zone I-any ROP, Zone II-stage 2 with Plus disease, or Zone II-stage 3) note that pre-threshold disease is extremely critical and repeat examinations should be performed every week until either threshold is reached or regression is unequivocally seen.
Threshold	Zone I or II with 5 contiguous clock hours or 8 accumulative clock hours of stage 3 (in the presence of Plus disease). Once threshold is reached, cryotherapy or laser therapy must be performed within 72 hours.
Stage 4	Retinal surgery may be indicated, but there is poor prognosis.
Stage 5	Retinal surgery may be indicated, but there is universally poor visual outcome.

to inform the patient's family and nurses of the ocular status and proposed follow-up after the examination.

Table 19-5 summarizes the protocol for examining immature infants. The frequency of follow-up eye examinations is determined by the ophthalmologist based on the retinal findings. If immature retina is found in Zone III on initial screening, but with no ROP, the eye examination is repeated every month until a normal regression pattern is established. Once normal regression is complete, plan a long-term follow-up in 6 months for an ocular examination including cycloplegic refraction. If stage 1 or stage 2 ROP is found, a repeat exam should be performed approximately every 2 weeks, depending on the severity and Zone, to monitor for progression. Once a normal regression pattern is identified, follow-up examinations can be spaced to approximately every month. Patients with stage 3 ROP or stage 2 ROP in Zone II with Plus disease must be monitored very closely, as this represents **pre-threshold disease.** The eye examination should be performed at least every week, since these patients are at significant risk for progressing to **threshold disease.** Patients who develop stage 3 ROP over 5 contiguous clock hours or 8 accumulative clock hours with Plus disease have reached threshold disease and require cryotherapy or laser therapy. Treatment should be given within 72 hours of identifying threshold disease.

Medical Treatments

The most important medical treatment, and also the most difficult, is to keep a low, stable tissue dose of oxygen during the infant's stay in the neonatal intensive care unit. Other treatment modalities include the administration of **surfactant** that reduces respiratory distress syndrome. A recent study examined the use of high-dose oxygen given after identification of severe ROP (**STOP-ROP**). The idea is that increased oxygen will down-regulate VEGF, thus causing regression of severe, active ROP. Results of this multi-center trial showed no advantage of high-dose oxygen after development of severe ROP and, in fact, showed adverse pulmonary outcomes. The most critical time period for careful and strict oxygen management appears to be early, before ROP develops. Low and stable oxygen saturation levels early in the post-natal course have shown to significantly decrease severe ROP (**Hong, 2002**).

Treatment of Active Retinopathy of Prematurity (Cryotherapy and Laser Therapy)

Cryotherapy and laser therapy act by obliterating peripheral hypoxic avascular retina, thus reducing the production of vaso-proliferative factor VEGF. Less VEGF results in regression of the abnormal shunt vessels and the neovascularization. Ablation therapy is given to the avascular retina, not directly to the shunt or the neovascularization. If left untreated, threshold disease is associated with an unfavorable outcome in approximately 45% of cases, whereas cryotherapy or laser therapy reduces these unfavorable outcomes to approximately 20%. Laser therapy has been shown to be effective and is less invasive, with possibly improved final visual acuity compaired to cryotherapy (**Ng, 2002**)

Treatment of Cicatricial Retinopathy of Prematurity (Vitreoretinal Surgery)

The surgical management of retinal detachments (stage 4 or 5 ROP) is controversial. Scleral buckling procedure may be indicated for some stage 4 cases. Stage 5 has an extremely poor prognosis even with modern vitreoretinal techniques, and postoperative visual function is universally poor. The "heroic" vitreoretinal surgery required to repair a stage 5 retinal detachment should be performed only after a full discussion with the parents to establish realistic expectations about the poor prognosis.

■ LATE COMPLICATIONS OF ROP

Retinopathy of prematurity holds an increased incidence for myopia, astigmatism, anisometropia, amblyopia, and strabismus. Infants with ROP should have follow-up appointments with an ophthalmologist for a full office examination. Late retinal detachment is a potential complication, especially in patients with high myopia.

■ DIFFERENTIAL DIAGNOSIS OF RETINOPATHY OF PREMATURITY

The differential diagnosis of ROP includes Persistent Hyperplastic Primary Vitreous (PHPV) (Chapter 22), Norrie disease (Chapter 6), incontinentia pigmenti (this chapter), FEVR (this chapter), and the causes of leukocoria (Chapter 22). The diagnosis of ROP usually is straightforward based on the history of prematurity, oxygen exposure, and characteristic fundus findings. Nonetheless, the following are rare diseases that can be confused with ROP.

Familial Exudative Vitreal Retinopathy (FEVR)

This is an autosomal dominant inherited peripheral retinopathy, that, in its early stage, looks very similar to ROP. Findings include peripheral neovascularization, avascular retina, and retinal exudates. The disease may evolve to produce retinal traction, macular dragging, retinal folds, retinal breaks, and retinal detachment.

Incontinentia Pigmenti

Incontinentia pigmenti is an X-linked dominant disorder (gestational death in males). Females have linear erythema with bullae and vesicles appearing over the skin of the torso and extremities within the first 2 weeks of life. Eosinophils in peripheral blood transiently occur, and intraepithelial eosinophils on skin biopsy are diagnostic. Verrucous plaques replace the bullae. Then, at 4 to 6 months, a pattern of brown splashes of pigment with jagged borders appears on the torso and extremities. Ocular involvement occurs in 30% of cases and consists of peripheral fibrovascular proliferation and eventually retinal detachment. Treatment with laser or cryotherapy to the peripheral retina may prevent retinal detachment. A dilated fundus examination with the indirect ophthalmoscope is required to document the peripheral retinal findings. Systemic findings are related to ectodermal components including hair, teeth, nails, and the central nervous system. Alopecia (40%), spoon-shaped nails (7%), and missing or pegged teeth (80%) are part of the syndrome. Neurological disorders include mental retardation (30%), seizures, and paralytic motor problems.

■ BIBLIOGRAPHY

1. Cryotherapy for Retinopathy of Prematurity Cooperative Group. Multicenter trial of cryotherapy for retinopathy of prematurity. $3\frac{1}{2}$-year outcome—structure and function. *Arch Ophthalmol.* 1993;111:339–344
2. Flynn JT, Bancalari E, Snyder ES, et al. A cohort study of transcutaneous oxygen tension and the incidence and severity of retinopathy of prematurity. *N Engl J Med.* 1992;326:1050–1054
3. Hong PH, Wright KW, Fillafer S, Sola A, Chow LC. Strict oxygen management is associated with decreased incidence of severe retinopathy of prematurity. Presented at: Annual Meeting of the Association for

Research in Vision and Ophthalmology, May 2002 Fort Lauderdale, FL
4. Ng EYJ, Connolly BP, McNamara A, et al. A comparison of laser photo-coagulation with cryotherapy for threshold retinopathy of prematurity at 10 years. *Ophthalmology.* 2002;109:928–934
5. Ober RR, Bird AC, Hamilton AM, Sehmi K. Autosomal dominant exudative vitreoretinopathy. *Br J Ophthalmol.* 1980;64:112–120
6. Palmer EA, Flynn JT, Hardy RJ, et al for the cryotherapy for Retinopathy of Prematurity Cooperative Group. Incidence and early course of retinopathy of prematurity. *Ophthalmology.* 1991;98:1628–1640
7. Patz A, Hoeck LE, DeLaCruz E. Studies on the effect of high oxygen administration in retrolental fibroplasia. Nursery observations. *Am J Ophthalmol.* 1952;27:1248–1253
8. Repka MX, Hardy RJ, Phelps DL, Summers CG. Surfactant prophylaxis and retinopathy of prematurity. *Arch Ophthalmol.* 1993;111: 618–620
9. The International Committee for the Classification of the Late Stages of Retinopathy of Prematurity. An international classification of retinopathy of prematurity. II. The classification of retinal detachment. *Arch Ophthalmol.* 1987;105:906–912
10. The Laser ROP Study Group. Laser therapy for retinopathy of prematurity. *Arch Ophthalmol.* 1994;112:154–156
11. The STOP-ROP Multicenter Study Group. Supplemental therapeutic oxygen for pre-threshold retinopathy of prematurity (STOP-ROP) randomized, controlled trial. I: primary outcomes. *Pediatrics.* 2000;105: 295–310

20 Dyslexia and Learning Disabilities

Dyslexia is a very difficult problem for the child, parents, and teachers alike. Since children with dyslexia often have normal or superior intelligence, the teachers and parents often look to visual defects as the cause for poor reading. In truth, there is no evidence of a relationship between visual abilities and reading problems (**Helveston 1985, Vellutino 1987**). Studies have consistently shown that normal readers and patients with dyslexia have similar incidences of visual defects. This concurs with the author's clinical experience, noting numerous patients with poor visual function, limited ocular rotations (Duane syndrome), strabismus, and even nystagmus, who still have excellent reading skills. On the other hand, the vast majority of children with dyslexia will have absolutely normal ocular examinations.

Even though the majority of children with dyslexia will have normal ophthalmologic examinations, they should have a complete eye examination, including dilating drops for a cycloplegic refraction. Convergence insufficiency and hypermetropia are conditions that may interfere with reading and lead to near fatigue and asthenopia, yet are not easily detected by routine screening examinations.

There are vision therapists who claim that children with dyslexia have an oculomotor deficit that disrupts the normal reading pattern. They go on to rationalize that eye exercises improve ocular coordination, thereby improving reading skills. Much of this thinking comes from early anecdotal publications in the 1950s. In contrast, studies by Drs Goldberg and Schiffman at Johns Hopkins University using electronystagmography clearly demonstrated that

285

ocular coordination and motility are normal in children with dys-lexia. Additionally, they showed that the degree of comprehension produces the pattern of ocular movement, not that the innate ocular motility potential determines the degree of comprehension. That is to say that children who have difficulty comprehending and reading have abnormal fixation and refixation movements as they read; however, their ocular motility is normal. A patient who can read French fluently has normal eye motility when reading French; how-ever, the patient has abnormal eye movements when reading English. These and other studies have shown that reading and learning disabilities in children are not caused by a lack of ocular coordination.

In a joint organizational statement, executive committees from the American Academy of Pediatrics and the American Academy of Ophthalmology have stated that children with learning disabilities have the same incidence of ocular abnormalities as children who are normal achievers and are reading at grade level. Visual training, eye muscle exercises, and reading therapy with tinted glasses fre-quently result in unwarranted expense and often misplace resources when they could be better used for reading education and tutors (**Metzger and Werner 1984**).

Not all children with learning disabilities have dyslexia. Neuro-psychology processes such as Attention-Deficit Disorder (ADD), autism, mental retardation, and syndromes such as William syndrome, can cause learning disabilities. A team approach with a neuropsychologist, pediatrician, educator, and ophthalmologist is indicated for children with learning disabilities.

■ BIBLIOGRAPHY

1. Goldberg HK. *Dyslexia/Learning Disabilities.* 2nd ed. Philadelphia PA: WB Saunders; 1983:1305–1318
2. Helveston EM, Weber JC, Miller K, et al. Visual function and academic performance. *Am J Ophthalmol.*1985;99:346–355
3. Metzger RL, Werner DB. Use of visual training for reading disabilities: a review. *Pediatrics.*1984;73:824–829
4. Vellutino FR. Dyslexia. *Sci Am.*1987;256:34–41

21 Ocular Pigmentation Abnormalities

■ ALBINISM (Also see Chapter 6.)

Albinism is a lack of melanin pigment that can occur primarily involving the eyes (ocular albinism) or systemically (oculocutaneous albinism).

Oculocutaneous Albinism

Oculocutaneous albinism can be divided into tyrosinase-positive and tyrosinase-negative types. With tyrosinase-positive oculocutaneous albinism, hair root studies show positive tyrosinase activity. Advances in molecular genetics have shown that there are many possible genetic defects that cause a specific albino phenotype. For example, tyrosinase-positive oculocutaneous albinism has been found to be secondary to abnormalities involving at least 3 separate genes: tyrosinase gene mutations, P gene mutations, and tyrosinase-related protein type 1 (TRP-1). In addition, a variety of mutations on a specific albinism gene may result in different phenotypes of tyrosinase-negative oculocutaneous albinism. Molecular genetics is the basis for a new classification of albinism; however, most clinicians still use the clinical classification of tyrosinase-negative and tyrosinase-positive oculocutaneous albinism. The eye findings associated with oculocutaneous albinism include nystagmus, hypopigmentation of the iris with transillumination defects, hypopigmented fundus, foveal hypoplasia, and poor visual acuity, usually 20/80 to

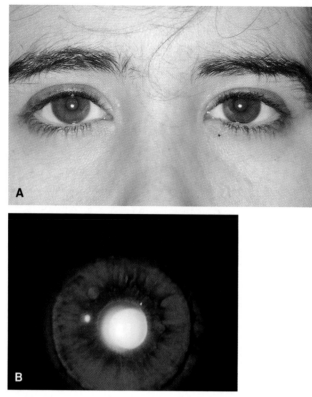

Figure 21-1.
A, Hermansky-Pudlak syndrome with ocular albinism, but irides are brown. **B,** Despite brown eyes, the iris transilluminates on slit-lamp examination, showing the hypopigmentation of the iris pigmented epithelium.

20/400. Patients with tyrosinase-positive oculocutaneous albinism show progressive increased pigmentation, as they are able to produce melanin. Tyrosinase-negative oculocutaneous albinism is a severe hypopigmentation disorder that tends to be static and is associated with very poor visual acuity and legal blindness. Both tyrosinase-positive and tyrosinase-negative oculocutaneous albinism are inherited as an autosomal recessive trait. Transillumination defects of the iris are important in distinguishing true albinism from otherwise normal patients with hypopigmentation (**Figure 21-1 A and B**).

Ocular Albinism

Ocular albinism is hypopigmentation that is localized to the eye. Patients with ocular albinism may have brown or dark hair and will not look like the typical patient with albinism. Ocular albinism is usually inherited as X-linked, or autosomal recessive trait. Typical findings of ocular albinism are transillumination defects of the iris, nystagmus, and hypopigmented fundus. Macular hypoplasia also can be associated with ocular albinism. Also, strabismus is commonly seen with both oculocutaneous and ocular albinism. Hemifield visual evoked potential (VEP) studies show excess of decussation at the chiasm, and patients with albinism show decreased binocularity. Decreased vision associated with albinism is related to macular hypoplasia. Vision tends to improve over time as pigmentation increases, especially in patients with tyrosinase-positive albinism.

Hermansky-Pudlak Syndrome

Hermansky-Pudlak syndrome is a tyrosinase-positive albinism with prolonged bleeding time secondary to abnormal platelet aggregation. Lung disease and ulcerative colitis develop at approximately 30 to 40 years of age. Because of the platelet abnormalities, patients show bruisability, increased nosebleeds, and increased bleeding after minor surgical procedures **(Figure 21-1)**.

Chédiak-Higashi Syndrome

Chédiak-Higashi syndrome is a tyrosinase-positive oculocutaneous albinism and is associated with defective degranulation of neutrophils that fails to prevent infections secondary to defective microtubule assembly. Bacterial infections are dangerous in these patients and can be fatal in childhood. A severe lymphoma-like syndrome may also occur.

Waardenburg Syndrome

Waardenburg syndrome is not a pigment dilution disease, but is associated with white forelocks, hypopigmented fundus, and heterochromia secondary to hypopigmentation of all or part of the iris. Other findings include telecanthus, confluent eyebrows, and sensorineural deafness.

■ NEVUS OF OTA

Nevus of Ota is congenital melanosis of the periocular skin and eye (melanosis oculi) that occurs unilaterally. Characteristics of melanosis oculi include increased pigmentation of the conjunctiva, sclera, and episclera. The mandible, oral and nasal mucosa, tympanic membrane, and dura may also have increased pigmentation. The condition is most commonly seen in females, often occurring in Asian or black people and almost all cases are unilateral, although bilateral cases have been reported. Skin lesions, which are simply areas of increased pigmentation, may be present at birth and often increase in pigment density during puberty. There is a slight, but significant, increased risk for malignant transformation of the nevus, with approximately 4% of cases evolving into melanomas. This is an important cosmetic problem, as the increased pigmentation is difficult to treat with cosmetic cover-ups.

Conjunctival Nevi (See Chapter 13 and Figure 13-17.)

Blue Sclera

Blue sclera is due to visibility of uveal tissue through thin sclera. The common ocular and systemic conditions associated with blue sclera are listed in **Table 21-1.**

Table 21-1.
Ocular and Systemic Conditions Associated With Blue Sclera

1. Myopia
2. Buphthalmos
3. Scleral staphyloma
4. Congenital ocular melanosis
5. Aniridia
6. Ehlers-Danlos syndrome
7. Marfan syndrome
8. Osteogenesis imperfecta
9. Paget syndrome
10. Pierre Robin syndrome

22 Leukocoria: Cataracts, Retinal Tumors, and Coats Disease

■ LEUKOCORIA "WHITE PUPIL"

Leukocoria is defined as a white pupil and indicates an opacity at or behind the pupil. A white pupil can be the result of a cataract, an opacity of the vitreous, or retinal disease (**Table 22-1**). Leukocoria implies that the cornea is clear. A corneal opacity will, however, result in an abnormal red reflex and obscure visualization of the pupil. If the details of the iris and pupil are clearly seen, the opacity is behind the pupil. If, on the other hand, visualization of the iris

Table 22-1.
Differential Diagnosis of Leukocoria

Cataract (this chapter)
Coats disease (this chapter)
Coloboma of macula and optic nerve (Chapter 6)
Corneal opacity (Chapter 15)
Familial Exudative Vitreoretinopathy (FEVR) (Chapter 19)
Incontinentia pigmenti (Chapter 19)
Leukemia with vitreous hemorrhage (this chapter)
Medulloepithelioma and retinal tumors (this chapter)
Myelinated nerve fibers (Chapter 9)
Norrie disease (Chapter 6)
Persistent Hyperplastic Primary Vitreous (PHPV) (this chapter)
Retinoblastoma (this chapter)
Retinopathy of prematurity (Chapter 19)
Toxocariasis (Chapter 14)

and pupil is obscured, the opacity is in front of the iris (ie, in the anterior chamber or cornea). Refer to Chapter 15 for a discussion of corneal abnormalities. Patients with leukocoria require an immediate referral for a full ophthalmic evaluation.

■ PEDIATRIC CATARACTS

In contrast to adults, cataracts in children present a special challenge, since early visual rehabilitation is critical to prevent irreversible amblyopia. Until the late 1980s, many ophthalmologists would not even attempt surgery on unilateral congenital cataracts because of the poor prognosis. Now ophthalmologists operate as early as the first week of life, and the prognosis is much improved.

Morphology of Infantile Cataracts

Infantile cataracts can be classified by the location of the lens opacity. The lens nucleus is the first part of the lens to develop and is demarcated by 2 "Y"- sutures, one on the anterior surface and one

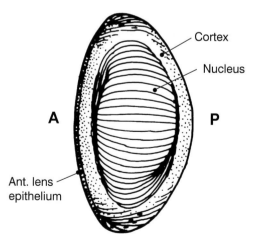

Figure 22-1.
Diagram of neonatal lens showing anterior lens epithelium and lens nucleus located between the Y-sutures and the cortex peripheral to the Y-sutures. A, anterior: P, posterior.

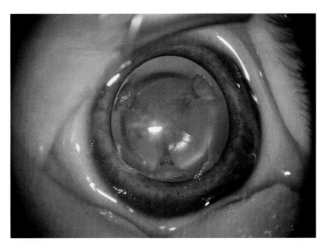

Figure 22-2.
Photograph of a 4-week-old infant with a congenital sutural nuclear cataract. Note the anterior Y-suture is oriented upright. The peripheral clear red reflex represents clear lens cortex, whereas the central opacity involves the sutures and nucleus.

on the posterior surface (**Figure 22-1**). Opacities at or within the Y-sutures are termed nuclear cataracts. This indicates that the cataract was present since birth (**Figure 22-2**). Cataracts located peripheral to the Y-sutures are called cortical cataracts. Cortical cataracts that are layered in an onionskin-like pattern with clear zones between the opacities are termed lamellar, or zonular, cataracts (**Figure 22-3**). The visual prognosis for lamellar cataracts is relatively good because they are acquired, and the lens is relatively clear during the early period of visual development. Cataracts are characterized as anterior or posterior.

Anterior Cataracts

Anterior Polar Cataracts
Anterior polar cataracts involve the anterior capsule and anterior cortex at the center or "pole" of the lens (**Figure 22-4**). Typically, anterior polar cataracts are small, nonprogressive, and usually do not interfere with visual acuity, although some will progress and eventually require surgery.

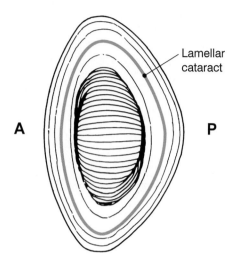

A   P

Lamellar cataract

Figure 22-3.
Drawing of lamellar cataract with the opacity (identified in red) occurring in the cortex just peripheral to the lens nucleus.

Anterior Subcapsular Cataracts

Anterior subcapsular cataracts are opacities located directly under the anterior capsule in the anterior lens cortex.

Alport Syndrome

Alport syndrome is classically described as being associated with **anterior lenticonus** (anterior bowing of the anterior capsule), with or without anterior polar subcapsular cataracts. Systemic findings include neurosensory hearing loss and hemorrhagic nephritis with late renal failure and renal hypertension. Alport syndrome is fairly common and accounts for approximately one sixth of familial glomerular nephritis. Only 15% of patients, however, have ocular abnormalities. Various modes of inheritance have been described, including X-linked dominant (most common), autosomal recessive, and autosomal dominant. There is no specific treatment, and management is directed to delaying renal failure.

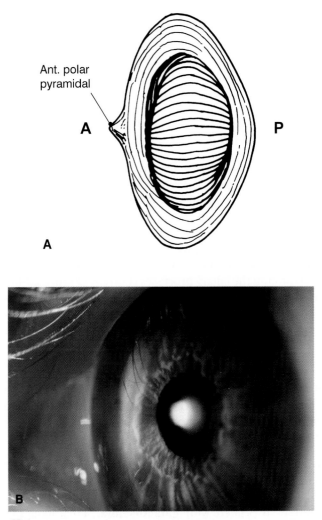

Figure 22-4.
Anterior polar cataract. **A,** Drawing of a pyramidal anterior polar cataract with anterior conical opacity consisting of fibrous tissue. **B,** Companion photograph showing white conical area of fibrosis coming off the anterior capsule, through the pupil, and protruding into the anterior chamber. Over time, progressive cortical changes occurred and this patient required cataract surgery. At the time of surgery, the fibrotic conical opacity was difficult to fragment and required removal with intraocular forceps.

Posterior Cataracts

Posterior lenticonus

Posterior lenticonus is a congenital thinning and posterior bowing of the posterior capsule (**Figure 22-5**). Early in infancy, the cortex is relatively clear. Over time, however, the area of cortex surrounding the abnormal posterior capsule opacifies and the cataract progresses. The visual prognosis for posterior lenticonus is relatively good, since the visual axis is fairly clear during the early visual developmental period and the opacity progresses later.

Persistent hyperplastic primary vitreous

Persistent hyperplastic primary vitreous (PHPV) represents abnormal regression of the primitive hyaloid vascular system. This produces a fibrovascular tissue that emanates from the optic disc as a stalk, and then courses to the back of the lens where it forms a retrolental membrane (**Figure 22-6A**). This membrane may extend to the ciliary processes. Over time, the fibrovascular membrane can contract, pulling the ciliary processes centrally (**Figure 22-6B**). Surgery is indicated to improve vision and prevent amblyopia, but also to save the eye. If left untreated, severe forms of PHPV can lead to shallowing of the anterior chamber, angle closure glaucoma, and eventual loss of the eye in late childhood. Overall, the surgical prognosis with PHPV is relatively good as long as the retina is normal.

Posterior subcapsular cataracts

Posterior subcapsular cataracts involve the posterior lens cortex are associated with Down syndrome, chronic steroid use, and blunt trauma. They also may be idiopathic.

Oil drop cataract

Oil drop cataract is the term typically given to a faint opacity in the central aspect of the posterior cortex that is seen on retro-illumination and is associated with **galactosemia.** Treatment of galactosemia is through dietary restriction. Treatment can result in reversal of the cataract if the galactosemia is diagnosed early and the dietary restriction is instituted prior to lenticular cortical scarring.

Christmas tree cataracts

Christmas tree cataracts consist of multiple small flecks of various colors that reflect light and give the appearance of a lighted Christmas tree. These cataracts can be associated with myotonic dystrophy, pseudohypoparathyroidism, and hypoparathyroidism.

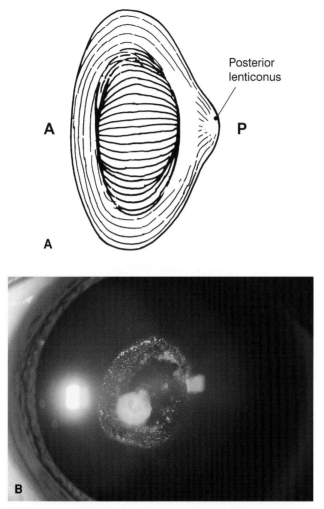

Figure 22-5.
Posterior lenticonus is a posterior bowing of the posterior capsule with capsular thinning. This capsular ectasia produces a progressive posterior capsular opacity. **A,** shows a diagram of posterior lenticonus with the posterior ectasia seen in red. **B,** is a slitlamp photograph of posterior lenticonus. The circular opacity represents the area of thinning and posterior bowing of the posterior capsule.

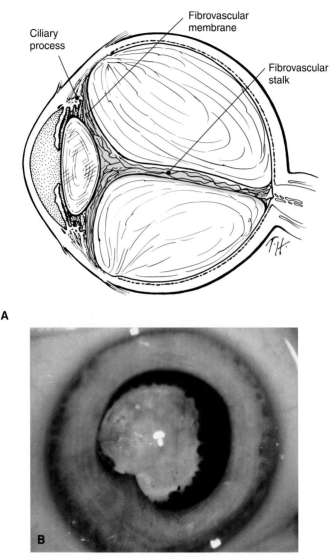

Figure 22-6.
Persistent hyperplastic primary vitreous (PHPV). **A,** Diagram of PHPV showing a
fibrovascular stalk, which emanates from the optic nerve and extends to the posterior
capsule of the lens to form a retrolental fibrovascular membrane. In severe forms
of PHPV, the fibrovascular membrane contracts with time, pulling the ciliary body
centrally, shallowing the anterior chamber, thus causing angle closure glaucoma. **B,**
is a clinical photograph of severe PHPV with the fibrovascular membrane pulling
the ciliary processes centrally. The dark black tissue with the scalloped border is the
ciliary body being pulled to the center of the pupil by the fibrovascular membrane.
The pink appearance of the membrane is secondary to vascularization of the
membrane.

Table 22-2.
Etiology of Congenital Cataracts

Unilateral Cataracts
1. Idiopathic (40%)
2. Posterior lenticonus (20%)
3. Persistent Hyperplastic Primary Vitreous (PHPV) (10%)
4. Anterior polar (10%)
5. Other (9%)
   a. Anterior segment dysgenesis
   b. Posterior pole tumors (rare)
6. Traumatic (10%)—consider child abuse
5. Intrauterine infection (rubella) (1%)
Note: Asymmetric bilateral lens opacities may be misinterpreted as a unilateral cataract.

Bilateral Cataracts
1. Idiopathic (50%)
2. Hereditary cataracts (40%) without systemic disease
   a. Autosomal dominant (most common)
   b. Autosomal recessive
   c. X-linked
3. Systemic diseases (5%)
   a. Hallermann-Streiff syndrome (midfacial hypoplasia, dwarfism)
   b. Lowe syndrome (oculocerebrorenal syndrome)
   c. Smith-Lemli-Optiz syndrome
   d. Galactosemia
   e. Hypoglycemia
   f. Trisomy
      1) Down syndrome (21)
      2) Edward syndrome (28)
      3) Patau syndrome (13)
   g. Alport syndrome
   h. Myotonic dystrophy
   i. Fabry disease (ceramide trihexosidase deficiency)
   j. Hypoparathyroidism
   k. Marfan syndrome
   l. Pseudohypoparathyroidism
   m. Conradi syndrome
   n. Diabetes mellitus
   o. Peroxisomal biogenesis disorder
   p. Wilson disease
4. Intrauterine infection (3%)
   a. Rubella
   b. Cytomegalovirus
   c. Varicella
   d. Syphilis
   e. Toxoplasmosis
   f. Herpes simplex
5. Ocular abnormalities (2%)
   a. Aniridia
   b. Anterior segment dysgenesis

Table 22-3.
Systemic Syndromes and Diseases Associated With Cataracts

A. Cataracts Associated With Skeletal Disease

Syndrome/Disease	Systemic Manifestations
Albright hereditary	Short stature, subcutaneous calcification, osteodystrophy, brachydactyly
Chondrodysplasia punctata	Dysplastic skeletal changes, dermatosis of the skin, saddle-nose deformity, pathognomonic radiologic findings in epiphysis
Majewski syndrome	Neonatal dwarfism, polydactyly, narrow thorax, cleft lip and palate, visceral deformities
Myotonic dystrophy	Muscle wasting, hypogonadism, cardiac changes, baldness
Osteogenesis imperfecta	Bone fractures, deafness, skull anomalies, ligament congenital hyperflexibility, discoloration of dentition

B. Cataracts Associated With Dermatological Disorders

Syndrome/Disease	Systemic Manifestations
Atopic dermatitis	Red, thickened, crusty skin, allergic history
Cockayne	Dwarfism, precocious senile appearance, deafness, retardation
Congenital ichthyosis	Fish-scale skin, hyperkeratosis, lack of hair
Incontinentia pigmenti	Skin pigmentation, hypodontia, skeletal defects, mental deficiency, microcephaly
Rothmund-Thomson syndrome	Telangiectasia, hypogonadism, vascular skin lesions, saddle-nose deformity, congenital bone defects

C. Cataracts Associated With Central Nervous System Syndromes

Syndrome/Disease	Systemic Manifestations
Laurence-Moon; Bardet-Biedl	Retinitis pigmentosa, nystagmus, strabismus, polydactyly, mental retardation
Marinesco-Sjögren	Oligophrenia, spinocerebellar ataxia, nystagmus, mental retardation
Sjögren-Larsson	Ichthyosis, spasticity, short stature, mental retardation, oligophrenia

(*continued*)

Table 22-3.
(continued)

D. Cataracts Associated With Craniofacial Syndromes

Syndrome/Disease	Systemic Manifestations
Hallermann-Streiff	More than 90% have congenital cataracts, small stature, malar hypoplasia, micrognathia, abnormal dentition, bird-like facies
Pierre Robin	Cataracts uncommon, micrognathia, cleft palate, glossoptosis
Alport	Cataracts uncommon, oxycephalic skull, normal intelligence, finger fusion, congenital heart defects, polycystic kidneys
Crouzon	Cataracts uncommon, brachycephaly, broadened nasal root, irregular dentition, mental retardation
Smith-Lemli-Opitz	Cataracts common, microcephaly, mental deficiency, syndactyly, hypospadias, cryptorchidism

E. Cataracts Associated With Multisystem Syndromes

Syndrome/Disease	Systemic Manifestations
Noonan	Webbed neck, low-set ears, typical facies, pulmonary stenosis
Werner	Arrested growth, premature graying, scleroderma-like changes, arteriosclerosis, diabetes mellitus, hypogonadism, osteoporosis, premature senility

Etiology of Infantile Cataracts

The etiologies of unilateral versus bilateral congenital cataracts are listed in **Table 22-2,** and systemic diseases associated with cataracts are listed in **Table 22-3.** The most common identifiable cause for bilateral cataracts is genetic with autosomal dominant inheritance; however, recessive and X-linked patterns have also been described.

Unilateral Cataracts

Unilateral infantile cataracts are rarely caused by a systemic disease, except in some cases of intrauterine infections such as rubella. Approximately 20% to 30% of rubella cataracts are unilateral. Thus, the presence of a unilateral cataract does not totally rule out the possibility of an associated systemic disease, but it is highly

Table 22-4.
Systemic Evaluation of Pediatric Cataracts

I. HISTORY
 A. Family history is critical
 B. Age of onset of cataract
 C. Developmental milestones
 D. Trauma (battered-child syndrome?)
II. PEDIATRIC PHYSICAL EXAMINATION
 Also consult geneticist or dysmorphologist
III. OCULAR PHYSICAL EXAMINATION
 Diagnose specific morphological features of the cataract (ie, PHPV, posterior lenticonus, anterior polar cataract)
IV. REQUIRED LABORATORY TESTS
 A. Unilateral cataracts
  1. TORCH titer and VDRL
 B. Bilateral cataracts
  1. ROUTINE
   a. TORCH titer and VDRL
   b. Urine for reducing substance (after milk feeding)
  2. OPTIONAL
   a. Red cell galactokinase (developmental cataracts)
   b. Serum for amino acids (developmental delay and glaucoma)
   c. Calcium and phosphorus (cataracts and metabolic disorders)

suggestive that the cataract is caused by local dysgenesis. The workup for a unilateral congenital cataract should include a full ophthalmic examination (**Table 22-4**). Some physicians prefer to obtain only antibody titers against the specific diseases suspected because of the cost of obtaining total serum TORCH (*t*oxoplasmosis, *o*ther infections, *r*ubella, *c*ytomegalovirus infection, and *h*erpes simplex) titers. However, if the examination does not clearly reveal a specific diagnosis, then serum TORCH titers should be obtained to rule out intrauterine infection. If a titer is positive, IgM assays should be performed, as IgM does not transfer across the placenta and IgM indicates fetal immunoglobulin and fetal infection.

Bilateral Cataracts

Bilateral cataracts are often inherited, with autosomal dominant being the most common inheritance pattern. Recent genetic studies have isolated chromosomal abnormalities associated with many types of cataracts. Approximately 5% to 10% of bilateral cataracts are associated with a systemic disorder. The workup for bilateral congenital or infantile cataracts should include a careful pediatric examination, a urine test for reducing substance (sugar) after a milk feeding, and TORCH titer (**Table 22-4**). Laboratory workup is not necessary if the cataracts can be positively defined as hereditary without other systemic abnormalities.

Cataracts and Infantile Glaucoma

The differential diagnosis of congenital cataracts with glaucoma includes Lowe syndrome, congenital rubella syndrome, anterior segment dysgenesis syndromes, and aniridia with cataract.

Lowe Syndrome (oculocerebrorenal syndrome)
This is an X-linked disorder that presents with bilateral congenital cataracts and often with bilateral congenital glaucoma. Infants show severe developmental delay, hypotonia, and renal failure with aminoaciduria. The prognosis is poor, as there is progressive neurological and renal deterioration with death occurring in late childhood. A dilated slit lamp examination of the patient's mother shows multiple punctate white snowflake opacities of the lens (check the lens periphery).

Congenital Rubella Syndrome
Systemic findings of congenital rubella syndrome include congenital heart defects, hearing loss, and mental retardation. Ocular findings include cataracts (15%), salt and pepper retinopathy (25%), strabismus (20%), microphthalmos (15%), optic atrophy (10%), corneal haze (10%), glaucoma (10%), and phthisis bulbi (2%). The retinopathy is stable and usually does not affect vision. Rubella cataracts are caused by invasion of the lens by the rubella virus, and are bilateral in 80% of all cases. These cataracts may present with a hazy cornea caused by either congenital glaucoma or keratitis. Treatment of the cataract involves removing all of the lens cortex, since the patient's tendency to postoperative inflammation is increased if residual cortex is left after surgery.

■ TREATMENT OF PEDIATRIC CATARACTS

The strategy for treating congenital cataracts is to provide a clear retinal image as soon as possible to avoid irreversible amblyopia. The most common cause for poor vision after pediatric cataract surgery is amblyopia, which can be unilateral or bilateral. Because of this, a unilateral or bilateral congenital cataract that is visually significant must be visually rehabilitated as soon as possible, even during the first week of life. Treatment is urgent—bilateral congenital cataracts that obscure the visual axis will often result in sensory nystagmus and a bilateral poor visual outcome if not treated by 2 months of age.

Surgical Technique

Pediatric cataracts and cataracts in young adults (younger than 30 years of age) can be removed by microinstrumentation using suction and suction-cutting modalities. Complications of cataract surgery are unusual, but late complications include retinal detachment (rare), immediate or late glaucoma (5%), retinal hemorrhages, secondary cortex growth (Elschnig pearls), and endophthalmitis.

Lens Implantation

Intraocular lenses have now become an accepted method for treating aphakia (absence of a natural lens) in children. One must be selective, however, when considering lens implantation in the pediatric age group. During the first year of life, there is a dramatic increase in eye length and consequent change in the lens power (approximately 10 to 14 diopters) needed to focus. Because of the significant change in eye size during the first year of life, implantation of intraocular lenses in infants is controversial. By 2 years of age, however, the eye is almost adult size. For the most part, intraocular lenses are becoming the standard in children older than 2 years of age. Since the posterior capsule invariably opacifies after a lens implantation, a secondary YAG capsulotomy or secondary procedure is usually necessary.

Spectacles and Contact Lenses

Spectacles

Spectacles are an option to correct bilateral aphakia in children. However, they are unsightly, do not provide constant correction, and are not used for monocular aphakia because of the unilateral magnification of the aphakic lens.

Contact Lenses

In newborns, **contact lenses** are the standard treatment for either unilateral or bilateral aphakia. Aphakic spectacles can be used as a backup for contact lenses in bilaterally aphakic children.

Occlusion Therapy

Monocular pediatric cataracts require occlusion therapy to treat amblyopia. There is some controversy about the amount of patching for patients with monocular cataracts. The amount of patching should be based on the severity of amblyopia. Critical to the management of monocular congenital cataracts is educating the parents about amblyopia, the importance of a clear retinal image, and the need for occlusion therapy.

Visual Prognosis of Pediatric Cataracts

Monocular Cataracts

If surgery and optical correction are provided early, by 2 months of age, visual acuity outcomes are relatively good even for monocular congenital cataracts. **Birch and Stager** reported that a mean visual acuity of 20/60 (range 20/800 to 20/30) was achieved if surgery was performed before 2 months of age, whereas surgery after 2 months of age resulted in poor visual acuity (ranging from hand motion to 20/160). Historically, patients with monocular cataracts have a very poor prognosis for obtaining fusion, and virtually all studies report that almost 100% of patients will develop strabismus. **Wright, et al,** and **Gregg and Parks** reported that good visual acuity and good binocularity with stereopsis are possible in patients with monocular cataracts. The key points to these cases were that very early surgery (less than 2 months of age and as early as the first week of life) was performed with immediate contact lens fitting, and part-time monocular occlusion (less than 50%) for amblyopia was initiated during the first few months of life.

Cataracts in children do not always present during the first few months of life. Often, the clinician is faced with the child who has a unilateral or bilateral cataract and the question is, "Should the cataract be operated upon or is there irreversible amblyopia?"

Reports by **Kushner** and **Wright, et al,** indicate that many older children with presumed congenital cataracts can show significant visual acuity improvement after surgical treatment. Lack of strabismus (straight eyes) is also a good prognostic sign for patients with unilateral cataracts.

Binocular Cataracts

It is sometimes said that binocular cataracts are less amblyogenic than monocular cataracts. This is misleading because, even though a monocular cataract causes a very dense amblyopia, binocular cataracts can also cause significant amblyopia. It is important that binocular cataracts are treated with urgency and are operated during the first few weeks of life. If a visually significant bilateral congenital cataract is not cleared by 2 months of age, patients will develop sensory nystagmus and very poor visual acuity (usually less than 20/200) in the majority of cases. Patients with non-operated bilateral cataracts and sensory nystagmus can show improvement in visual acuity and improvement of the nystagmus, even if surgery is performed late, after the critical period of visual development. This author has reported that visual acuity as good as 20/50 to 20/70 can be achieved even when late surgery is performed. Surgery by 2 months of age is definitely the treatment of choice; however, older children who present late should be considered for cataract surgery even though they present with bilateral cataracts and nystagmus. The exception to this are those patients with an abnormality of the retina or optic nerve, such as aniridia. In patients with aniridia, cataract surgery usually does not improve vision because macular hypoplasia limits the visual acuity potential.

■ RETINOBLASTOMA

Retinoblastoma is a malignant tumor of the sensory retina and is the most common ocular malignancy in childhood. Critical to the treatment of retinoblastoma is early identification, as cure rates are higher than 90% if the tumor is localized within the eye. A white reflex within the pupil (**leukocoria**) is a serious sign that could suggest retinoblastoma and deserves immediate referral (**Figure 22-7A**).

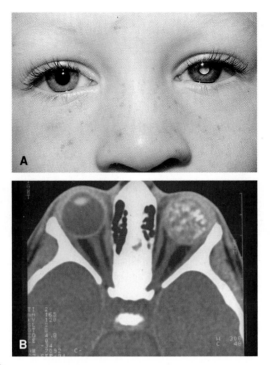

Figure 22-7.
A, photograph of a 19-month-old child with leukocoria in the left eye secondary to retinoblastoma. **B,** CT scan showing extensive intraocular calcification associated with retinoblastoma. Calcification represents area of tumor necrosis.

Clinical Signs of Retinoblastoma

The most common presenting signs of retinoblastoma are leukocoria and strabismus. Retinoblastoma also may present with findings that mimic other ophthalmic disorders such as primary angle closure glaucoma, vitreous hemorrhage, retinal detachment, hyphema, hypopyon, and even preseptal cellulitis. Usually, retinoblastoma presents with a quiet eye; however, tumor necrosis can lead to intraocular hemorrhage, inflammation, and a red, painful eye. Angle closure glaucoma occurs when the posterior pole fills with tumor, thus pushing the lens-iris diaphragm anteriorly. Even though retinoblastoma is rare (estimated at 1:20,000 live births), the pediatrician must hold high suspicion for this disease in any child with leukocoria.

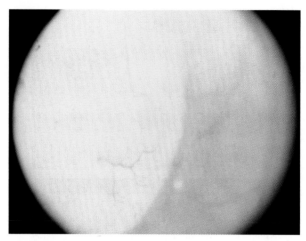

Figure 22-8.
Fundus photograph of endophytic retinoblastoma. Note the yellow-white appearance of the domed mass. Normal attached retina is seen in the background to the right.

Retinoblastoma tumors have a yellow or slightly pink gelatinous appearance (**Figure 22-8**). There may be white areas within the tumor that represent calcification. **Calcification** is a hallmark of retinoblastoma and is best detected by CT scan (**Figure 22-7B**) or ocular ultrasound. Calcification is associated with tumor necrosis that occurs as the tumor outgrows its blood supply. The presence of calcium in a retinal mass is highly suggestive of retinoblastoma, although in rare cases, retinoblastoma tumors will not be calcified. Also, some ocular diseases such as Coats disease have tissue necrosis and can show calcifications as well.

Genetics of Retinoblastoma

Retinoblastoma is caused by a mutation in a growth suppressor gene. The site of the gene for retinoblastoma is chromosome 13q14, and the gene has been sequenced. Both the paternal and maternal alleles must be affected for the development of a retinoblastoma tumor, because a single intact suppressor gene is all that is necessary to regulate retinal cell growth. **Knudson** was the first to suggest this "2 hit" hypothesis. Retinoblastoma can be inherited or be secondary to a sporadic mutation. Inherited cases are often cited as an autosomal dominant disorder. It is the mutation of one allele (first hit) that is inherited as an autosomal dominant trait. The second allele mutation occurs after conception and is a somatic mutation. Retinoblastoma is actually an autosomal recessive trait since both alleles must be affected to express the disease. There are 2 recognized mechanisms that cause a mutation of both alleles, resulting in **hereditary retinoblastoma** and **sporadic retinoblastoma.**

Hereditary Retinoblastoma

In the hereditary form of retinoblastoma, a mutation of both retinoblastoma genes occurs by inheriting an abnormal gene from one parent (germinal mutation) and then acquiring a spontaneous mutation of the other allelic gene at the retinal cell level later in development (somatic mutation). Patients with hereditary retinoblastoma have a defective retinoblastoma gene in virtually all cells in their body. Because of this, patients with hereditary retinoblastoma are predisposed to acquiring secondary non-ocular tumors, such as osteosarcoma, in late childhood and adulthood.

All the retinal cells in the inherited form have an abnormal gene (1 hit) at conception, and the second mutation occurs after conception in approximately 80% of cases. Thus, almost all patients who have inherited the abnormal allele will develop the second mutation and develop retinoblastoma. Most inherited retinoblastomas are bilateral, with only 15% being unilateral. Hereditary retinoblastoma is often multifocal, with multiple tumors developing in each eye. Patients with the hereditary form present early, around 12 months of age on the average. The inherited form can come from a parent with known retinoblastoma, from a germinal mutation in the egg or sperm, or from a mutation at the time of conception. In these latter cases, the family history is negative for retinoblastoma. In fact, the majority of new cases of bilateral hereditary retinoblastoma are due to a new germinal mutation, as only 10% have a positive family history. If a parent has retinoblastoma, there is a 50% chance of passing the predisposition (a retinoblastoma gene) to the child. Because not all children with one mutated allele develop a mutation in the second allele, the chance of a child developing retinoblastoma from a parent with retinoblastoma is 40%, rather than 50%. If there is no family history of retinoblastoma and a child is born with bilateral retinoblastoma, the chance that another sibling will develop retinoblastoma is approximately 8%. Remember that most germinal mutations are not present in the germinal stem cells of the parents, so subsequent children are at low risk. With DNA testing, carriers of a germinal mutation of the retinoblastoma gene can be identified in most cases. A large deletion in the area of the retinoblastoma gene will delete other local genes and cause an identifiable defect in the karyotype at chromosome 13q14. Patients with this deletion may have the clinical characteristics of facial dysmorphism, developmental delay, mental retardation, and low-set ears. This phenotype only occurs in 3% of retinoblastoma cases where multiple genes are deleted in addition to the retinoblastoma gene.

Sporadic Retinoblastoma

The sporadic form of retinoblastoma is caused by a spontaneous mutation of both alleles at the retinal cell level (2 somatic mutations). This requires 2 independent mutational events that are not inherited. Sporadic retinoblastoma presents as a unilateral-unifocal tumor. It must be noted, however, that 15% of hereditary retinoblastomas occur as a unilateral tumor, albeit usually multifocal. Approximately 60% of all retinoblastoma cases are the nonhereditary form.

Staging of Retinoblastoma

Retinoblastoma has been classified by **Reese Ellsworth** by determining the prognosis of the eye. This classification has been mistakenly extrapolated to estimate the prognosis for patient survival. The extrapolation states that small tumors located posterior to the equator have a favorable outcome. Any tumor at or anterior to the equator, or a tumor larger than 10 disc diameters in size, has an unfavorable prognosis. Massive tumors involving more than half the retina or the presence of vitreous seeding indicates a very unfavorable prognosis for salvaging the eye.

The classic histologic findings of retinoblastoma are **Flexner-Wintersteiner rosettes.** Less commonly seen are **fleurettes.** Pathological signs of poor systemic prognosis may include choroidal involvement, but most often seen is extrascleral extension and extension of the tumor into the optic nerve posterior to the lamina cribrosa. Local extension into the orbit and metastasis through the subarachnoid space into the brain are the most common routes of tumor spread. Bone marrow, liver, and lungs are also distant sites for metastasis.

Pinealoblastoma (trilateral retinoblastoma)

Pinealoma associated with bilateral retinoblastoma has been termed trilateral retinoblastoma and is a rare occurrence with an extremely poor prognosis. The pineal body is considered a third eye because it has embryological links to the retinal tissue.

Treatment of Retinoblastoma

Large tumors involving the macula are associated with a poor visual prognosis and generally are treated by enucleation. Smaller tumors can be treated with external beam radiation (approximately 4,000 rad) or chemo reduction. If the tumor is bilateral, then every attempt should be made to save at least one eye. External beam radiation is most useful for posteriorly located tumors. Radioactive plaque treatment, which involves attaching a radioactive "button" directly over the site of the tumor, has also been used and has the advantage of minimizing radiation to normal tissue. External beam radiation may have the disadvantage of inducing or speeding up the development of secondary tumors in patients with the hereditary form of retinoblastoma. The use of chemotherapy to decrease the size of the tumor, followed by laser or cryotherapy, has been effective in eyes with salvageable vision. Small peripheral tumors can be treated with cryotherapy or laser photocoagulation.

Infants who present with unilateral retinoblastoma must be followed closely, since 20% will develop a new tumor in the "good eye." This risk diminishes greatly after 2 years of age. In cases of hereditary retinoblastoma, siblings are at risk for developing the tumor. They should be followed with serial retinal examinations using scleral depression (use of a special instrument to view the peripheral retina).

Prognosis of Retinoblastoma

Unilateral retinoblastoma without extrascleral extension and without extension past the lamina cribrosa, having been treated by enucleation, is associated with long-term survival of over 90%. If the tumor cells extend posterior to the lamina cribrosa, the survival rate lowers to approximately 60%, even if the cut end of the optic nerve is free of tumor. Extrascleral extension of tumor cells beyond the surgical transection site of the optic nerve is associated with a long-term survival rate of less than 20%. The use of eye-saving therapies such as external beam radiation, radioactive plaque, and chemo reduction performed in patients without extrascleral extension results in a cure in approximately 85% of patients. Patients with hereditary retinoblastoma are at risk for developing secondary malignant tumors later in life. These tumors are often in the area of the external beam radiation, but can also occur in remote sites. Secondary tumors include malignant melanoma, fibrosarcoma, leiomyosarcoma, osteosarcoma, and renal cell carcinoma. Patients who have had radiation therapy develop secondary tumors earlier than patients who have not had radiation. The incidence for developing a secondary tumor in patients with hereditary retinoblastoma is probably higher than 50% with a long-term follow-up of over 30 years.

■ MEDULLOEPITHELIOMA

Medulloepithelioma is a tumor that arises from the ciliary body or iris. It occurs sporadically and at virtually any time during life, but most commonly presents in early childhood between 4 and 8 years of age. The tumor probably stems from non-pigmented ciliary epithelium.

The tumor is slow growing and tends to stay localized within the eye. Survival rates are excellent if the tumor is localized to the eye. The tumor usually arises from the ciliary body, however, rare reports of optic nerve and retinal involvement have been described. Because the tumors arise from the ciliary body, they usually are not detected until they are quite large. Often, patients present with angle closure glaucoma, pain, poor vision, or an anterior chamber cyst or mass. Cataract, rubeosis, and PHPV have also been associated with medulloepitheliomas. The treatment for medulloepitheliomas is usually enucleation; however, iridocyclectomy can be curative if the entire lesion is removed.

■ UVEAL MELANOMA

Uveal melanomas are extremely rare in children. Tumors may involve the iris, ciliary body, or choroid. The diagnosis of melanoma should be entertained in patients with an enlarging pigmented mass. Other causes of a pigmented intraocular mass in children include melanocytoma, choroidal nevus, iris cysts, pigmented neurofibroma, juvenile xanthogranuloma, and a retinal pigment epithelial hamartoma. Uveal melanomas may arise from ocular and oculodermal melanocytosis. Ocular ultrasound is an important tool for establishing the proper diagnosis in children, just as it is in adults.

The prognosis of uveal melanomas in children parallels that of adults. A review by **Barr, McLean, and Zimmermann** of choroidal and ciliary body tumors in children showed that of 42 patients, 13 died of metastatic disease, an incidence similar to the adult population. Poor prognostic features include extraocular extension, large basal diameter (greater than 10 mm), aggressive cell type, and red painful eye with tumor necrosis at the time of presentation. The treatment is usually enucleation.

■ LEUKEMIA

Leukemia can involve all ocular structures; however, the retina is the most commonly involved site. Acute lymphoblastic leukemia (ALL) is the most common leukemic cell type in children. Retinal involvement includes cotton-wool spots, exudates, dilated veins, and, most commonly, retinal hemorrhages. Hemorrhages may take on the appearance of a Roth spot, with white centers and surrounding hemorrhage. Other ocular manifestations include retinal infiltrates, vitreous involvement, exudative detachment, optic nerve involvement, iris infiltrate, hypopyon, ring corneal ulcers, and conjunctiva and perilimbal infiltrates. Treatment, for the most part, is directed toward the systemic disease by the oncology team. However, local ocular radiation to anterior lesions (conjunctiva, anterior chamber, or iris) with low-dose external beam radiation has been found to be effective.

■ COATS DISEASE

Coats disease is a unilateral sporadic congenital vasculopathy of the retina of unknown cause. It is characterized by the presence of telangiectatic vessels with aneurysmal buds that leak exudate into the retina (**Figure 22-9**). Coats disease presents as leukocoria in childhood, usually before 10 years of age. Retinal fluorescein angiography shows intense leakage from the untreated telangiectatic vessels. The disease is progressive and can lead to retinal detachment and blindness. Treatment is laser photocoagulation or cryotherapy to ablate the abnormal vessels. Multiple treatment sessions are usually necessary.

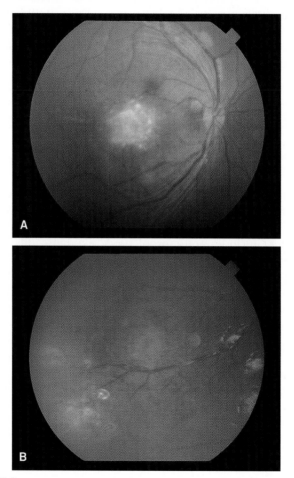

Figure 22-9.
Coats disease in a 6-year-old child. Color photographs show massive exudation with cystic change in the fovea **(A),** and numerous bulb-shaped arterial and venous aneurysms **(B).**

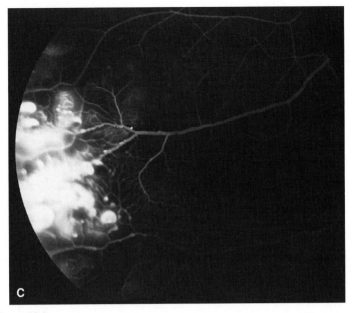

Figure 22-9.
(continued) Fluorescein angiography shows blockage of choroidal fluorescence by foveal exudates with intense leakage from telangiectatic vessels temporal to the macula **(C)**.

■ BIBLIOGRAPHY

1. Abramson DH, Ellsworth RM, Kitchin FD, Tung G. Second nonocular tumors in retinoblastoma survivors: Are they radiation-induced? *Ophthalmology.* 1984;91:1351–1355
2. Abramson DH, Ellsworth RM, Tretter P, Javitt J, Kitchin FD. Treatment of bilateral groups I through III: retinoblastoma with bilateral radiation. *Arch Ophthalmol.*1981;99:1761–1762
3. Abramson DH, Wachtel A, Watson CW, Jereb B, Wollner N. Leukemic hypopyon. *J Pediatr Ophthalmol Strabismus.* May-June 1981;18:42–44
4. Bader JL, Meadows AT, Zimmerman LE. Bilateral reintoblastoma with ectopic intracranial retinoblastoma: trilateral retinoblastoma. *Cancer Genet Cytogenet.* 1982;5:203–213
5. Barr CC, McLean IW, Zimmerman LE. Uveal melanoma in children and adolescents. *Arch Ophthalmol.* 1981;99:2133–2136
6. Birch EE, Stager DR. Prevalence of good visual acuity following surgery for congenital unilateral cataract. *Arch Ophthalmol.* 1988;106:40–43

7. Canning CR, McCartney AC, Hungerford J. Medulloepithelioma (diktyoma). *Br J Ophthalmol.* 1988;72:764–767

8. Cavenee WK, Dryja TP, Phillips RA, et al. Expression of recessive alleles by chromosomal mechanisms in retinoblastoma. *Nature.* 1983; 305:779–784

9. Cordes FC. Galactosemia cataract: a review. *Am J Ophthalmol.* 1960;50: 1151–1158

10. Friend SH, Bernards R, Rogelj S, et al. A human DNA segment with properties of the gene that predisposes to retinoblastoma and osteosarcoma. *Nature.* 1986;323:643–646

11. Ginsberg J, Bove KE, Fogelson MH. Pathological features of the eye in the oculocerebrorenal (Lowe) syndrome. *J Pediatr Ophthalmol Strabismus.* July-August 1981;18:16–24

12. Gregg FM, Parks MM. Stereopsis after congenital monocular cataract extraction. *Am J Ophthalmol.* 1992;114:314–317

13. Guyer DR, Schachat AP, Vitale S, et al. Leukemic retinopathy. Relationship between fundus lesions and hematologic parameters at diagnosis. *Ophthalmology.* 1989;96:860–864

14. Kincaid MC and Green WR: Ocular and orbital involvement in leukemia. *Surv Ophthalmol.* Jan-Feb 1983;27:211–232

15. Knudson AG Jr. Hereditary cancer, oncogenes, and antioncogenes. *Cancer Res.* 1985;45:1437–1443

16. Kushner BJ. Visual results after surgery for monocular juvenile cataracts of undetermined onset. *Am J Ophthalmol.* October 1986;102: 468–472

17. Nelson SC, Friedman HS, Oakes WJ, et al. Successful therapy for trilateral retinoblastoma. *Am J Ophthalmol.* 1992;114:23–29

18. Rosenbaum PS, Boniuk M, Font RL. Diffuse uveal melanoma in a 5-year-old child. *Am J Ophthalmol.* 1988;106:601–606

19. Scheie HG, Schaffer DB, Plotkin SA, Kertesz ED. Congenital rubella cataracts. Surgical results and virus recovery from intraocular tissue. *Arch Ophthalmol.* 1967;77:440–444

20. Shields CL, Shields JA, Milite J, De Potter P, Sabbagh R, Menduke H. Uveal melanoma in teenagers and children. A report of 40 cases. *Ophthalmology.* 1991;98:1662–1666

21. Streeten BW, Robinson MR, Wallace R, Jones DB. Lens capsule abnormalities in Alport's syndrome. *Arch Ophthalmol.* 1987:105;1693–1697

22. Wright KW, Christensen LE, Noguchi BA. Results of late surgery for presumed congenital cataracts. *Am J Ophthalmol.* 1992;114:409–415

23. Wright KW, Matsumoto E, Edelman PM. Binocular fusion and stereopsis associated with early surgery for monocular congenital cataracts. *Arch Ophthalmol.* 1992;110:1607–1609

23 Ocular Trauma

■ GENERAL APPROACH

Children are especially vulnerable to ocular trauma. Eye injuries can occur at virtually any age, even in utero secondary to perforation of the globe by amniocentesis. It is especially important to take a good history when evaluating ocular trauma: clarify exactly what, when, and how the trauma occurred. Is it possible that a foreign body is involved? Document the timetable of events and whether there was an antecedent ocular disease. Other important history includes coexisting systemic disease, allergy, prior injuries, bleeding diathesis, and previous tetanus prophylaxis. Ocular trauma is often associated with head trauma. Amnesia, headache, change in mental status, or loss of consciousness should prompt further neurological workup and neuro-imaging.

Use the **"I-ARM"** (**I**nspection, **A**cuity, **R**ed reflex, and **M**otility) formula to direct the ocular examination (Chapter 3). The first goal of the ocular examination is to determine the extent of the trauma and to rule out a ruptured globe (later in this chapter). If a ruptured globe is identified or suspected, then stop the examination, place a protective shield over the eye to avoid extrusion of intraocular contents, and obtain an emergency ophthalmology consultation. When testing the vision of a patient who does not have his or her glasses, use a pinhole as a substitute for glasses to test best-corrected vision. Create a pinhole by simply taking a 3″ × 5″ card and using a safety pin to punch a hole. Have the child look through the pin-

317

Table 23-1.

Minor Trauma Signs

Send patient home without treatment if

- Vision is good (20/40 or better)
- Good red reflex
- No pain
- No hyphema
- No significant conjunctival hemorrhage

hole to test visual acuity. The pinhole will focus the image and give an estimate of best-corrected visual acuity.

Pediatric ocular trauma can be quite alarming but, if the findings of a careful ocular examination is normal, the patient and family can be reassured. The features of minor trauma without significant ocular damage and not requiring treatment are listed in **Table 23-1.** If these criteria are met, it is safe to send the patient home without treatment.

A computed tomography (CT) scan of the head and orbits is indicated in patients who sustain a penetrating injury to the eye or orbit with a possibility of an ocular or orbital foreign body. A CT scan is preferable over MRI because the magnetic field associated with MRI can move a metallic intraocular foreign body, possibly resulting in further ocular trauma.

■ CHILD ABUSE (BATTERED-CHILD SYNDROME)

Unfortunately, **child abuse,** or **battered-child syndrome,** is a significant cause of pediatric ocular trauma. Warning signs of child abuse include an injury that is not consistent with the alleged accident, multiple trauma admissions at different hospitals, delay in presentation to the physician, multiple fractures and soft tissue injuries at different stages of healing, and skin burns that may be related to a cigarette or submersion in hot liquid. If child abuse is suspected, the workup should consist of a complete pediatric examination with genital examination and a skeletal X-ray series to evaluate for past and present fractures. Neuro-imaging should be considered if there are central nervous system signs such as lethargy or irritability. A complete ocular examination, including a dilated fundus examination to rule out retinal hemorrhages, is critical to the evaluation of a child with possible battered-child syndrome.

Early Detection of Child Abuse Is Critical

It is the physician's responsibility to immediately report all suspected cases of battered-child syndrome to social services or the police department. Most states have laws that require physicians and health care professionals to report all suspected cases of battered-child syndrome. Battered-child syndrome is almost always a recurrent problem. Without early intervention, children continue to be abused, suffering physical and psychological devastation, which all too often results in death.

Retinal Hemorrhages

Retinal hemorrhages in infants are highly suggestive of battered-child syndrome and include dot and blot hemorrhages, pre-retinal (boat-shaped) hemorrhages, and vitreous hemorrhages (**Figure 23-1**). Other retinal findings are chorioretinal scars, optic atrophy, reti-

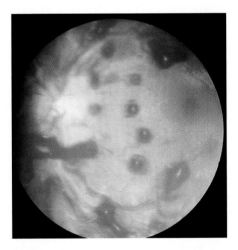

Figure 23-1.
Fundus photograph of a battered infant. Just inferior to the optic disc is a preretinal boat-shaped hemorrhage. Note the presence of multiple preretinal hemorrhages with white light reflexes off the dome of the hemorrhage giving the appearance of **Roth spots.** These are not true Roth spots, which are localized hemorrhages with a central white spot, representing an accumulation of white blood cells or an area of ischemia (cotton-wool spot). Roth spots are usually associated with subacute bacterial endocarditis, leukemia, or anemia.

noschisis, and cotton-wool spots. Infants who present with lethargy, subdural hematomas or subdural effusions, and/or retinal hemorrhages of unknown cause should be evaluated for child abuse. Birth trauma, leukemia, increased intracranial pressure, malignant hypertension, bacterial endocarditis, idiopathic thrombocytopenia, Purtscher's retinopathy (discussed in this chapter), Terson's retinopathy (discussed in this chapter), and, rarely, cardiopulmonary resuscitation are other causes of pediatric retinal hemorrhages.

Purtscher's Retinopathy

Purtscher's retinopathy is a cause of retinal hemorrhages. It occurs secondary to mechanical injury elsewhere in the body. It may be the result of a microembolism (such as fat or blood aggregate) that causes ischemia and hemorrhage, or from increased venous pressure secondary to chest compression. Purtscher's retinopathy is associated with soft exudates throughout the posterior pole, which are often concentrated around the optic disc. Nerve fiber layer hemorrhages and preretinal hemorrhages are often present. The treatment of Purtscher's retinopathy is conservative observation, as the retinal lesions disappear within a few weeks to a few months after the injury.

Terson's Retinopathy

Terson's retinopathy is a hemorrhagic retinopathy caused by an intracranial subarachnoid hemorrhage with increased intracranial pressure. Blood dissects anteriorly through the lamina cribrosa into the eye. Nerve fiber layer and preretinal hemorrhages are typically seen emanating from the optic nerve.

■ RUPTURED GLOBE

A ruptured globe is defined as a perforating injury of the cornea and/or sclera that violates the integrity of the eye. This can be caused by blunt trauma, a sharp object, or a missile. Injuries can be divided into anterior segment trauma (injuries to the cornea, anterior chamber, iris, and lens) and posterior segment trauma (perforation of sclera, retina, and vitreous). Posterior segment trauma carries a much higher risk of postoperative retinal detachment and has a

Table 23-2.
Signs of a Ruptured Globe

Anterior Perforating Injury (Figure 23–2)
Peaked or irregular pupil
Iris prolapse
Shallow anterior chamber
Corneal laceration
Hyphema
Posterior Perforating Injury (Figures 23–3 and 23–4)
Poor red reflex (vitreous hemorrhage)
Decreased vision
Uveal prolapse (black tissue under conjunctiva)
Subconjunctival hemorrhage and chemosis (fluid under the conjunctiva)
Deep anterior chamber
Hyphema

poorer prognosis than anterior segment trauma, especially if a vitreous hemorrhage is present. The poor prognosis of posterior perforating injuries is secondary to cellular proliferation and retinal fibrosis, which can lead to retinal scarring and detachment.

Signs of a ruptured globe include chemosis (edema and swelling of the conjunctiva), pigment under the conjunctiva, peaked pupil (anterior rupture), vitreous hemorrhage (posterior rupture), and low intraocular pressure (**Table 23-2, Figures 23-2 and 23-3**). These are the classic features that are usually present; however, the findings of a ruptured globe may be subtle, especially with sharp, posterior penetrating injuries (**Figure 23-4**). The areas of the eye wall most susceptible to rupture are the sclera posterior to the rectus muscle insertions, the corneoscleral limbus, and areas of previous surgical incisions (previous cataract surgery, corneal graft, and radial keratotomy incisions). Blunt trauma often produces lacerations that extend posteriorly behind a rectus muscle insertion, because the sclera is thinnest directly behind the rectus muscles.

Scleral and Corneal Wound Healing

Since the sclera and the cornea are essentially avascular, wound healing is slow, often requiring 3 to 6 months to heal completely. The anterior aspect of the corneal wound heals in a manner similar to skin, with the epithelium being a major contributor. A posterior wound may heal by endothelial cell fibrous metaplasia. Histological

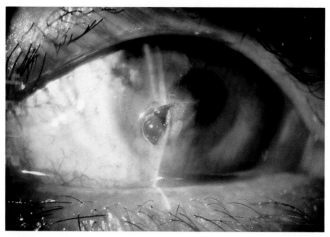

Figure 23-2.
Corneal laceration with iris prolapse through the wound. The iris prolapse is the brownish bubble of tissue at the line of the slit lamp beam. This child cut himself with a kitchen knife.

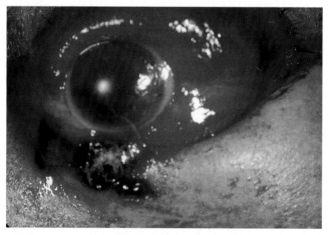

Figure 23-3.
Ruptured globe secondary to a posterior scleral laceration. The black tissue at the 6-o'clock position is choroidal tissue (ie, uveal tissue) that has prolapsed out of the scleral laceration. Note the presence of a subconjunctival hemorrhage, chemosis (swollen conjunctiva), and poor visualization of the iris because of a diffuse hyphema.

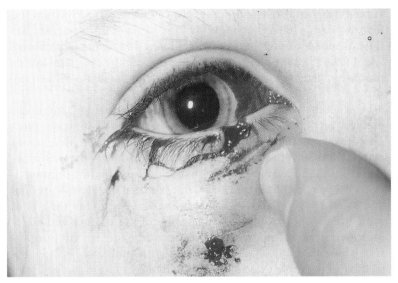

Figure 23-4.
Lower lid margin laceration caused by children who were playing with knives. Lid margin laceration requires special surgical techniques to properly repair the wound, which is usually done by an ophthalmologist. Also note the subconjunctival hemorrhage on the nasal half of the eyeball. This patient also has a posterior scleral laceration and a ruptured globe.

healing occurs as fibrous tissue fills the corneal or scleral wound, with the fibrous tissue oriented perpendicular to the stromal lamellae.

Management of a Ruptured Globe

After surgical closure of the ruptured globe by an ophthalmologist, broad-spectrum IV antibiotics (ciprofloxacin) and an aminoglycoside (gentamicin or tobramycin) should be continued for at least 3 days. Clindamycin should be considered if there is a possibility of a *Bacillus cereus* contamination (organic foreign body). The incidence of posttraumatic endophthalmitis after a ruptured globe is approximately 10%.

Lacerations that involve the retina and are associated with a vitreous hemorrhage usually require a posterior vitrectomy to remove the vitreous, thereby reducing the possibility of cellular proliferation, intraocular fibrosis, and retinal detachment. The timing of the vitrectomy is controversial; some advocate early surgery within the first few days while others wait for 7 to 14 days. Early surgery has the advantage of preventing irreversible retinal damage. Delaying 7 to 14 days lessens inflammation, lessens hemorrhage, and avoids posterior vitreous separation. These effects facilitate vitrectomy surgery.

A severely traumatized globe with uveal prolapse and documented no light perception (NLP) has no visual function postoperatively. There is a small, but significant, risk of developing **sympathetic ophthalmia** and losing vision in the good eye. Sympathetic ophthalmia is a rare inflammatory disease of the nontraumatized eye caused by exposure of the lymphatic system to retinal and uveal antigen from the traumatized eye. Because of the risk of sympathetic ophthalmia, an enucleation of the traumatized eye is indicated if no light perception persists after the primary surgical repair. Enucleation should be performed within 2 weeks after the trauma to prevent sympathetic ophthalmia.

■ PHTHISIS BULBI

A blind, scarred eye that is shrunken and hypotonic is termed phthisis bulbi. This end-stage eye is often painful. A blind, painful eye usually is treated with enucleation.

■ NONPERFORATING ANTERIOR SEGMENT TRAUMA

Corneal Abrasion

A corneal abrasion occurs when the corneal epithelium is removed. This creates severe pain, tearing, and photophobia. Patients usually feel there is something in the affected eye, even in the absence of a foreign body. Corneal abrasions heal by the sliding of existing epithelium to fill in the areas of abraded epithelium. After careful examination to rule out corneal foreign body or infiltrate, antibiotic ointment and a pressure patch is placed on the eye. Place the tape obliquely in parallel strips from the forehead to the cheek. In most cases, a corneal abrasion will heal after 24 to 48 hours of being patched. Antibiotic ointment is typically used for 2 to 3 days after the patch is removed and then discontinued.

If the abrasion is associated with contact lens use, then an oph-thalmology consult is indicated to rule out a bacterial corneal infec-tion. The differential diagnosis of a corneal abrasion includes herpes keratitis, bacterial ulcer, or retained corneal foreign body.

Conjunctival and Corneal Foreign Body

Common conjunctival and corneal foreign bodies include dust, dirt, or metallic slivers. Metallic foreign bodies usually are the result of a hammer or a hand tool made of forged steel striking something hard, like a rock. Metal from forged steel is under stress and, when it cracks, a metal sliver explodes off at high speed. Retained metallic foreign bodies will cause a rust ring in the cornea. To remove a foreign body, first anesthetize the eye with topical drops (eg, tetra-caine). If the foreign body is visualized, remove it with a sterile cotton-tipped applicator. Even superficial corneal foreign bodies can be removed in this manner. Deep corneal foreign bodies or foreign bodies that cannot be removed easily should be removed by an ophthalmologist. Once the foreign body is removed, irrigate the conjunctiva by everting the lid to flush the conjunctival fornix, and then instill a topical antibiotic ointment. Often the patient will continue to feel a foreign body sensation even after the foreign body is removed, because of an associated abrasion. If an abrasion is present, pressure-patch the eye as described previously. If a specific foreign body cannot be found, try irrigating the eye and conjuncti-val fornix.

Corneal Hydrops

Traumatic corneal hydrops is localized corneal edema caused by blunt trauma that produces breaks in Descemet's membrane. **Birth trauma,** with the forceps being placed on the infant's eyes, can cause corneal hydrops. Traumatic forceps breaks tend to be verti-cally aligned, in contrast to **Haab's striae** (in congenital glaucoma) that are usually horizontal.

Subconjunctival Hemorrhage

A **traumatic subconjunctival hemorrhage** can occur even after mild trauma without significant damage to the eye, and often makes things look worse than they are. Even so, a subconjunctival hemorrhage is an important sign, as it may indicate the presence of significant ocular trauma and even a ruptured globe (**Figures 23-3 and 23-4**). **Spontaneous subconjunctival hemorrhage,** usually of unknown cause, may occur without trauma. There is no treatment for subconjunctival hemorrhages except to reassure the patient that the hemorrhage will resolve spontaneously in approximately 2 weeks. If the hemorrhages are recurrent, a systemic evaluation is indicated. In rare cases, a spontaneous subconjunctival hemorrhage is associated with a systemic disease such as systemic hypertension, a bleeding diathesis, or diabetes mellitus. In the vast majority of cases, however, no systemic evaluation is necessary. Conjunctivitis caused by adenovirus or *Haemophilus influenzae* can cause subconjunctival hemorrhage.

Hyphema

A hyphema is blood in the anterior chamber (**Figure 23-5**). Hyphemas are most frequently caused by blunt ocular trauma; however, non-traumatic causes (**spontaneous hyphemas**) include iris neovascularization (associated with diabetes, intraocular tumors, or retinal vascular occlusive disease) or iris tumors such as **juvenile xanthogranuloma**. The skin lesions are much more obvious than the iris lesions (**Figure 23-6**). The mechanism of bleeding associated with blunt trauma is thought to be external compression and secondary expansion of the angle with tearing of the iris root. This results in rupture of the vascular arcade of the iris. Since a hyphema indicates severe ocular trauma, and concurrent injuries to the retina or other ocular tissues can occur, an ophthalmology consultation is required.

The most important complications of a hyphema include late rebleeds into the anterior chamber, increased intraocular pressure, and corneal blood staining. Increased intraocular pressure can occur from red blood cells, red blood cell remnants (ghost cells) or sickled erythrocytes in patients with sickle cell anemia that block the trabecular meshwork outflow, or from pupillary block glaucoma secondary to a large central blood clot that occludes the pupil. Damage to the trabecular meshwork associated with angle recession can cause glaucoma that presents acutely or late (ie, months or even years after the trauma).

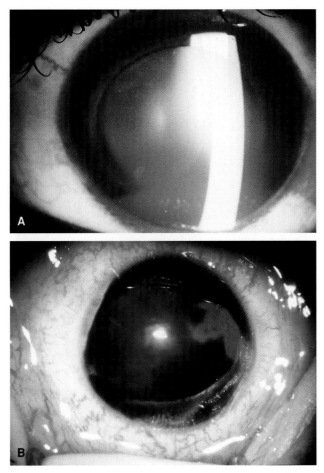

Figure 23-5.
A, Photograph of a small hyphema that is layered inferiorly, plus some diffuse blood. A small hyphema is a hyphema that occupies less than or equal to one third of the anterior chamber. **B,** Total hyphema secondary to blunt trauma. The anterior chamber is full of clot and takes on a black or "eight ball" appearance. This patient required surgical evacuation of the clot.

Corneal Blood Staining

Corneal blood staining may occur in association with large hyphemas that occupy the entire anterior chamber. Hemoglobin and hemosiderin from the hyphema infiltrate through the endothelial cells into the posterior aspect of the corneal stroma and produce an

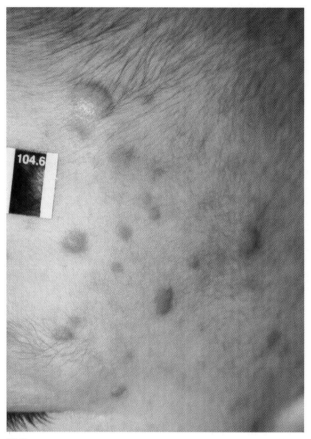

Figure 23-6.
Juvenile xanthogranuloma of scalp: multiple raised, orange nodules that later regressed.

amber opacity (**Figure 23-7**). In children, it is important to avoid the complication of corneal blood staining, since this can produce a severely blurred retinal image, resulting in amblyopia.

Another important complication of hyphema is optic neuropathy associated with **sickle cell hemoglobinopathies.** Even slightly elevated intraocular pressures (greater than 25 mm Hg) will cause optic neuropathy in patients with SC, SS, or S-Thal disease. A sickle cell prep or hemoglobin electrophoresis should be part of the workup of patients with hyphemas who are at risk for having a sickle cell hemoglobinopathy. The ischemic optic neuropathy can be avoided if the intraocular pressure is kept under 25 mm Hg. If the hyphema is causing increased intraocular pressure, the pressure may be low-

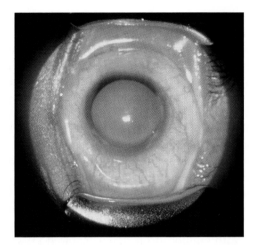

Figure 23-7.
Photograph of corneal blood staining several weeks after removal of an "eight ball" hyphema. Note the yellowish-amber appearance of the cornea that represents iron deposition in the posterior corneal stroma.

ered with topical or oral glaucoma medications. Oral methazolamide is preferred over acetazolamide for patients with sickle cell disease, because methazolamide slightly raises the pH within the eye, while acetazolamide lowers the pH, thus predisposing it to sickling.

Medical Management of Traumatic Hyphemas

Controversy persists as to the medical management of traumatic hyphemas. The classic treatment is hospitalization with bed rest for at least 5 days. Hyphemas resolve as blood is absorbed via the iris and trabecular meshwork. Since hyphema clots contract approximately 3 to 5 days posttrauma, the greatest incidence of re-bleeds occur at this time. An alternative to hospitalization is treatment with bed rest at home. This outpatient treatment has been shown to be safe; however, it should be only used for patients who are reliable and can return to the office for daily checkups. In general, patients with small hyphemas (hyphemas less than one third of the anterior chamber) have a good prognosis, with re-bleed rates of 7% to 14%. These cases are often followed as outpatients. Hyphemas larger than one third of the anterior chamber, however, have an increased risk of developing re-bleeds. Patients with large hyphemas may benefit from hospitalization and bed rest. Some authorities advocate no medical treatment, not even topical drops, while others suggest long-acting cycloplegic agents to minimize ciliary spasm and pre-scribe topical corticosteroids to reduce inflammation. The use of systemic antifibrinolytic agents, such as aminocaproic acid, may decrease the incidence of re-bleeding. This is controversial because adverse effects such as nausea, emesis, hypotension, and prolonged absorption of the clot can occur. Those who advocate the use of fibrinolytic agents restrict their use to small hyphemas less than one third of the anterior chamber in size. These agents are contraindicated in patients who are pregnant, have renal failure, blood dyscrasia, coagulopathies, and thrombotic disease. Previous reports have stated that antifibrinolytic agents reduce the re-bleed rate in patients with small hyphemas from 33% to 4%. Others, however, have shown that the re-bleed rate of small hyphemas is similar without antifibrinolytic agents. Still, in other cases, patients who were treated with aminocaproic agents showed no significant improvement in the re-bleed rate.

Surgical Management of Hyphemas

In most cases, hyphemas can be managed medically, with the hyphema resolving within 3 to 5 days after trauma. Indications for surgery include increased intraocular pressure (IOP), unresolved clot, and corneal blood staining. The timing of the surgery is somewhat arbitrary, and each case must be individualized. Surgery should be considered in the following situations:

• Total hyphema with IOP greater than 25 mm Hg for 6 days
• Large hyphema with IOP greater than 50 mm Hg for 2 days
• Sickle cell disease or trait with IOP greater than 25 mm Hg for 1 day
• Intermittent IOP greater than 30 mm Hg

The surgical procedure should depend on the type of hyphema. This author prefers the closed vitrectomy instrumentation for clot evacuation.

Traumatic Iritis

Blunt, nonperforating ocular trauma can result in an acute iritis. Symptoms usually last for 1 to 2 weeks and include tearing, photophobia, and eye pain. Topical cycloplegics, usually used with a topical corticosteroid, are the treatment for traumatic iritis.

Angle Recession

An angle recession occurs when blunt trauma pushes the lens-iris diaphragm posteriorly, thus tearing the ciliary body. If the angle recession is more than 50% of the circumference of the angle, then the patient is at risk for developing posttraumatic glaucoma. Since glaucoma can occur months, or even years, after the trauma, these patients must be followed closely long-term. Angle recession can only be diagnosed by gonioscopy, which is the use of a special mirrored instrument to view the entire 360° angle.

Traumatic Cataracts

Traumatic cataracts can occur after blunt or penetrating injuries to the anterior segment. Blunt trauma can result in a cataract, which may occur several weeks or even months after the injury. If there is a large rupture of the lens capsule, the lens usually will need to be removed. In rare cases, a small anterior capsule tear will heal, leaving a local opacity that will not require removal of the lens.

Traumatic Subluxation of the Lens

See Chapter 18.

Retinal Trauma

Commotio Retinae (Berlin's Edema)

Commotio retinae is a retinal contusion caused by pressure waves emanating from blunt anterior trauma. Commotio retinae appears grayish-white and often involves the macula. There also may be associated retinal hemorrhages or a choriodal rupture. After the acute edema episode, the retina may scar with pigment clumping. Macular commotio retinae will reduce central vision, but vision usually improves as the edema resolves, unless there is a macular hole or retinal pigment epithelial disruption of the fovea. Animal studies have shown the cause of commotio retinae is probably due to a disruption of photoreceptor outer segments, not true extracellular edema. Fluorescein angiograms of humans show early blockage in areas of white retina, and no alteration of retinal vascular permeability.

Choroidal Rupture

Choroidal rupture can occur with blunt anterior trauma. These represent crescent-shaped curvilinear lines that usually transect the macula. They are deep and gray in appearance. Hemorrhages may be associated with an acute choroidal rupture, representing a break in Bruch's membrane. Subretinal neovascular membranes may develop months or years after a traumatic choroidal rupture occurs.

Traumatic Retinal Breaks

Retinal breaks can occur from direct retinal perforation, vitreous traction, or retinal contusion (see Commotio Retinae described earlier). Blunt injury can cause retinal breaks directly in the area of trauma, most often located at the equator in the inferior temporal quadrant (this is the most exposed area). Retinal detachment after trauma usually occurs late, with most detachments appearing between 1 month and 2 years after trauma.

■ OPTIC NERVE INJURY

Traumatic Optic Neuropathy

Traumatic optic neuropathy is an acute optic nerve injury that occurs after blunt head trauma, usually after a frontal blow. Decreased vision is associated with an afferent pupillary defect and a relatively normal fundus appearance. The head trauma is usually quite severe, associated with loss of consciousness or amnesia. Most authorities recommend a short course of high-dose corticosteroids. If this treatment plan does not improve vision, then optic nerve decompression may be considered in selective cases. Patients who have no light perception have a poor prognosis for visual recovery regardless of treatment. Frontal head trauma can also cause injury to the chiasm, resulting in a bitemporal visual field defect. This is an unusual complication of severe closed head trauma and often is associated with diabetes insipidus or a skull fracture.

Optic Nerve Avulsion

Optic nerve avulsion is caused by severe blunt anterior trauma to the eye that produces a pressure wave, pushing the optic disc posteriorly behind the lamina cribrosa. Visual acuity is usually no light perception (NLP). On fundus examination, the optic disc may be recessed or absent.

■ CHEMICAL BURNS

Acid or alkaline solutions that come into direct contact with the surface of the eye can cause severe damage. A chemical burn is a true ophthalmic emergency and deserves immediate irrigation and lavage in the field prior to the patient arriving at the emergency room. Once in the emergency room, lavage should be continued using at least 3L of normal saline. Litmus paper can be used to check the pH of the conjunctival fornix.

Alkaline Burns

Alkaline burns are especially damaging because the base will denature proteins and lyse cell membranes. This enhances the alkaline penetration into the eye and increases the damage. Surface damage includes removal of the corneal epithelium and obliteration of conjunctival blood vessels. The prognosis is proportional to the clock hours of avascular conjunctiva and sclera whitening. If more than 50% of the limbus is blanched, the prognosis is very poor. After the acute burn, damage and corneal breakdown continues. Collagenase is released from regenerating tissue, producing even more destruction. Over time, symblepharon and cicatricial entropion may occur. In severe cases, the cornea undergoes progressive degeneration and melt, leading to eventual perforation. The treatment for late alkaline burns includes anti-collagenases such as acetylcysteine, artificial tears for dry eye, and topical antibiotics to prevent infection. In addition, a conformer (a plastic shield placed directly on the cornea under the eyelids) is used to prevent symblepharon and preserve the conjunctival fornix.

Acid Burns

Acid burns can cause severe damage; however, because the acid tends to precipitate proteins, the area and depth of necrosis are more limited than with alkaline burns. The treatment is generally the same as for alkaline burns.

■ RADIATION INJURY

Radiation therapy of ocular tumors (eg, retinoblastoma and choroidal melanoma), and orbital tumors (eg, rhabdomyosarcoma and lymphoma) can cause ocular injury. **Radiation cataracts** can form with a single fraction dose as low as 200 rad, but they are usually not progressive and are not visually significant. Doses over 800 rad, however, can cause a progressive cataract that develops over 2 to 3 years. Doses over 5,000 rad can cause injury to the **lacrimal gland,** resulting in a dry-eye syndrome that occurs within 3 months to a year after radiation therapy. **Radiation keratopathy** and conjunctivitis can occur as a consequence of dry-eye syndrome and also from direct epithelial damage. This keratopathy is characterized by superficial punctate epithelial erosions that may become confluent, and form a large epithelial defect. The use of artificial tears is critical for successful treatment of the keratitis.

Radiation retinopathy is caused by retinal vascular ischemia initiated by damage to retinal capillary endothelial cells. Radiation retinopathy develops 2 to 3 years after high-dose radiation therapy (usually over 5,000 rad). The majority of patients receiving over 8,000 rad develop retinopathy. The retinopathy begins with areas of cotton-wool spots, the first sign of radiation retinopathy, representing early retinal ischemia. As the retinal ischemia progresses, large areas of capillary nonperfusion develop. Next, microaneurysms and telangiectatic neovascularization occur. Late changes include iris rubeosis, glaucoma, hyphema, and vitreous hemorrhage. The retinal appearance is similar to diabetic retinopathy. **Radiation optic neuropathy** is uncommon, but can occur with doses over 6,000 rad.

■ LID LACERATION

Lid lacerations that involve the eyelid margin (**Figure 23-4**) should be repaired by an ophthalmologist or someone familiar with the complex anatomy of the lid (tarsus, canaliculus, and canthal tendons). Lid margin lacerations that involve the tarsus must be apposed properly to avoid lid notching (**Figure 23-8**). Improper

——————————————————————————▶

Figure 23-8.
Technique for repairing a lid margin laceration that involves the tarsal plate. **A,** 5-0 Vicryl sutures uniting the tarsal plate. **B,** Vertical mattress 6-0 silk suture to align the lid margin. **C,** Eyelash margin is aligned with a 7-0 nylon suture.

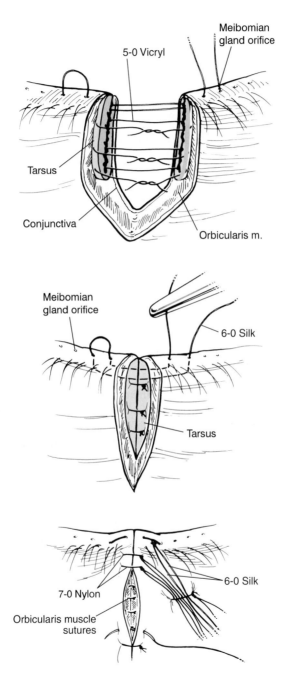

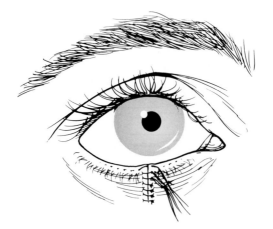

Figure 23-8.
(continued) **D,** Skin closure is achieved with 7-0 nylon sutures. The lid margin sutures can be secured away from the corneal surface.

repair of medial and lateral canthal tears will cause a loose lid with poor lid margin apposition. Lacerations of the medial canthal area may be subtle, and patients with trauma to the medial area should be examined closely. Even minor lacerations of the medial canthal area may involve the canaliculus (see Chapter 1, Figure 14, for anatomy of canalicular system). Canalicular lacerations need to be repaired with special surgical techniques and a silicone tube stent used to preserve canalicular patency and prevent posttrauma tearing (**Figure 23-9**). Lacerations of the superficial lid skin, away from the lid margin, can be safely closed by standard wound closure techniques (**Figure 23-10**). The lid skin is very thin and if careful closure with small gauge suture (6-0 to 7-0) is accomplished, there is usually little scarring and a good cosmetic result. After repair of the laceration, apply topical corticosteroid-antibiotic combination ointment, 2 to 3 times a day for 3 to 5 days.

■ ORBITAL TRAUMA

Orbital Foreign Body

If there is a possibility of an orbital foreign body after a penetrating injury to the orbit, a CT scan of the eye and orbit is indicated. Blunt orbital trauma may also require a CT scan to diagnose orbital fractures, since plain X-ray films miss approximately 50% of floor fractures.

Orbital Floor Fracture

An orbital floor fracture (blow-out fracture) results from blunt trauma to the eye or orbital rim. The orbital floor is thin and prone to fracture. If a floor fracture is suspected, a CT scan should be

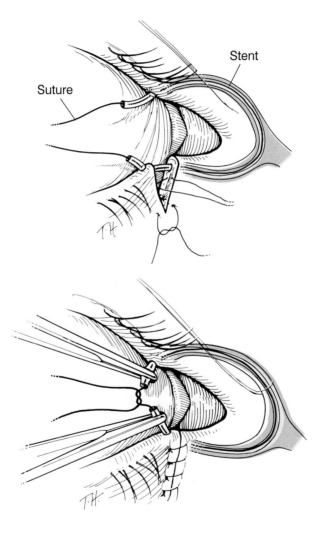

Figure 23-9.
Technique for repairing a canalicular laceration showing silicone tube stent. **A,** A silicone stent bridging the wound. **B,** The ends of the Prolene sutures are tied to tie the ends of the silicone stent.

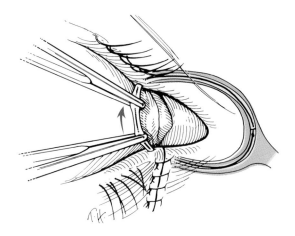

Figure 23-9.
(continued) **C,** The doughnut stent is rotated 180° to position the anastomosis within the common caniliculus.

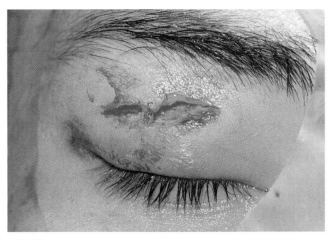

Figure 23-10.
Superficial laceration of the upper lid not involving the lid margin or canthal areas. This laceration can be nicely closed by standard wound closure techniques, after the integrity of the eye is examined.

obtained. Signs of a blow-out fracture include diplopia, due to restricted vertical eye movement, and enophthalmos, resulting from displacement of orbital fat into the maxillary sinus. The presence of strabismus after an orbital floor fracture is due to entrapment of fat and, possibly, inferior rectus muscle in the fracture, thus causing restricted elevation of the globe (**Figure 23-11**). Numbness of the cheek below the traumatized orbit and along the upper teeth can occur if the infraorbital nerve is damaged. If a floor fracture is sus-

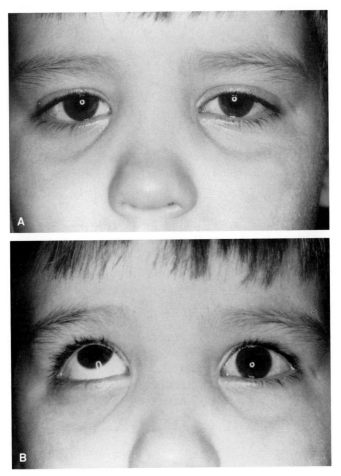

Figure 23-11.
Left orbital floor fracture with enophthalmos (sunken, retracted eye) with narrow lid fissure. **A,** In primary gaze, there is no significant deviation. **B,** Restricted elevation of the left eye in upgaze.

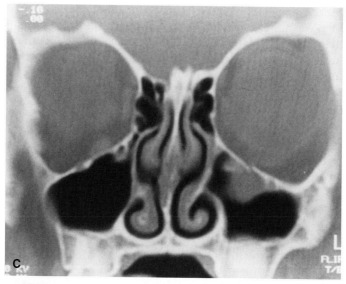

Figure 23-11.
(continued) **C,** Computed tomography scan shows herniation and entrapment of inferior orbital fat into the maxillary antrum. Note the inferior rectus is not entrapped and is within the orbit.

pected, a CT scan should be obtained. Acute treatment includes oral antibiotics (eg, amoxicillin) to prevent an orbital infectious contamination from the maxillary sinus. Immediate surgical intervention is needed in small trapdoor fractures to prevent strangulation and necrosis of entrapped orbital fat and extraocular muscle. Other floor fractures do not necessarily need to be surgically repaired unless there is persistent diplopia after 2 to 4 weeks, or if there is significant enophthalmos. Surgical repair consists of removing the herniated orbital fat from the maxillary sinus and placing a silicone or Teflon plate to cover the fracture site. Medial wall fracture often occurs with blunt trauma. Nose blowing should be avoided to prevent orbital emphysema and infection.

■ BIBLIOGRAPHY

1. Friendly DS. Ocular manifestations of physical child abuse. *Trans Am Acad Ophthalmol Otolaryngol.* 1971;75:318–332
2. Goldberg MF. Sickled erythrocytes, hyphema, and secondary glaucoma: I. The diagnosis and treatment of sickled erythrocytes in human hyphemas. *Ophthalmic Surg.* 1979;10:17–31
3. Greenwald MJ, Weiss A, Oesterle CS, Friendly DS. Traumatic retinoschisis in battered babies. *Ophthalmology.* 1986;93:618–625
4. Harcourt B, Hopkins D. Permanent chorio-retinal lesions in childhood of suspected traumatic origin. *Trans Ophthalmol Soc UK.* 1973;93: 199–205
5. Joseph MP, Lessell S, Rizzo J, Momose KJ. Extracranial optic nerve decompression for traumatic optic neuropathy. *Arch Ophthalmol.* 1990; 108: 1091–1093
6. Kanter RK. Retinal hemorrhage after cardiopulmonary resuscitation or child abuse. *J Pediatr.* 1986;108:430–432
7. Kraft SP, Christianson MD, Crawford JS, Wagman RD, Antoszyk JH. Traumatic hyphema in children. Treatment with epsilon-aminocaproic acid. *Ophthalmology.* 1987;94:1232–1237
8. Ober RR. Hemorrhagic retinopathy in infancy: a clinicopathologic report. *J Pediatr Ophthalmol Strabismus.* 1980;17:17–20
9. Spoor TC, Hartel WC, Lensink DB, Wilkinson MJ. Treatment of traumatic optic neuropathy with corticosteroids. *Am J Ophthalmol.* 1990; 110: 665–669
10. Wright KW, Sunalp M, Urrea P. Bed rest versus activity ad lib in the treatment of small hyphemas. *Ann Ophthalmol.* 1988;20:143–145

24 Pediatric Ophthalmology Syndromes

This chapter discusses the following categories of syndromes associated with pediatric ophthalmology:

- Phakomatoses
- Craniofacial Abnormalities
- Connective Tissue Disorders
- Metabolic Storage Diseases
- Chromosomal Abnormalities

■ PHAKOMATOSES

The phakomatoses (or "birth marks") disorders involve the formation of hamartomas that typically involve the skin and nervous system. The term "phakos" is Greek for birthmark or mole. There are many diseases that fall in the phakomatoses group of disorders; however, 6 conditions commonly associated with ocular manifestations are covered in this chapter.

Neurofibromatosis (von Recklinghausen Disease)

Neurofibromatosis is an autosomal dominant inherited disease and has 2 forms: neurofibromatosis 1 (NF1) (von Recklinghausen disease) and neurofibromatosis 2 (NF2) (bilateral acoustic neurofibromatosis, or central NF). Prenatal diagnosis is available primarily

Table 24-1.
Genetics of Neurofibromatosis 1

- Long arm of chromosome 17 (17q11.2)
- Large gene related to GAP protein
- GAP regulates cell growth
- Incidence 1:3000
- Autosomal dominant with complete penetrance
- High mutation rate: 50% of new cases are new mutations

through linkage analysis or occasionally by direct mutation detection. NF1 results from a mutation in the gene encoding neurofibromin, a GTPase activating protein of the ras family of proto-oncogenes, while NF2 is associated with abnormalities in merlin, a tumor-suppressor gene of the moesin-ezrin-radixin family of cytoskeletal proteins.

Neurofibromatosis 1

Neurofibromatosis 1 (NF1) is the classic form of neurofibromatosis described by von Recklinghausen. It is the most common of the phakomatoses, occurring in 1 of every 3,000 to 4,000 individuals in the general population. The most outstanding clinical features include cutaneous nevi called café-au-lait macules, plexiform neurofibromas of the lids, pigmented freckling around the axillary or inguinal areas, optic nerve glioma, Lisch iris nodules and bone lesions including sphenoid dysplasia or thinning of the long bone cortex. Mapping studies identify that the gene maps to the proximal portion of the long arm of chromosome 17 (chromosome band 17q11.2) (**Table 24-1**). The primary embryologic defect involves primitive neural crest cells and neuroectoderm.

The clinical diagnostic criterion for NF1 is the presence of 2 or more of the characteristics listed in **Table 24-2.**

Ophthalmic Findings of Neurofibromatosis 1
One of the most consistent findings of NF1 is the presence of **Lisch nodules** of the iris. These are iris hamartomas composed of melanocytes. They appear as well-circumscribed small nodules in the iris that are slightly raised and have a brownish appearance (**Figure 24-1**). They are present in approximately 30% of children under age 6, and in more than 90% of patients who are adults or in late childhood. Plexiform neurofibromas can occur in the eyelid and

Table 24-2.
Neurofibromatosis 1—Diagnostic Criteria

The presence of 2 or more of the following:
- Six or more café-au-lait spots (>5 mm prepubertal; >15 mm postpubertal)
- Two or more neurofibromas or 1 plexiform neurofibroma
- Optic nerve glioma
- Axillary or inguinal freckling
- Two or more Lisch nodules
- A characteristic bone lesion
- First degree relative with NF1

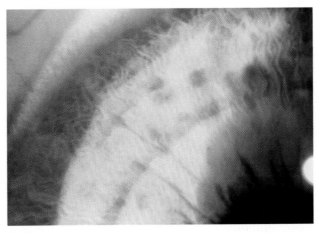

Figure 24-1.
Lisch nodules on iris in neurofibromatosis type 1. They are brownish raised nodules.

orbit. The eyelid tumors often cause an S-shaped deformity of the lid margin. Facial asymmetry and hemihypertrophy can also be associated with NF1. Neurofibromas of the conjunctiva, corneal nerve thickening, and glaucoma secondary to trabecular meshwork outflow obstruction also may occur. Retinal findings include small glial tumors. Optic nerve pallor or proptosis may occur secondary to an optic nerve glioma.

Optic nerve gliomas occur in approximately 15% of patients with NF1; however, almost 30% to 70% of all patients with optic nerve gliomas have NF1. These tumors tend to be slow growing and usually are conservatively managed by observation. Computed tomography scan and magnetic resonance imaging findings illustrate the characteristic fusiform shape of the optic nerve glioma. Gliomas of the chiasm have a worse prognosis and should be suspected in a patient having NF1 with optic nerve pallor and no proptosis.

Systemic Findings of Neurofibromatosis 1

Patients with NF1 can develop intracranial tumors at any time, including gliomas, meningiomas, and ependymomas. Benign tumors can undergo malignant transformation into neurofibrosarcoma and malignant schwannomas. Other malignant transformations include pheochromocytoma, medullary carcinoma, and chronic myelogenous leukemia. Other systemic findings include cystic lesions of the lung, cardiac rhabdomyoma, and neurofibromas of virtually any organ.

Neurofibromatosis 2

Neurofibromatosis 2 (NF2) consists of bilateral vestibular schwannomas and posterior subcapsular cataracts. The vestibular schwannomas develop during the second to third decade of life. Other tumors associated with NF2 include brain or spinal chord tumors, meningiomas, astrocytomas, and neurofibromas. Unlike NF1, where cutaneous involvement is prominent, NF2 presents with minimal cutaneous involvement. NF2 is inherited as an autosomal dominant trait and has been mapped to chromosome 22.

NF2 is a rare disorder, affecting approximately 1 out of 40,000 individuals. Auditory symptoms at clinical presentation include hearing loss, tinnitus, dizziness, and/or headache. The diagnostic criteria for NF2 are described in **Table 24-3.**

Table 24-3.
Criteria for Diagnosing Neurofibromatosis 2

1. Bilateral *vestibular schwannomas* (acoustic neuromas) or eighth nerve mass on MRI or CT scan
   OR
2. Family history of NF2 (first-degree relative) and patient with a unilateral vestibular schwannoma
   OR
3. Two of the following:
   • Juvenile posterior subcapsular cataract
   • Neurofibroma
   • Meningioma

Von Hippel-Lindau Disease

Von Hippel-Lindau disease consists of a vascular lesion, such as a hemangioblastoma, classically affecting the retina (angiomatosis retinae) and the cerebellum. Patients can present with signs of cerebellar dysfunction or vision loss. Angiomas can occur in the kidney, pancreas, liver, and spleen with renal cell carcinoma occurring in approximately one third of patients. Cutaneous involvement is unusual; however, some patients may develop pigmented macular lesions of the skin in the third or fourth decade of life. Patients most commonly die of either cerebellar hemangioblastomas or retinal cell carcinomas. Fortunately, this is a rare disorder, occurring in less than 1 in 40,000 patients. The inheritance is autosomal dominant with incomplete penetrance. The gene has been mapped to 3p25 and is the result of a mutation in a tumor suppressor gene.

Ocular findings are mainly hemangioblastomas of the retina (**Figure 24-2**). The retinal vascular tumors can be found in patients between the ages of 10 and 40 years, which is earlier than the cerebellar presentation. Initially, the tumor is extremely small and appears to be no more than a slight aneurysmal dilation of peripheral retinal vessels. Over time, the vascular tumor increases in size to form a smooth, domed tumor that is fed by a tortuous dilated tumor vessel emanating from the optic nerve. This creates an arteriove-

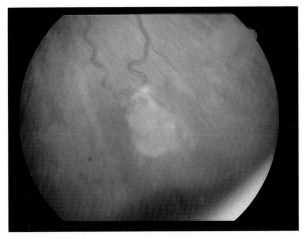

Figure 24-2.
Retinal hemangioblastoma in von Hippel-Lindau. Note the 2 feeder vessels that connect with the yellowish vascularized retinal mass.

nous shunt. Tumors may involve the optic disc and be present anywhere in the retina, but are most commonly seen in the midperiphery. Leakage from the tumor can cause lipid exudates of the retina and may take on the appearance of Coats disease. Involvement may be bilateral or multi-focal in one eye. Almost 100% of patients with von Hippel-Lindau disease will have retinal involvement.

Tuberous Sclerosis (Bourneville Disease)

Tuberous sclerosis is a neurocutaneous disease in which tumors, including astrocytic hamartomas and angiofibromas, involve multiple organs. The classical presentation includes the triad of seizures, mental retardation, and facial angiomas. These features have variable expressivity; however, seizures are the most common manifestation, occurring in almost 20% of patients.

Ocular findings include astrocytic hamartomas of the retina or optic disc and retinal pigment epithelial defects. The astrocytic hamartomas classically appear as a smooth white or gray mass with a mulberry or tapioca texture (**Figure 24-3**). Retinal lesions do not require treatment. In addition to retinal findings, angiofibromas of the eyelid can also occur.

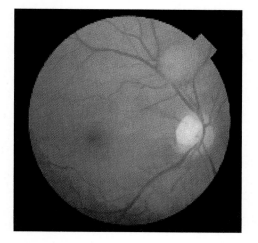

Figure 24-3.
Retinal astrocytic hamartoma in a patient with tuberous sclerosis. The lesion is seen just superior to the optic disc.

Table 24-4.
Associated Findings of Tuberous Sclerosis

Ocular findings
1. Ocular astrocytic hamartomas of the retina
2. Retinal pigmentary abnormalities
3. Sector iris hypopigmentations
4. Angiomas of the lid

Systemic findings
1. Seizures
2. Facial cutaneous angiofibromas (butterfly distribution)
3. Subungual fibromas of the fingernails and toenails
4. Ash-leaf spots
5. Fibrous plaques of the forehead and scalp
6. Dental enamel pits
7. Renal cysts or tumors
8. Pulmonary involvement
9. Cardiac rhabdomyoma
10. Mental retardation

Systemic findings of tuberous sclerosis include angiofibromas over the nose and cheeks, which are often termed adenoma sebaceum. Depigmented macules or ash-leaf spots and cafe-au-lait spots can also been present. Ash-leaf spots are best identified by illumination with a blue light or fluorescent lamp. Cerebral lesions include white-matter abnormalities, subependymal nodules, cortical tubers, and subependymal giant cell astrocytoma. These lesions may be present in up to 50% of affected individuals. **Table 24-4** lists associated findings of tuberous sclerosis.

Tuberous sclerosis is a rare disorder inherited as an autosomal dominant trait with variable penetrance. More than 80% of patients present as a new mutation without a family history of tuberous sclerosis. Tuberous sclerosis has been found in 2 genes: **type 1**—mapped to 9q34—and **type 2**—linked to chromosome 16p13.3. Type 1 is associated with a mutation of the gene responsible for a protein called hamartin, which acts as a tumor suppressor. In Type 2, tuberin protein, which has similar but separate functions as hamartin, is defective. There is phenotypic overlap between type 1 and type 2 tuberous sclerosis. Patients with tuberous sclerosis should be followed with neuro-imaging, renal ultrasound, and cardiac workup. Genetic counseling is important, and accurate communication to the patient and family is essential for treatment and disease management.

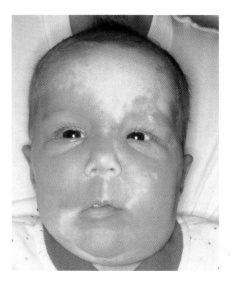

Figure 24-4.
Sturge-Weber Syndrome: a child with a facial hemangioma (port wine stain) in the trigeminal distribution. This child also had glaucoma and a large choroidal hemangioma in the left eye.

Sturge-Weber Syndrome

Sturge-Weber syndrome is an angiomatosis causing a facial cutaneous hemangioma (port-wine stain) that may be unilateral or bilateral and involves the first and second division of the trigeminal nerve (**Figure 24-4**). Leptomeningeal angiomatosis, childhood seizures (contralateral side), hemifacial hypertrophy, and mental retardation may also occur. Expressivity is variable, and most patients do not manifest the entire syndrome.

Ocular findings include eyelid hemangiomas (nevus flammeus or port-wine stain), conjunctival tortuous vessels with episcleral vascular plexi, and choroidal hemangiomas. The choroidal hemangiomas are diffuse with a tomato catsup appearance and are found in approximately 40% of patients. It is often difficult to see the choroidal hemangioma because of its diffuse nature, and comparison of one eye to the other is helpful in making the diagnosis. In addition, heterochromia of the iris can be noted in patients with unilateral cutaneous hemangiomatosis.

Glaucoma occurs in approximately 30% of patients with Sturge-Weber syndrome and is probably secondary to increased episcleral venous pressure. Upper eyelid involvement is thought to be an indicator that glaucoma may develop. Glaucoma associated with Sturge-Weber syndrome is difficult to manage medically and has potential surgical risks; most importantly, intraoperative or postoperative choroidal effusion or choroidal hemorrhage. Other systemic findings include focal or generalized motor seizures. Approximately 80% of affected individuals have hemangiomatous involvement of the mouth and lips and the classic radiologic finding of railroad track calcifications in the leptomeninges.

Sturge-Weber syndrome is not associated with a recognized mendelian inheritance pattern, so a positive family history is unusual.

Klippel-Trénaunay-Weber Syndrome

Klippel-Trénaunay-Weber syndrome appears to be related to Sturge-Weber syndrome in that it is not inherited by classical mendelian patterns and is associated with cutaneous hemangiomas. The cutaneous hemangiomas can be quite large and are extremely difficult to remove surgically because of the danger of massive blood loss. The syndrome also includes hypertrophy of bones and soft tissue, ipsilateral varicosities, and arterial venous fistula.

Ataxia-Telangiectasia (Louis-Bar Syndrome)

Louis-Bar syndrome is characterized by cerebellar ataxia and ocular and cutaneous telangiectasia. The ocular telangiectasias involve the conjunctiva and appear between 4 and 7 years of age. Diffuse cerebellar atrophy occurs and the patient develops ocular-motor apraxia with deficient saccadic generation, cerebellar nystagmus, and strabismus. Systemic manifestations caused by cerebellar atrophy include choreoathetosis, dysarthria, hypotonia, and ataxia. Immunologic compromise occurs and may be secondary to thymus gland hypoplasia. Pulmonary infections are common and hematological cancer, such as leukemia, lymphoma, lymphosarcoma, and Hodgkin's disease, are associated with Louis-Bar syndrome.

Louis-Bar syndrome is inherited as an autosomal recessive trait and is caused by a gene that functions to repair DNA. Patients with Louis-Bar syndrome are, therefore, susceptible to radiation.

Wyburn-Mason Syndrome (Racemose Angiomatosis)

Wyburn-Mason syndrome consists of arteriovenous malformations that involve the retina, midbrain, and thalamus. Ocular characteristics include dilated tortuous retinal vessels often occurring in the inferior temporal quadrant of the retina. The tortuous vessels represent a large arteriovenous shunt. Presence of an angioma can also involve the orbit and cause proptosis. Systemic findings include cavernous sinus angiomata or angiomata along the basilar or posterior cerebellar artery. Intracranial hemorrhage or compression of surrounding structures can cause headaches and neurological symptoms.

■ CRANIOFACIAL ABNORMALITIES

Hypertelorism

Hypertelorism is an increased distance between the orbits. Clinical estimate of hypertelorism can be determined by measuring interpupillary distance; however, radiologic measurements are the most accurate.

Telecanthus

A wide intercanthal distance with normal interpupillary distance is termed telecanthus. This is caused by redundant skin and soft tissue. Telecanthus often improves in late childhood as the nose develops and the nasal bridge skin is pulled forward.

Craniosynostosis

Craniosynostosis results from premature closure of the cranial sutures. Premature closure of a suture results in inhibited skull growth perpendicular to the closed suture. Increased growth occurs at the opened sutures. Since the pattern of premature closure is quite variable, there is a large spectrum of presentations with varying skull shapes. Craniosynostosis is often associated with strabismus and can be associated with missing or congenitally displaced extraocular muscles. The most common manifestations of craniosynostosis, including Crouzon, Apert, and Pfeiffer syndromes, are inherited as autosomal dominant traits. In addition to cranial and facial abnormalities, patients with Apert and Pfeiffer syndromes have syndactyly. In many cases, these conditions have been associated with abnormalities in fibroblast growth factor receptor genes. The causative genes for these conditions have been identified, but the genetic aspects are complex.

Apert Syndrome

Apert syndrome is caused by a synostosis of the coronal suture. Associated findings include midfacial hypoplasia, protrusion of the lower jaw, high-arched or cleft palate, and syndactyly of the fingers and toes, usually in a "mitten glove" pattern. Other features include proptosis, antimongoloid slant of the palpebral fissures, strabismus, and hypertelorism. The strabismus is often characterized by esotropia with a V-pattern. Shallow orbits can cause severe proptosis, optic nerve atrophy, and subluxation of the globes. Apert syndrome is probably autosomal dominant inheritance, but most present as sporadic events, probably due to new mutations.

Pfeiffer Syndrome

Pfeiffer syndrome is similar to Apert syndrome; however, in Pfeiffer syndrome there are characteristic broad, short thumbs and great toes. The orbits are extremely shallow, and there is severe proptosis often with corneal exposure, and strabismus is common.

Crouzon Disease

Crouzon disease is similar to Apert syndrome and other types of craniosynostosis, with the coronal suture being most frequently involved. It has autosomal dominant inheritance and 67% of cases are familial. However, other combinations of suture synostosis are commonly present. With Crouzon disease, there are no anomalies of the hands or feet as seen in Apert and Pfeiffer syndromes. Proptosis can be severe and vision threatening due to optic nerve compression or corneal exposure secondary to the proptosis (**Figure 24-5**). Abnormal extraocular muscles and the absence of extraocular muscles are frequently reported in Crouzon disease as they are in Apert syndrome. There is maxillary hypoplasia, hook-shaped nose, and flat forehead. Other associated abnormalities include deafness

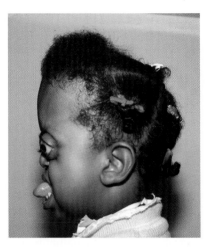

Figure 24-5.
Facial features showing severe proptosis, flattening of forehead, and micrognathia in Crouzon disease.

and delayed development. Iris coloboma, microcornea, and ectopia lentis have also been reported.

First and Second Brachial Arch Defects

The mandibulofacial dysostoses represents abnormal differentiation of the first brachial arch and includes Goldenhar syndrome, Treacher Collins syndrome, and several rare conditions.

Oculoauriculovertebral-spectrum (Goldenhar Syndrome)

Oculoauriculovertebral-spectrum (OAV) includes Goldenhar syndrome and hemifacial microsomia. It most commonly presents as a sporadic occurrence and it is estimated that 2% to 3% of future siblings are at risk for developing Goldenhar syndrome. Typical findings include facial asymmetry with mandibular hypoplasia, usually involving the right side of the face. Preauricular appendages or ear tags, malformation of the ear, and hearing loss due to external ear lesions or middle or inner ear malformations are also present (**Figure 24-6A**). Vertebral abnormalities include fusional defects, scoliosis, and spina bifida. Microsomia is common and is associated with mandibular hypoplasia. Ocular findings include epibulbar or conjunctival lipodermoids often associated with vertebral

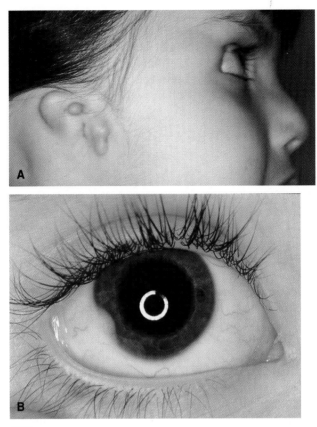

Figure 24-6.
A, Microtia with preauricular tags in Goldenhar syndrome. **B,** Limbal dermoid.

abnormalities, limbal dermoids, eyelid colobomas, and subcutaneous dermoids of the lids (**Figure 24-6B**). When the features are bilateral and include epibulbar lipodermoids, the condition is commonly referred to as **Goldenhar syndrome.** Although relatively uncommon, other systemic findings may include heart, lung, and kidney malformations.

Treacher Collins Syndrome (Mandibulofacial dysostosis)

Treacher Collins syndrome is inherited as an autosomal dominant trait with incomplete penetrance and variable expressivity. Ocular manifestations include eyelid coloboma, or notching of the lower lid, and the lacrimal punctum may be absent. Other, less frequently

encountered ocular anomalies include upper-lid coloboma and ptosis. Systemic signs include hypoplasia of the malar and mandibular
bones, malformations of the external ear, atypical hair line with
projections toward the cheek, antimongoloid slant of the palpebral
fissures, cleft palate, and a blind fistula between the angles of the
mouth and ears. Treacher Collins syndrome is bilateral.

Other Disorders With Ocular Findings

Aicardi Syndrome

Aicardi syndrome is caused by an X-linked dominant gene that is
lethal if it occurs in males; therefore, it is seen almost exclusively
in females. Aicardi syndrome consists of infantile spasms or seizures,
absence of the corpus callosum, progressive mental retardation, and
characteristic chorioretinal lacunae. Initial neurological evaluations
may yield normal results during early infancy; however, progressive
mental retardation, hypotonia, and seizures usually occur within 4
to 6 months after birth. The disease is generally fatal, with death
occurring during childhood. Multiple skeletal anomalies have been
described including scoliosis, spina bifida, vertebral abnormalities,
cleft lip and palate, and fused ribs. Ocular abnormalities include
chorioretinal lacunae of the fundus, microphthalmos, colobomas of
the choroid and optic nerve, optic nerve hypoplasia, peripapillary
glial tissue, and the morning glory anomaly. The fundus appearance is specific to Aicardi syndrome and consists of bilateral circum-
scribed chorioretinal lesions with pigmented borders. The central
aspect of these lesions is hypopigmented. Strabismus, nystagmus,
and ptosis occur along with deterioration of the neurological status.
There is no specific treatment for this disorder except for suppor-
tive measures.

Cockayne Syndrome

Cockayne syndrome consists of premature aging, dwarfism, bird-
like facies, and retinal degeneration. Mental retardation, seizures,
cerebellar ataxia, nystagmus, muscle rigidity, and neurosensory
deafness are part of the neurological sequelae. The disease is progressive, usually becoming evident by 2 years of age, with death
often occurring during late adolescence.

   Retinal findings include a retinitis pigmentosa picture with a
"salt and pepper" retinal pigment epithelial degeneration, waxy

optic disc pallor, and attenuated retinal vessels. Other ocular findings include corneal opacification, band keratopathy, cataracts, nystagmus, and poor pupillary response with hypoplastic irides. There is no specific treatment.

Rubinstein-Taybi Syndrome

Mental retardation, broad toes and thumbs, short stature, and an antimongoloid slant of the palpebral fissures are characteristics of Rubinstein-Taybi syndrome. In addition, more than 90% will have a high-arched palate and a beaked or straight nose. Rubinstein-Taybi syndrome is sporadic, and laboratory studies of muscle biopsies show a pattern consistent with denervation atrophy of the muscle. Some affected individuals have a deletion of chromosome 16p, while others have mutation in the gene for CREB-binding protein located in this region. There is no specific treatment for the syndrome.

Hallermann-Streiff Syndrome

Hallermann-Streiff syndrome is a sporadic, midfacial hypoplasia and is associated with congenital cataracts in 100% of cases. The presence of microcornea makes aphakic contact lens fitting difficult. Other characteristics include severe mandibular hypoplasia, beaked nose, and dwarfism.

Fetal Alcohol Syndrome

Fetal alcohol syndrome is associated with maternal ingestion of large amounts of alcohol during the first trimester. The most obvious findings of fetal alcohol syndrome are facial abnormalities including flat philtrum, thin vermilion border of the upper lid, flat facies, and large epicanthal folds. Newborns are usually of low birth weight, have developmental delay, and often show signs of mild to moderate mental retardation. Ocular manifestations include telecanthus, ptosis, strabismus, optic nerve hypoplasia, and anomalies of the anterior segment, including anterior chamber dysgenesis syndromes. Patients diagnosed with fetal alcohol syndrome should be referred for an ophthalmology consultation.

■ CONNECTIVE TISSUE DISORDERS

Marfan Syndrome

Marfan syndrome is a connective tissue disorder that is inherited as an autosomal dominant trait and is the most common cause of subluxed lenses. See Chapter 18 on subluxed lens for further discussion.

Stickler Syndrome

Stickler syndrome is a heterogenous autosomal dominant collagen disorder with high penetrance and is associated with facial and skeletal abnormalities, high myopia, and a high incidence of retinal detachment. The vitreous is liquefied with optically empty areas of vitreous veils and condensations. Other ocular findings include glaucoma and cataracts. The classic facial appearance includes malar hypoplasia with flattened midface, flattened nasal bridge, micrognathia, and cleft or high-arched palate. The cleft palate is part of the **Pierre Robin sequence,** and may also occur in other syndromes. Mitral valve prolapse occurs in approximately 50% of cases. A progressive arthropathy is present in almost all patients, but it may be subtle and only show up on X-ray films as flattening of the epiphyseal centers.

Ehlers-Danlos Syndrome

There are various forms of Ehlers-Danlos syndrome. The ocular form, or form VI, consists of blue, fragile sclera with spontaneous perforation of the globe, keratoconus, and **angioid streaks.** Angioid streaks are breaks in Bruch's membrane (the layer under the retinal pigment epithelium). Patients with Ehlers-Danlos syndrome have thin, extensible skin, hyperextensibility of joints, and skin that scars easily.

Pseudoxanthoma Elasticum

Pseudoxanthoma elasticum is an autosomal dominant or autosomal recessive disease that affects the elastic component of connective tissue. There is calcification of the elastic component of vessels and of Bruch's membrane. Because of the vasculopathy, multiple systems are affected. Resultant systemic problems include coronary heart disease, renal failure and hypertension, neurological disease, and gastrointestinal hemorrhages. Mitral valve prolapse occurs in more than 70% of cases. Skin is elastic and hyperextensible.

Ocular findings include angioid streaks that radiate peripherally from the optic disc. The elastic layer of Bruch's membrane is replaced by calcific changes and subretinal neovascularization occurs as vessels grow through the breaks in Bruch's membrane. There is no specific treatment except for addressing complications of the vasculopathy and retinal neovascularization.

Osteogenesis Imperfecta

Osteogenesis imperfecta has at least 5 clinical subtypes. This is a disease of alpha type 1 collagen and affects connective tissue. Ocular signs include blue sclera resulting from visualization of the choroid through thin sclera. The scleral thickness in these patients is approximately half that of normal patients. Other ocular findings include keratoconus, megalocornea, and posterior embryotoxon. Rarely patients will have cataracts, glaucoma, and spontaneous rupture of the globe. Patients are prone to fractures of the long bones and spine.

■ METABOLIC AND STORAGE DISEASES

Mucopolysaccharidosis

Mucopolysaccharidoses (MPSs) are a group of storage diseases caused by an error of carbohydrate metabolism. At present, there are 6 types of MPS syndromes: 5 recessively inherited and 1, Hunter syndrome, which is X-linked. The classification of MPS into groups I-VI is based on the type of enzyme deficiency. Type V is presently vacant, as the former type V has been identified as a subtype of type I. Type I is subdivided into 3 categories based on the severity of the disease: type I-H (Hurler syndrome), type I-S (Scheie syndrome), and type I-H/S (Hurler-Scheie syndrome).

Table 24-5 summarizes the clinical features of the MPS syndromes. Systemic and ocular features are variable and subtype specific. Typical systemic abnormalities include coarse facial features, short stature, and mental retardation (**Figure 24-7**). Depending on the enzyme deficiency, various types of mucopolysaccharides can be found in the urine. Common ocular findings include corneal stromal clouding, pigmentary retinal degeneration, and optic nerve atrophy. Corneal clouding usually coexists with skeletal

Table 24-5
Features of Mucolipidoses

Type and Syndrome	Ocular Features			Systemic Features			Prognosis
	Corneal clouding	Retinal degeneration	Optic nerve atrophy	Coarse facial features	Mental retardation	Skeletal dysplasia	
I H (Hurler)	+, by 6 mos	+	+, frequent	+	+	+	death by 10 years
I S (Scheie)	+, by 12–24 mos	+	+	+	variable	+	may live to middle age
I H/S (Hurler-Scheie)	+	+	–	+	variable	+	better than I-H
II (Hunter)	rare	+	+	+	+	+	death by 15 years
III (Sanfilippo)	–	+	+	+	variable	+	death by second or third decade
IV (Morquio)	by age 10	rare	–	+	mild	+	may survive to sixth decade
VI (Maroteaux-Lamy)	after age 5	–	+	+	–	+	death in second decade
VII (Sly)	mild	–	–	variable	+	+	may live to middle age

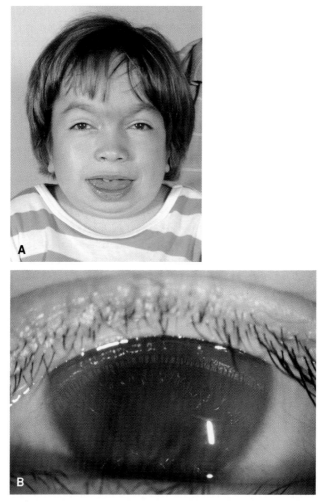

Figure 24-7.
A, Typical Hurler facies. **B,** Slit-lamp photo of cloudy cornea in mucopolysaccharidosis.

abnormalities and is present in all types except type III. Pigmentary retinopathy is associated with the presence of mental retardation.

Depending on the type, MPS are progressive diseases with variable prognosis. Usually, patients live well into middle age except for patients with Type I and Type VI who develop respiratory infection and heart failure at an earlier age. Patients with visually significant corneal opacities may benefit from corneal transplantation.

There may, in fact, be clearing of the surrounding recipient corneal bed 1 or 2 years after transplantation. Early data from enzyme replacement trials suggests some benefits of systemic treatment for MPS.

Tyrosinemia

An error in tyrosine metabolism leads to high serum levels and increased urinary excretion of tyrosine and parahydroxyphenylpyruvate.

Tyrosinemia Type 1 and neonatal tyrosinemia have no characteristic skin or eye lesions.

Tyrosinemia Type 2, or Richner-Hanhart syndrome, has a clinical triad of skin lesions, ocular manifestations, and mental retardation. The ocular features are typically seen as corneal lesions and appear early in childhood. Painful, erosive, or hyperkeratotic skin lesions over palms and soles coexist with, or precede, ocular lesions. Pseudodendritic corneal erosions, culture-negative ulcers, and intraepithelial linear or stellate opacities have been described.

Estimation of serum tyrosine levels is imperative in a child with bilateral photophobia and pseudodendritic corneal lesions. Early detection and dietary restriction of phenylalanine and tyrosine lead to reversal of ocular and skin changes and even prevention of mental retardation.

Mucolipidosis

Some of the clinical features seen in this group of conditions overlap those found in mucopolysaccharidoses and sphingolipidoses. Mucolipidosis is characterized by the presence of peculiar inclusion cells (I-cells) in cultured fibroblasts. A conjunctival biopsy is diagnostic. **Table 24-6** lists the clinical features of the subtypes.

Gangliosidosis

This rare group of storage disorders represents errors of sphingolipid metabolism. These are characterized by intracellular storage of phospholipids and glycolipids in the ganglion cell layer of retina, as well as other tissues of the body. The macula, being devoid of ganglion cells, presents a characteristic "cherry red" appearance

Table 24-6.
Clinical Features of Mucolipidoses

Type	Enzyme Deficiency	Ocular Features	Systemic Features	Prognosis
I	α-N acetylneuraminidase	corneal clouding, cherry red spot, optic atrophy	mental retardation, dysostosis multiplex	uncertain, no known treatment
II	multiple lysosomal enzymes	late corneal clouding correlating with survival, no cherry red spot	Hurler-like facies, dysostosis multiplex, mental retardation	early death
III	multiple lysosomal enzymes	ground glass corneal clouding, hyperopic astigmatism	Hurler-like facies, skeletal dysplasias, aortic valve disease	progressive joint stiffness, hyperopia should be corrected
IV	ganglioside neuraminidase	corneal clouding, retinal degeneration, optic nerve atrophy	progressive psychomotor retardation, no skeletal dysplasia or facial dysmorphism	poor visual prognosis due to retinal degeneration

Table 24-7.
Differential Diagnosis of a Cherry Red Spot

Gangliosidosis
Niemann-Pick disease
Farber disease
Sialidosis
Mucolipidosis
Ocular trauma
Central retinal artery occlusion

against a white background of lipid-laden ganglion cells and indicates the initial stage of the disease. **Table 24-7** lists the differential diagnosis of a cherry red spot. **Table 24-8** describes the salient features of the different subtypes of gangliosidoses.

Niemann-Pick Disease

Niemann-Pick disease is a disorder of sphingomyelin metabolism and is characterised by the presence of "foam cells" (intracellular deposits of sphingomyelin) in bone marrow, peripheral blood smear, liver, spleen, and brain. These are classified into Types A–E on biochemical and clinical basis and all present with a cherry red spot.

Type A: Most common (85%) and 80% are Ashkenazi Jews. They have early and severe central nervous system (CNS) involvement.
Type B: Visceral involvement with apparently normal CNS involvement.
Type C: Moderate CNS involvement. Ocular features also include supranuclear paralysis of extraocular muscles.
Type D: Has later onset but severe involvement of CNS.
Type E: Mild, chronic adult onset with no CNS involvement.

Sialidosis

In this condition, enzyme neuraminidase is deficient. It exists as 2 types.

Type I: Myoclonus syndrome begins in the second decade of life in patients who otherwise have a normal appearance and normal intelligence.

Table 24-8.
Gangliosidoses

Type/Disease	Deficient Enzyme	Ocular Features	Systemic Features	Prognosis
GM$_1$ Type 1 (Landing)	A-, B-, and C-Beta galactosidase	Cherry red spot in 50% of cases. Tortuous conjunctival vessels, cloudy cornea, optic atrophy, myopia.	Psychomotor retardation, Hurler-like facial features, hepatosplenomegaly and congestive heart failure	Death by 2 years
GM$_1$ Type 2 (Derry)	B and C galactosidase	No cherry red spot, nystagmus, esotropia, pigmentary retinopathy.	Ataxia, psychomotor retardation	Death by 3 to 10 years
GM$_2$ Type 1 (Tay-Sachs Disease)	Isoenzyme hexosaminidase A (autosomal recessive- typically affecting European Jews)	Cherry red spot in 90% by 6 months, nystagmus, optic atrophy, attenuation of retinal vasculature.	Hypotony, abnormal sensitivity to sound, seizures	Death by 2 to 5 years
GM$_2$ Type 2 (Sandhoff Disease)	Hexosaminidase A and B	Cherry red spot, strabismus, minimal corneal clouding, normal optic nerve.	Progressive psychomotor retardation	Death by 2 to 12 years
GM$_2$ Type 3 (Bernheimer-Seitelberger Disease)	Partial deficiency-hexosaminidase A	No cherry red spot.	Psychomotor retardation	Death by 15 years

Type II: Patients have a more severe and progressive systemic involvement. Corneal clouding, as well as cherry red spots, has been reported in this subtype.

Farber Disease

Deficiency of ceramidase has been demonstrated in patients with Farber disease. They are known to also present with cherry red spots, in addition to the systemic features of lumps on wrists, ankles, and joints. In the infantile form of the disease, death occurs due to pulmonary complications. The adult onset group develops progressive neurological disease.

Metachromatic Leukodystrophy

Metachromatic leukodystrophy is an autosomal recessive condition with deficiency of arylsulfatase A, leading to widespread demyelination of the brain and spinal cord. A classic cherry red spot has been described in addition to the finding of optic atrophy. Of the infantile, juvenile, adolescent, and adult forms, the infantile form is most common and has the worst prognosis.

Wilson Disease

Wilson disease is a rare condition that is characterized by widespread deposition of copper due to the deficiency of alpha 2 ceruloplasmin. It is associated with mutations in the gene ATP7B, a copper transporting ATPase. The genetic defect has been mapped to chromosome 13q near esterase D locus and is the named gene for Wilson disease. **Kayser-Fleischer ring,** a golden brown ring of copper deposits at the level of Descemet's membrane in the cornea, is the most specific ocular finding and is present in all cases, although its appearance may be delayed in some children. Typically, it develops superiorly, then inferiorly, and finally in the horizontal meridian. It recedes in an identical manner after penicillamine therapy or liver transplantation.

Some patients also present with a green "sunflower" cataract. This is actually an anterior subcapsular deposit of granular pigment rather than a cataract. Copper deposition in the liver, spleen, and CNS can cause a wide spectrum of clinical presentations such as jaundice, hepatosplenomegaly, cerebral degeneration, and mental instability.

Fabry Disease

Fabry disease is inherited in an X-linked recessive fashion and is due to the deficiency of the enzyme alpha-galactosidase A. In most cases, the patients present with angiokeratomas of skin and have episodes of excruciating pain in the fingers and toes. The most common ocular features are corneal verticillata, or whorl dystrophy of cornea, and a "Fabry cataract." Corneal verticillata are bilateral, brownish deposits at the level of Bowman's membrane located inferiorly on the cornea. Corneal verticillata have also been described in patients on antiarrhythmic drugs such as indomethacin, chloroquine, and meperidine.

Fabry cataract is unique with spokelike granular lens opacities. Aneurysmal dilatation of inferior bulbar conjunctival vessels has also been reported in 78% of cases. Common systemic features include angiokeratomas and cardiac and renal lesions.

Cystinosis

Widespread systemic and ocular cystine crystal deposition occurs in this autosomal recessive disease. Cystinosis has been mapped to gene locus 17p13. This gene encodes an integral membrane protein, which has features of a lysosomal membrane protein. The gene was strongly expressed in pancreas, kidneys (mature and fetal), and skeletal muscle; to a lesser extent in placenta and heart; and weakly in lung and liver. The common sites include the kidneys, leukocytes, and bone marrow. The ocular tissues affected are the conjunctiva, cornea, iris, lens, and retina. Photophobia and pain may result from corneal deposits that initially appear in the periphery and then progress to involve full thickness of the central cornea. Pigmentary retinopathy has also been reported in some cases. Depending upon the age at onset, 3 forms have been described.

1. The *infantile form*, also known as Fanconi syndrome, presents with progressive renal failure, growth retardation, and renal rickets.
2. In the *adolescent form*, the symptoms of renal failure are variable

and generally appear in the second decade of life. Retinopathy is typically absent in this group.

3. The *adult form* is asymptomatic, with normal renal function and normal life expectancy.

While treatment with oral cysteamine prevents additional deposits in ocular tissue and the kidney, it does not reverse preexisting damage. Children with renal transplantation do well, but survive only to the second or third decade. Topical cysteamine and corneal grafts have been tried with some success.

Alkaptonuria (Ochronosis)

Alkaptonuria is the deficiency of the enzyme homogentisic acid oxidase. The characteristic features include the presence of homogentisic acid in the urine, widespread cartilage and connective tissue pigmentation, cardiac valvular sclerosis, premature arterial sclerosis, and degenerative arthritis involving large peripheral joints. Tissue pigmentation is due to the presence of benzoquinoacetic acid and its polymers, which are indistinguishable from melanin.

Ocular involvement in the form of ochronotic pigment deposition in the conjunctiva limbus or cornea is seen in 80% of patients. Typically, the scleral patches are triangular and anterior to the insertion of the horizontal recti. The treatment is purely symptomatic, as dietary restriction is not helpful.

Diabetes

Juvenile onset diabetes (Type 1 diabetes) results from autoimmune destruction of insulin-producing beta cells on the pancreatic islets of Langerhans. The major ocular complication of diabetes is diabetic retinopathy. Severe diabetic retinopathy is unusual in children, as the disease progresses over time. Approximately 50% of patients with diabetes will show some degree of retinopathy 7 years after the onset of the disease. Ninety percent (90%) of patients will show retinopathy after 20 years.

Diabetes affects the microvascular circulation of the retinal vessels. Small retinal vessels and capillaries break down and lose the integrity of their tight junction and leak exudates into the surrounding retina. Abnormalities in the precapillaries produce microaneurysms. Leakage from the microaneurysms produce retinal edema, lipid exudates, and intraretinal hemorrhages (**Figure 24-8**). As the vasculopathy progresses, capillaries are lost and cause areas of capillary non-perfusion. Areas of capillary non-perfusion produce hypoxic retina and stimulate vascular endothelial growth factor (**Figure 24-9**). To this point, the diabetic retinopathy is classified as nonproliferative diabetic retinopathy (NPDR). Vascular endothelial growth factor (VEGF) produced from hypoxic retina stimulates neovascularization, which is abnormal vascular retinal vessel proliferation.

Retinal neovascularization is an important sign, as it indicates severe diabetic retinopathy that may require laser treatment

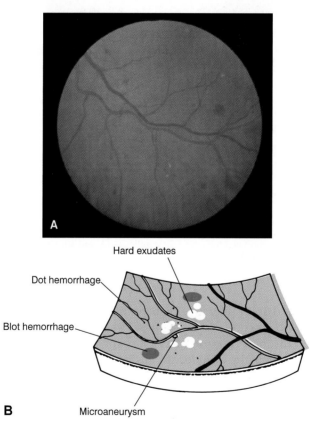

Figure 24-8.
Among the earliest microvascular changes in diabetes is the formation of microaneurysms, and dot and blot hemorrhages (**A and B**). Microaneurysms may leak fluid and may sometimes be identified at the center of a ring of exudates.

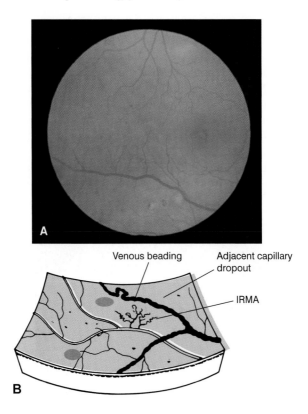

Figure 24-9.
In areas of capillary droupout, intraretinal microvascular abnormalities (IRMAs) form, representing dilated telangiectatic capillaries (**A and B**). Unlike extraretinal neovascularization, IRMAs do not leak on fluorescein angiography.

(**Figure 24-10**). Proliferative diabetic retinopathy (PDR) must be followed closely, since early treatment with laser can reduce unfavorable outcomes (**Figure 24-11**). Complications of proliferative diabetic retinopathy include vitreous hemorrhage, retinal detachment, macular edema, and neovascular glaucoma. The risk in children for developing proliferative diabetic retinopathy increases dramatically after puberty, and it is rare for children to have retinal changes before 10 years of age. Children with diabetes should have an initial baseline ophthalmic examination before puberty, then followed every year until puberty, and then twice a year or as is indicated per the retinal findings.

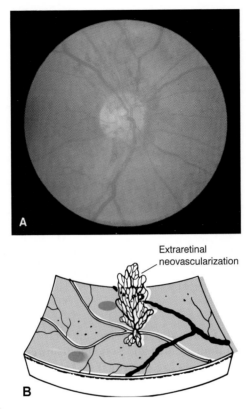

Extraretinal
neovascularization

Figure 24-10.
Extraretinal neovascularization my form at the optic disc (**A**) or elsewhere in the retina (**B**). These new vessels extend from the retina into the vitreous. Extraretinal neovascularization is associated with vitreous hemorrhage and production of fibrovascular traction.

Panretinal photocoagulation (PRP) obliterates the hypoxic retina and reduces the vascular endothelial growth factor, thereby reducing the stimulus for neovascularization.

■ CHROMOSOMAL ANOMALIES

The common ocular manifestations exhibited by many of the identifiable chromosomal anomalies include hypertelorism, epicanthus, blepharoptosis, up- or down-slanting of palpebral fissures, strabismus, and microphthalmia. Nearly all patients with autosomal de-

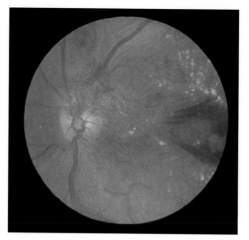

Figure 24-11.
Proliferative diabetic retinopathy. In this color photograph, several high-risk characteristics are apparent—severe neovascularization of the disc and preretinal hemorrhage. Immediate panretinal photocoagulation is indicated to induce regression of the new vessels.

fects present with some degree of mental retardation. The more specific and common ocular and systemic features of well-known chromosomal anomalies are described in **Table 24-9.**

Alagille Syndrome

Alagille syndrome is an autosomal dominant condition that also has been associated with a deletion of the short arm of chromosome 20. The major features include peculiar facies, chronic cholestasis, butterfly-like vertebral defects, peripheral pulmonary arterial hypoplasia, and an ocular anomaly of the cornea called **posterior embryotoxon.** Posterior embryotoxon represents an anterior displacement and thickening of Schwalbe's line, and delineates the posterior aspect of the cornea from the trabecular meshwork and the sclera. Schwalbe's line indicates the change from clear cornea to white sclera. Approximately 90% of patients with Alagille syndrome will have posterior embryotoxon, which is difficult to see and requires a slit-lamp examination. Other ocular anomalies include pigmentary retinopathy, iris hypoplasia, optic nerve anomalies, strabismus, and microcornea. Associated systemic findings may include growth retardation (50%), mental retardation (16%), renal problems, congenital heart disease, bone abnormalities, high-

Table 24-9.
Features of Chromosomal Anomalies

Syndromes	Ocular Features	Systemic Features
TRISOMY SYNDROMES		
Trisomy 13 or Patau syndrome	Microphthalmia, coloboma, cataract, PHPV, intraocular cartilage, retinal dysplasia, optic nerve hypoplasia and cyclopia.	Cleft lip/palate, polydactyly, cardiac, and CNS malformation.
Trisomy 18 or Edward syndrome	Corneal opacities, coloboma, microphthalmia, cornea opacity, congenital glaucoma, cyclopia.	Characteristic facies, rocker bottom feet, renal and cardiac abnormalities, apneic spells, failure to thrive.
Trisomy 21 or Down syndrome	Epicanthus, upward slanting of palpebral fissures (mongoloid slant), myopia, strabismus, keratoconus, cataract, ectropion of eyelid, increased number of vessels at disc margin, Brushfield spots, congenital glaucoma, optic atrophy. Blepharitis can be quite severe.	Characteristic mongoloid facies, protruding tongue, Simian palmar crease, hypotonia, cardiac malformations, stunted growth.
DELETION SYNDROMES		
4p deletion (Wolf-Hirschhorn syndrome)	Coloboma, coarse iris, exophthalmos.	Scalp defects, cleft or high arched palate, deformed nose, hemangiomas of forehead, internal hydrocephalus.
5p deletion (cri du chat syndrome)	Cataract, glaucoma, foveal hypoplasia, optic atrophy, coloboma, microphthalmia.	"Cat-like cry" (abnormality in the larynx), hypotonia, microcephaly, cardiac malformation.

(continued)

Table 24-9.
(continued)

Syndromes	Ocular Features	Systemic Features
11p13 deletion WAGR Syndrome (Wilms' tumor, aniridia, gonadoblastoma, retardation syndrome)	Aniridia, cataract, glaucoma, corneal dystrophy, macula hypoplasia, strabismus.	Mental retardation, predisposition to Wilms' tumor, genitourinary abnormalities (cryptorchidism and hypospadias in males). Pseudohermaphroditism and renal anomalies.
13 q deletion	Retinoblastoma (band q14), cataract, coloboma, microphthalmia.	Dysmorphic features, microcephaly, cardiac and renal malformation.
DUPLICATION SYNDROMES		
Duplicated 22 q "Cat eye syndrome"	Coloboma of uveal tract, microphthalmia.	Imperforate anus/anal atresia with rectovesical or rectovaginal fistula.
ANEUPLOIDY SYNDROMES		
Turner syndrome 45,X	Ptosis, cataract, refractive errors, corneal scar, blue sclera, color blindness (same incidence as in normal males).	Sexual infantilism, short stature, webbed neck, broad shield chest, multiple pigmented nevi, coarctation of aorta, high risk of diabetes and Hashimoto thyroiditis.
Klinefelter syndrome 47, XXX 47, XXY 48 XXXX 48, XXXY 49, XXXXX 49, XXXXY	Brushfield spots, myopia, choroidal atrophy, coloboma, microphthalmia.	Mental retardation increasing with number of X chromosomes, radio-ulnar synostosis, microcephaly, cardiac malformations.

pitched voice, and decreased deep tendon reflexes. Patients who are suspected of having Alagille syndrome should be referred for an ophthalmologic examination.

Prader-Willi Syndrome

Prader-Willi syndrome is characterized by hypogonadism, hypotonia, obesity, small hands and feet, mental retardation, strabismus and, occasionally, hypopigmentation or albinism. Patients with Prader-Willi syndrome have an insatiable appetite and will eat virtually anything. Their appetite increases with age and parents are often forced to lock the refrigerator to prevent malignant obesity. Microdeletion of the long arm of chromosome 15 and maternal uniparental disarray for chromosome 15 are the most common causes of Prader-Willi syndrome.

Index

Note: Page numbers followed by "f" refer to figures; page numbers followed by "t" refer to tables.